Textbook of Bone Marrow Failure

Mahmoud Aljurf • Régis Peffault de Latour
Antonio M. Risitano • Andrea Bacigalupo
Carlo Dufour
Editors

Textbook of Bone Marrow Failure

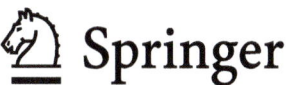 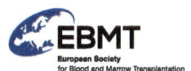

Editors
Mahmoud Aljurf
Cancer Centre of Excellence, MBC-64
King Faisal Specialist Hospital &
Research Centre
Riyadh, Saudi Arabia

Antonio M. Risitano
Hematology and Hematopoietic
Transplant Unit
Azienda Ospedaliera di Rilievo
Nazionale San Giuseppe Moscati
Avellino, Italy

Carlo Dufour
Hematology Unit
IRCCS Istituto Giannina Gaslini
Genoa, Italy

Régis Peffault de Latour
Hematology and Transplant Unit
Saint-Louis Hospital, AP-HP and Université
Paris Cité
Paris, France

Andrea Bacigalupo
Dipartimento di Scienze di Laboratorio ed
Ematologiche
Fondazione Policlinico Universitario
A. Gemelli IRCCS
Rome, Italy

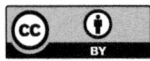

ISBN 978-3-032-02385-8   ISBN 978-3-032-02386-5   (eBook)
https://doi.org/10.1007/978-3-032-02386-5

This work was supported by the Mahmoud Aljurf

© The Editor(s) (if applicable) and The Author(s) 2026. This book is an open access publication.
Open Access   This book is licensed under the terms of the Creative Commons Attribution 4.0 International License (http://creativecommons.org/licenses/by/4.0/), which permits use, sharing, adaptation, distribution and reproduction in any medium or format, as long as you give appropriate credit to the original author(s) and the source, provide a link to the Creative Commons license and indicate if changes were made.
The images or other third party material in this book are included in the book's Creative Commons license, unless indicated otherwise in a credit line to the material. If material is not included in the book's Creative Commons license and your intended use is not permitted by statutory regulation or exceeds the permitted use, you will need to obtain permission directly from the copyright holder.
The use of general descriptive names, registered names, trademarks, service marks, etc. in this publication does not imply, even in the absence of a specific statement, that such names are exempt from the relevant protective laws and regulations and therefore free for general use.
The publisher, the authors and the editors are safe to assume that the advice and information in this book are believed to be true and accurate at the date of publication. Neither the publisher nor the authors or the editors give a warranty, expressed or implied, with respect to the material contained herein or for any errors or omissions that may have been made. The publisher remains neutral with regard to jurisdictional claims in published maps and institutional affiliations.

This Springer imprint is published by the registered company Springer Nature Switzerland AG
The registered company address is: Gewerbestrasse 11, 6330 Cham, Switzerland

If disposing of this product, please recycle the paper.

Contents

1 **Introduction**... 1
   Mahmoud Aljurf, Régis Peffault de Latour, Antonio M. Risitano,
   Andrea Bacigalupo, and Carlo Dufour

Part I Epidemiology and Pathophysiology

2 **Epidemiology of Acquired Bone Marrow Failure**................. 7
   Beatrice Drexler, Francesco Grimaldi, and Jakob R. Passweg

3 **Pathophysiology of Acquired Bone Marrow Failure**.............. 21
   Nicholas C. Lee and Neal S. Young

Part II Diagnosis and Classification

4 **Diagnosis of Acquired Aplastic Anemia with Figures**........... 55
   Alicia Rovó, Carlo Dufour, André Tichelli,
   and On behalf of the SAA-WP EBMT

5 **Acquired Overlap Bone Marrow Failure Disorders**............... 77
   Jakob R. Passweg and Beatrice Drexler

Part III Non-transplant Treatment and Supportive Care

6 **Non-transplant Treatments for Acquired Bone
   Marrow Failure Disorders**...................................... 87
   Pedro H. Prata, Camilla Frieri, Antonio M. Risitano,
   and Régis Peffault de Latour

7 **Supportive Care in Severe and Very Severe Aplastic Anemia**.... 99
   Britta Höchsmann, Mahmoud Aljurf, Hubert Schrezenmeier,
   and Shaykhah AlOtaibi

Part IV Management of Aplastic Anemia in Children and Elderly

8 Management of Acquired Aplastic Anemia in Children 117
Maurizio Miano, Gianluca Dell'Orso, and Carlo Dufour

9 Treatment of Elderly Patients with Aplastic Anemia.............. 133
André Tichelli, Alicia Rovó, Constantijn J. M. Halkes,
and Austin Kulasekararaj

Part V Hematopoietic Stem Cell Transplantation for Aplastic Anemia

10 Matched Sibling Donor Transplantation in Aplastic Anemia....... 145
Ali. D. Alahmari, Riad El Fakih, Constantijn J. M. Halkes,
Simone Cesaro, and Mahmoud Aljurf

**11 Unrelated Bone Marrow Transplantation for Acquired
Aplastic Anemia**... 159
Andrea Bacigalupo and Rainer Storb

**12 Haploidentical Donor Bone Marrow Transplantation
for Acquired Severe Aplastic Anemia** 169
Amy E. DeZern, Carmem Bonfim, and Andrea Bacigalupo

**13 Umbilical Cord Blood Transplantation for Patients
with Idiopathic and Inherited Bone Marrow Failure Disorders** 185
Simona Pagliuca and Arthur Sterin

Part VI Paroxysmal Nocturnal Hemoglobinuria (PNH) and Bone Marrow Failure

**14 Paroxysmal Nocturnal Hemoglobinuria: Bone Marrow
Failure and Beyond**.. 203
Antonio M. Risitano, Camilla Frieri, Pedro H. Prata,
and Régis Peffault de Latour

Part VII Constitutional Bone Marrow Failure Syndromes

**15 Constitutional Bone Marrow Failure due to Immune
Dysregulation Disorders**..................................... 227
Maurizio Miano, Francesca Tucci, and Alessandro Aiuti

16 Fanconi Anemia... 237
Filomena Pierri, Thierry Leblanc, Carlo Dufour, Jean Soulier,
Jean-Hugues Dalle, and Régis Peffault de Latour

17 Telomere Biology.. 249
Joshua Glass, Emma Groarke, and Neal S. Young

18	**Dyskeratosis Congenita** 267
	Mouhab Ayas and Syed Osman Ahmed
19	**Pathophysiology of Ribosomal Disorders** 281
	Lydie Da Costa and Alan J. Warren
20	**Clinical Management of Diamond–Blackfan Anemia Syndromes and Other Inherited Ribosomal Disorders** 309
	Thierry Leblanc and Maurizio Miano
21	**Chronic Neutropenias**.. 327
	Francesca Fioredda and Helen A. Papadaki
22	**Amegakaryocytic Thrombocytopenia** 337
	Chokri Ben Lamine, Thierry Leblanc, Mahmoud Aljurf, and Jean-Hugues Dalle
23	**Newly Recognized Inherited Bone Marrow Failure Syndromes** 345
	Alfadil Haroon, Marcin W. Wlodarski, Régis Peffault de Latour, and Mahmoud Aljurf

Part VIII Challenges in Global Management

24	**Managing Bone Marrow Failure in Countries with Restricted Resources** 361
	Raheel Iftikhar, Carmem Bonfim, Moosa Patel, Hazza Alzahrani, Adetola Kassim, and Mahmoud Aljurf

Index.. 373

Contributors

Syed Osman Ahmed Department of Hematology, Stem Cell Transplant & Cellular Therapy, Cancer Center of Excellence, King Faisal Specialist Hospital and Research Center, Riyadh, Saudi Arabia

Alessandro Aiuti Pediatric Immunohematology and Bone Marrow Transplantation Unit, San Raffaele Telethon Institute for Gene Therapy (SR-Tiget), IRCCS San Raffaele Scientific Institute, Milan, Italy

Ali. D. Alahmari Department of Hematology, Stem Cell Transplant & Cellular Therapy, Cancer Centre of Excellence, King Faisal Specialist Hospital & Research Centre, Riyadh, Saudi Arabia

Mahmoud Aljurf Department of Hematology, Stem Cell Transplant & Cellular Therapy, Cancer Centre of Excellence, King Faisal Specialist Hospital & Research Centre, Riyadh, Saudi Arabia

Shaykhah AlOtaibi Department of Hematology, Stem Cell Transplant & Cellular Therapy, Cancer Centre of Excellence, King Faisal Specialist Hospital & Research Centre, Riyadh, Saudi Arabia

Hazza Alzahrani Department of Hematology, Stem Cell Transplant & Cellular Therapy, Cancer Centre of Excellence, King Faisal Specialist Hospital & Research Centre, Riyadh, Saudi Arabia

Mouhab Ayas Department of Pediatric Hematology/Oncology, King Faisal Specialist Hospital and Research Center, Riyadh, Saudi Arabia

Andrea Bacigalupo Dipartimento di Scienze di Laboratorio ed Ematologiche, Fondazione Policlinico Universitario A. Gemelli IRCCS, Rome, Italy

Carmem Bonfim Division of Pediatric Transplantation and Cellular Therapy, Duke University, Durham, NC, USA

Simone Cesaro Pediatric Hematology and Oncology, Department of the Mother and the Child, Azienda Ospedaliera Universitaria Integrata, Verona, Italy

Lydie Da Costa Laboratory of Hematology, Bicêtre University Hospital, Le Kremlin-Bicêtre, France

Jean-Hugues Dalle Department of Pediatric Hematology and Immunology, Robert Debré Academic Hospital, GHU AP-HP Nord Université Paris Cité, Paris, France

Régis Peffault de Latour Hematology and Transplant Unit, Saint-Louis Hospital, AP-HP and Université Paris Cité, Paris, France

Gianluca Dell'Orso Hematology Unit, IRCCS Istituto Giannina Gaslini, Genoa, Italy

Amy E. DeZern Sidney Kimmel Comprehensive Cancer Center, Johns Hopkins University School of Medicine, Baltimore, MD, USA

Beatrice Drexler Division of Hematology, University Hospital Basel, Basel, Switzerland

Carlo Dufour Hematology Unit, IRCCS Istituto Giannina Gaslini, Genoa, Italy

Riad El Fakih Department of Hematology, Stem Cell Transplant & Cellular Therapy, Cancer Centre of Excellence, King Faisal Specialist Hospital & Research Centre, Riyadh, Saudi Arabia

Francesca Fioredda Hematology Unit-IRCCS Istituto Giannina Gaslini, Genoa, Italy

Camilla Frieri Hematology and Hematopoietic Transplant Unit, Azienda Ospedaliera di Rilievo Nazionale San Giuseppe Moscati, Avellino, Italy

Joshua Glass Hematology Branch, National Heart, Lung, and Blood Institute, National Institutes of Health, Bethesda, MD, USA

Francesco Grimaldi Department of Clinical Medicine and Surgery, Hematology Unit, University of Naples Federico II, Naples, Italy

Emma Groarke Hematology Branch, National Heart, Lung, and Blood Institute, National Institutes of Health, Bethesda, MD, USA

Constantijn J. M. Halkes Department of Hematology, Leiden University Medical Centre, Leiden, The Netherlands

Alfadil Haroon Department of Hematology, Stem Cell Transplant & Cellular Therapy, Cancer Centre of Excellence, King Faisal Specialist Hospital & Research Centre, Riyadh, Saudi Arabia

Britta Höchsmann Institute of Clinical Transfusion Medicine and Immunogenetics Ulm, German Red Cross Blood Transfusion Service Baden-Württemberg – Hessen and University Hospital Ulm, Ulm, Germany

Raheel Iftikhar Armed Forces Bone Marrow Transplant Center, Rawalpindi, Pakistan

Contributors

Adetola Kassim Department of Medicine, Division of Hematology/Oncology, Vanderbilt University Medical Center, Nashville, TN, USA

Austin Kulasekararaj Department of Hematological Medicine, King's College Hospital NHS Foundation Trust, London, UK

Chokri Ben Lamine Department of Hematology, Stem Cell Transplant & Cellular Therapy, Cancer Centre of Excellence, King Faisal Specialist Hospital & Research Centre, Riyadh, Saudi Arabia

Thierry Leblanc Department of Pediatric Hematology and Immunology, Robert Debré Academic Hospital, GHU AP-HP Nord Université Paris Cité, Paris, France

Nicholas C. Lee Hematology Branch, National Heart, Lung, and Blood Institutes, National Institutes of Health, Bethesda, MD, USA

Maurizio Miano Hematology Unit, IRCCS Istituto Giannina Gaslini, Genoa, Italy

Simona Pagliuca Department of Hematology, Nancy University Hospital, and UMR 7365, University of Lorraine, Vandoeuvre-lès-Nancy, France

Helen A. Papadaki Department of Hematology & Hemopoiesis Research Laboratory, School of Medicine, University of Crete, Greece and University Hospital of Heraklion, Heraklion, Greece

Jakob R. Passweg Division of Hematology, University Hospital Basel, Basel, Switzerland

Moosa Patel Department of Clinical Hematology, Faculty of Health Sciences, School of Clinical Medicine, University of the Witwatersrand, Johannesburg, South Africa

Filomena Pierri Hematopoietic Stem Cell Transplantation Unit, IRCSS Istituto Giannina Gaslini, Genoa, Italy

Pedro H. Prata Hematology and Cellular Therapy Department, CHU de Limoges, France

Antonio M. Risitano Hematology and Hematopoietic Transplant Unit, Azienda Ospedaliera di Rilievo Nazionale San Giuseppe Moscati, Avellino, Italy

Alicia Rovó Department of Hematology and Central Hematology Laboratory, Inselspital, Bern University Hospital, University of Bern, Bern, Switzerland

Hubert Schrezenmeier Institute of Transfusion Medicine, University of Ulm and German Red Cross, Ulm, Germany

Jean Soulier Hematology Laboratory, Saint Louis Hospital, APHP, Inserm, Saint Louis Research Institute, Université Paris Cité, Paris, France

Arthur Sterin Service D'hématologie Immunologie Oncologie Pédiatrique, CHU de Marseille, France

Rainer Storb Clinical Research Division, Fred Hutchinson Cancer Center and Division of Hematology and Oncology, University of Washington School of Medicine, Seattle, WA, USA

André Tichelli Division of Hematology, University Hospital Basel, Basel, Switzerland

Francesca Tucci Pediatric Immunohematology and Bone Marrow Transplantation Unit, San Raffaele Telethon Institute for Gene Therapy (SR-Tiget), IRCCS San Raffaele Scientific Institute, Milan, Italy

Alan J. Warren Department of Hematology, Cambridge Institute for Medical Research, University of Cambridge, Cambridge, UK

Department of Hematology, Cambridge Stem Cell Institute, University of Cambridge, Cambridge, UK

Marcin W. Wlodarski St. Jude Children's Research Hospital, Memphis, TN, USA

Neal S. Young Hematology Branch, National Heart, Lung, and Blood Institutes, National Institutes of Health, Bethesda, MD, USA

Chapter 1
Introduction

Mahmoud Aljurf, Régis Peffault de Latour, Antonio M. Risitano, Andrea Bacigalupo, and Carlo Dufour

Bone marrow failure syndromes encompass a diverse and complex group of hematologic disorders that pose significant diagnostic and therapeutic challenges. These conditions, whether acquired or inherited, often result in severe cytopenias, leading to life-threatening complications such as infections, hemorrhage, and progression to myelodysplastic syndromes (MDS) or leukemia. This *Textbook of Bone Marrow Failure* serves as a comprehensive resource for clinicians, hematologists, transplant physicians, pathologists, researchers, and allied healthcare professionals by providing an in-depth synthesis of knowledge on the epidemiology, pathophysiology, diagnosis, and management of these disorders.

The primary objective of this textbook is to bridge the gap between evolving research and clinical practice. With rapid advancements in molecular diagnostics, genetic screening, and novel therapeutic strategies, there is a pressing need for an integrated resource that translates these innovations into practical applications. This book explores current and emerging therapeutic approaches, including

---

M. Aljurf (✉)
Department of Hematology, Stem Cell Transplant & Cellular Therapy, Cancer Centre of Excellence, King Faisal Specialist Hospital & Research Centre, Riyadh, Saudi Arabia
e-mail: maljurf@kfshrc.edu.sa

R. Peffault de Latour
Hematology and Transplant Unit, Saint-Louis Hospital, AP-HP and Université Paris Cité, Paris, France

A. M. Risitano
Hematology and Hematopoietic Transplant Unit, Azienda Ospedaliera di Rilievo Nazionale San Giuseppe Moscati, Avellino, Italy

A. Bacigalupo
Dipartimento di Scienze di Laboratorio ed Ematologiche, Fondazione Policlinico Universitario A. Gemelli IRCCS, Rome, Italy

C. Dufour
Hematology Unit, IRCCS Istituto Giannina Gaslini, Genoa, Italy

immunosuppressive therapy, hematopoietic stem cell transplantation (HSCT), and targeted pharmacologic interventions, with a focus on optimizing patient outcomes.

The textbook is structured to provide a logical progression of topics, beginning with foundational concepts and advancing into disease-specific discussions and treatment modalities. The initial chapters focus on epidemiology and pathophysiology, detailing the mechanisms driving acquired and inherited bone marrow failure syndromes. Acquired aplastic anemia is discussed extensively, including its association with infections, toxins, immune dysregulation, and genetic predispositions. The evolving role of next-generation sequencing (NGS) in diagnosing both inherited and acquired forms of bone marrow failure is highlighted, reflecting its increasing impact on clinical decision-making.

Diagnostic considerations are explored in detail, covering disease classification, severity assessment, and differential diagnosis. Special attention is given to overlap syndromes, including hypoplastic MDS, pure red cell aplasia, large granular lymphocytic leukemia, and paroxysmal nocturnal hemoglobinuria (PNH), emphasizing their unique diagnostic and therapeutic challenges.

Advancements in supportive care and non-transplant treatment strategies are reviewed, including transfusion support, infection prophylaxis, and immunosuppressive therapy (IST) with antithymocyte globulin (ATG), cyclosporine, and thrombopoietin receptor agonists such as eltrombopag. The risks of clonal evolution and secondary MDS/AML following IST are discussed, along with strategies to mitigate these risks.

For patients requiring definitive treatment, hematopoietic stem cell transplantation (HSCT) remains the only curative approach for many bone marrow failure syndromes. This textbook provides a thorough review of transplantation strategies, including matched sibling donor transplantation, unrelated donor transplantation, haploidentical transplantation, and umbilical cord blood transplantation. Advances in transplantation techniques, such as post-transplant cyclophosphamide for graft-versus-host disease (GVHD) prophylaxis, are highlighted. Additionally, considerations for pediatric and elderly patients are discussed, emphasizing individualized approaches to patient selection and post-transplant management.

A dedicated chapter focuses on PNH, a unique disorder at the intersection of bone marrow failure and complement-mediated hemolysis. This section provides insights into the pathogenesis of PNH, its association with aplastic anemia, and advances in treatment, including complement inhibitors.

The textbook also extensively covers inherited bone marrow failure syndromes (IBMFS), including Fanconi anemia, dyskeratosis congenita, Diamond-Blackfan anemia, Shwachman-Diamond syndrome, and newly recognized genetic syndromes. These chapters explore molecular pathogenesis, clinical manifestations, diagnostic algorithms, and evolving treatment options such as gene therapy and stem cell transplantation. The significance of telomere biology and ribosomopathies in hematologic dysfunction and malignancy is also emphasized.

While significant progress has been made in understanding and treating bone marrow failure syndromes, substantial challenges remain, particularly in resource-limited settings. A dedicated section addresses disparities in global healthcare access, including the management of bone marrow failure syndromes in countries with restricted healthcare infrastructure. Strategies to improve access to transplantation, supportive care, and novel therapies in these settings are discussed.

This *Textbook of Bone Marrow Failure* integrates clinical expertise, translational research, and state-of-the-art therapeutic advancements to serve as an essential resource for healthcare professionals. With a multidisciplinary approach, it provides a comprehensive, evidence-based framework for diagnosing and managing these complex disorders. By fostering a deeper understanding of bone marrow failure syndromes and promoting innovative treatment strategies, this textbook aims to advance the field and improve patient outcomes worldwide.

Open Access This chapter is licensed under the terms of the Creative Commons Attribution 4.0 International License (http://creativecommons.org/licenses/by/4.0/), which permits use, sharing, adaptation, distribution and reproduction in any medium or format, as long as you give appropriate credit to the original author(s) and the source, provide a link to the Creative Commons license and indicate if changes were made.

The images or other third party material in this chapter are included in the chapter's Creative Commons license, unless indicated otherwise in a credit line to the material. If material is not included in the chapter's Creative Commons license and your intended use is not permitted by statutory regulation or exceeds the permitted use, you will need to obtain permission directly from the copyright holder.

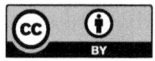

Part I
Epidemiology and Pathophysiology

Chapter 2
Epidemiology of Acquired Bone Marrow Failure

Beatrice Drexler, Francesco Grimaldi, and Jakob R. Passweg

Introduction

Paul Ehrlich, in 1888, gave the first seminal description of Aplastic Anemia in a pregnant woman, where the normal hemopoietic tissue was replaced by a fatty marrow and empty spaces, the "hypocellular" marrow that resulted in pancytopenia. Acquired Aplastic Anemia (AA) is a rare immune-mediated form of bone marrow failure [1]. Several retrospective studies from Europe, the United States, South America, and Asia suggest an incidence of about 0.6–6.1 cases per million population. The incidence of AA shows geographical variability, with lower rates reported in Europe, North America, and Brazil, and higher rates in Asia. Based on the two epidemiological studies carried out in Europe and Asia with a similar methodology, a 2- to three-fold higher incidence was reported in Asia than in the West [2–12]. This variability in incidence rates may reflect differences in exposure to environmental factors, including viruses, drugs, and chemicals, but also a different genetic background, diagnostic criteria, and study designs.

In the following, we discuss the studies performed and available in the literature, including case series and reports, to determine the epidemiology and demographics of acquired AA across different centers of the world.

B. Drexler (✉) · J. R. Passweg
Division of Hematology, University Hospital Basel, Basel, Switzerland
e-mail: beatrice.drexler@usb.ch; jakob.passweg@usb.ch

F. Grimaldi
Department of Clinical Medicine and Surgery, Hematology Unit, University of Naples Federico II, Naples, Italy

© The Author(s) 2026
M. Aljurf et al. (eds.), *Textbook of Bone Marrow Failure*,
https://doi.org/10.1007/978-3-032-02386-5_2

Incidence of AA in Different Geographical Regions and Races

The annual incidence of AA varies from 0.6 to 6 per million population per annum across centers in different continents. Most findings are from retrospective studies, including retrospective reviews of death registries. However, this incidence masks the variability that is seen across continents and different ethnic groups; e.g., reports from the Barcelona group (2008), which was a detailed prospective study by Montane et al. [2] had an incidence of 2.34 per million population. This incidence rate is similar to the 2.0/million reported by the International Agranulocytosis and Aplastic Anemia Study (IAAAS)[3], which was conducted in Europe and Israel from 1980 to 1984, and to rates reported in smaller national studies in Europe, which included the United Kingdom [4], France [5], Scandinavia [6], and in South America and Brazil [7]. A recent Swedish study, analyzing the national patient registry, reported a similar overall incidence of 2.35 (Vaht K et al.). The higher incidence was accurately determined to be four cases per million population in Bangkok [8], but based on prospective studies, it may actually be closer to 5.6 cases per million population in the rural areas of Thailand (Khonkaen region) [9]. In the prospective Chinese Epidemiologic Study Group of Leukemia and Aplastic Anemia survey, 7.4 per million was reported as a national incidence, which clearly is much on the higher side but may have been overestimated, as stringent criteria for the diagnosis of AA, such as bone marrow study, were not strictly applied [10]. Increased incidence in Eastern countries may be related to environmental factors, such as increased exposure to toxic chemicals and pesticides on agricultural farms, practiced in the Far East and South Asia. However, the incidence of AA in children of immigrants from East Asia in a pediatric population from the ages of 0 to 14 years, in a study from British Columbia (Canada), was significantly higher at 6.9/million, as compared to children of white/mixed ethnic descent at 1.7/million [11]. Children of immigrants from South Asia, in this study, were found to have an incidence even higher than their counterparts from East Asia, at 7.3/million [13]. This study suggested that Asian children have an increased incidence of AA, possibly due to a different genetic background. Indeed, in a hospital-based case-control study from Lucknow (India), the annual incidence of childhood AA was determined to be 6.8/million [14].

Benzene has been found to be toxic to the hemopoietic progenitor cells in a dose-dependent and direct manner. In large collaborative studies between the National Cancer Institute and American and Chinese institutions [15], hematologic susceptibility to benzene has been correlated to nucleotide polymorphism in key drug metabolic patways [16]. Although the AA incidence reported in a multicenter Latin American study remains very low at 1.6/million, this study also corroborated the association between risk of exposure to benzene, chloramphenicol, and also azithromycin and predisposition to AA in this area [17, 18]. Benzene has been a long-standing risk factor for AA in the past but seems to be less influential in recent times, contributing to fewer cases of bone marrow failures in many countries (Issaragrisil S et al. Thailand, Blood).

Age- and Gender-Related Demographics of AA

In nearly all modern studies of AA, the sex ratio has been close to 1:1, which is unusual for immune-mediated diseases [2, 19]. An exception to this has been a study from the Sabah province in Malaysia [12], where an unusually high male-to-female ratio was noted at 3.4. Similarly, a male predominance was also noted in studies from Thailand [9], India [20] and Pakistan [21]. This may reflect the under-reporting of cases of AA among females and access to adequate healthcare services in Asia. However, it remains unclear why a female predominance is not seen in a quintessential autoimmune disorder like AA among studies in Europe and the United States. In all the largest studies available, including a series of 300 patients reported by the Clinical Center at NIH by Young et al. [22], the Barcelona report [2], and an epidemiologic study from Thailand [9], two patient age peaks of incidence are constantly observed, one among young adults and the second in the elderly. This characteristic biphasic distribution shows two peaks, one from 10 to 25 years and the second above 60 years. Within the younger age group, a small peak in the incidence is observed in childhood, probably due to overlap with inherited marrow-failure syndromes featured by a less penetrating phenotype, where classical physical anomalies of the inherited marrow-failure syndromes are not obvious. On the other hand, the second incidence peak of AA seen above 60 years may reflect the smaller pool of hematopoietic stem cell reserve left with age-related telomeric attrition and its capacity to maintain normal hemopoiesis in the face of an immune insult against the hematopoietic precursor cells [23].

Post-hepatitis AA and AA Occurring After Viral Infections

Post-hepatitis AA is a stereotypical syndrome, where pancytopenia often presents two to three months after an acute attack of severe but self-limited seronegative liver inflammation. This distinct variant has been commonly seen in 5–10% of "classical" AA cases, typically occurring in adolescent boys and young men [24]. Severe imbalance of the T-cell immune system, as seen with "classical" AA, Human leukocyte antigen (HLA) association, and effective response to immunosuppressive therapy strongly suggest an immune-mediated mechanism. As for other forms of AA, a higher incidence is noted in East Asia (4–10%) when compared to Western countries and Europe, where recently an incidence of 5.4%, stable across the years, has been reported in a large registry study from EBMT [25].

Cases of AA associated with HAV, HBV, HGV, parvovirus B19 [26–29], Epstein-Barr virus (EBV) [30], transfusion-transmitted virus (TTV) [31], or echovirus [32] infections have been reported. In a German-Austrian study of 213 pediatric cases aged 17 years or less of AA, 80% of cases were idiopathic, 9% followed post-hepatitis AA, 7% followed viral infections, and 4% were associated with drugs/toxins [33].

Parvovirus B19 is the causative agent for fifth disease, usually in the immunocompetent host. However, transient aplastic crises have been reported in chronic hemolytic anemias such as sickle cell disease owing to reticulocytopenia, and cases of severe AA have also been reported in normal individuals during an acute episode of infection [34]. The actual incidence of acute parvovirus B19 infection at presentation in AA is not known, but in a single-case series of 27 patients with AA from India, parvovirus B19 IgM and viral DNA were detected in nearly 40% of the cases [35]. This may be an important etiological factor, especially in immunocompromised hosts or patients with chronic hemolytic anemias.

Very recently, retrospective observations about eight AA cases occurring during HIV infection have been reported [36]. Even if AA appears to be a late, rare complication in HIV patients, a report from Pagliuca et al. [36] highlights that immunosuppressive therapy is a feasible strategy in AA patients and that a better outcome is observed in patients eligible for transplant, while death from infection remains the principal cause of mortality in undertreated patients.

As seen with other infections, the worldwide pandemic with severe acute respiratory syndrome coronavirus 2 (SARS-CoV-2) was presumably associated with subsequent cases of new-onset marrow failure reported from several countries (Lee NCJ et al., Wu X et al.). COVID-19 is a hyperinflammatory and immune dysregulated state, which strengthens the hypothesis that SARS-CoV may also mediate an immunologic response with resulting marrow failure.

AA and Association with Toxins/Drugs

There is no discernible difference in the demographics or clinical behavior, including response to immunosuppressive therapy, between patients classified as having "drug or toxin induced" versus "idiopathic" AA [37].

Benzene is the most widely studied and implicated among toxins causing AA. The relationship was initially brought to light by a case series of workers exposed through their specific occupations [15] and has since been detected in some, but not all, population-based case-control studies. An association has been seen in some case-control studies, but even when present, the proportion of cases that can be attributed to this chemical has been small. Studies on American workers earlier in this century suggested that the risk of AA was about 3% in men exposed to concentrations higher than 300 ppm, and in the more recent IAAAS study [3], benzene accounted for about 1–3% of AA recorded cases. Similarly, in the Thai population, benzene carried a relative risk of 3.5 but accounted for an etiologic fraction of only 1% [9].

Pesticides have been associated with AA in a large number of medical records. In the Indian cohort of pediatric AA, although significantly higher blood levels of organochlorine compounds were detected, suggesting an association, they were not entirely supported by statistical methods [14]. Anecdotal case reports of AA following use of pesticides such as Dichloro-diethyly-trichlorthane (DDT), Chlordane, or Lindane, or

Table 2.1 Exposures to drugs reported to be associated with Aplastic Anemia in the 2–6 months prior to hospital admission among 235 cases

Drug	N (%)
Allopurinol	9 (3.8)
Indomethacin	9 (3.8)
Gold salts	9 (3.8)
Sulfonamides	9 (3.8)
Carbamazepine	5 (2.1)
Ticlopidine	4 (1.7)
Chloramphenicol	3 (1.2)
Oxyphenbutazone	3 (1.2)
Phenylbutazone	3 (1.2)
Penicillamine	3 (1.2)
Clopidogrel	2 (0.8)
Methimazole	2 (0.8)

Montane et al. [2]

following exposure to organic solvents such as toluene and other molecules resembling benzene or containing a benzene ring, again point merely to an association. Unfortunately, systematic population case-control studies correlating the level and duration of exposure to these identified toxins and AA onset are lacking.

Initially suggested by the accumulation of case reports, specific drug associations have been established in different population-based studies and have changed across time, mainly due to changes in drug diffusion and utilization. Chloramphenicol, for example, which gained notoriety for its prominent association with AA in the 1950s and for decades was considered the commonest cause of the disease, has progressively declined to the point that it has not been reported as a significant risk factor in any recent systematic epidemiologic study of AA in Western countries. Even in Thailand, where the need for such an effective and inexpensive antibiotic is substantial, and usage is reported 100 times greater than in the West, association with AA is infrequent, probably due to lower-dose prescriptions [9].

In the IAAAS study [3] approximately 25% of the identified AA cases were related to drug use. Major drug associations were with gold salt (Relative Risk, RR of 29), antithyroid drugs (RR of 11), and nonsteroidal anti-inflammatory agents (RR of 8.2 for indomethacin). Similarly, in 235 patients with AA prospectively followed by the Barcelona group [2], 67 cases (28.5%) had a history of exposure to drugs or toxic agents that have been associated with AA sometime in the preceding 6 months. Forty-nine (20.8%) cases had been exposed to the following drugs (Table 2.1). In addition, 21 (8.9%) cases had been exposed to toxic agents: insecticides ($n = 8$), benzene ($n = 6$), and other solvents ($n = 10$).

Finally, the incidence of drug-associated AA appears to be lower in East Asia [8, 9].

Recently, several cases of AA have been reported after therapy with immune-checkpoint inhibitors (Dasari S et al.). In an analysis of 52,303 treated patients, 0.15% of cases with a median onset of 126 days were reported. Another analysis of 5923 patients from 19 clinical trials calculated an overall rate of 0.6% for

Aplastic Anemia. In these cases, treatment with immune-checkpoint inhibitors should be held while starting supportive therapy (transfusions, G-CSF) and providing immunosuppressive treatment +/− eltrombopag in severe cases (Kroll MH et al).

Ultimately, with the introduction of CAR T-cell therapy, hematotoxicity has been reported as a well-known complication, which predisposes patients to severe infections and high non-relapse mortality. To further understand the pathomechanisms of CAR T cell-related hematotoxicity, the group by M. Subklewe and N. Young performed a detailed immunological analysis of a patient with diffuse large B-cell lymphoma receiving CD19-directing CAR T (Rejeski K et al). They first observed an oligoclonal T-cell expansion, which might have been stimulated by high-grade cytokine release syndrome and an inflammatory micromilieu and could also play a role in other cases of hematotoxicity. Future studies are needed to further elaborate this potential pathomechanism.

AA and Association with HLA Genes

The Human leukocyte antigen (HLA) system is a crucial group of genes responsible for starting and regulating the immune response. Since antigen presentation and T-cell activation through HLA may represent the early step that precedes global hematopoietic stem cell destruction in AA, HLA polymorphism may contribute to the pathogenesis of the disease by (i) increasing or decreasing susceptibility to AA, particularly for specific ethnic or age groups, (ii) facilitating activity of drugs or viral antigens to break immune tolerance, (iii) influencing response to immunosuppressive therapy.

As for other autoimmune diseases, a large number of studies demonstrated an association between polymorphism of HLA class II genes and AA susceptibility (Table 2.2, a).

An increased frequency of HLA-DR2 was first described in several studies for European and American Caucasian patients [38], and finally confirmed in a multi-ethnic cohort by Nimer et al. [39] Subsequently, a positive association between HLA-DR2 (precisely DRB1*15 allele) and AA was confirmed in Chinese [40], Japanese [41], Turkish [42], Pakistani [43], and Malaysian [44] series. These data depict a clear role for the HLA-DR2 gene as a risk factor for AA, and the different distribution of this gene across the human population probably accounts for the different incidence seen for AA in specific geographical areas and ethnic groups. Interestingly, when Maciejewski et al. [45] analyzed the distribution of HLA-DR2 (mainly DRB1*15 allele) across disease subgroups (i.e., AA, hemolytic PNH, and AA/PNH), they found an increased frequency in those where bone marrow failure was associated with a PNH clone. Other DR2 alleles have been correlated with AA; in a single-case report, Nakao et al. [46] showed a specific T-cell cytotoxic response associated with the DRB1*0405 allele. The DRB1*07 allele has been reported in a single cohort of Iranian subjects [47], and DRB1*0901 in Chinese children [48].

Table 2.2 Summary table of AA and incidence of specific HLA genes or alleles

a. HLA and increased risk of AA (Class II)	b. HLA and reduced risk of AA (Class I)	c. HLA and reduced risk of AA	d. HLA and onset age of AA	e. HLA and drug/viral related AA	f. HLA and AA outcome
HLA-DRB1*1501	HLA-A2	HLA-DRB1*13	HLA-DRB*09	Haplotype: −B38, − DR4, −DQ3	HLA-DR2
HLA-DRB1*0405	HLA-A*0206	HLA-DRB1*03:01	HLA-A26	Haplotype: −DRB1*0402, −DQB1*0302	HLA-DRB1*1501
HLA-DRB1*07	HLA-B7	HLA-DRB1*11:01	HLA-B14	Haplotype: −DRB1*1601, −DQB1*0502	HLA-DR4-Ala74
HLA-DRB1*0901	HLA-B14	HLA-DRB1*51:01	HLA-B48	HLA-DRB1*08	
HLA-Dpw3	HLA-B*4002	HLA-DRB1*03			
HLA-DR4		HLA-DRB1*13:02			

Finally, evidence available correlates AA even with other HLA-II class genes like Dpw3 [49] and DR4 [22].

Less data are available for HLA class I genes. Early reports suggested a correlation with the HLA-A2 gene [50, 51] and with HLA-B7 and HLA-B14 genes, at least in European patients [52, 53]. Moreover, the association between HLA-B14 alleles, HLA-Cw7, and AA has been confirmed by Maciejewski et al. [45] in a multiethnic cohort of 212 American individuals. Finally, Shichishima et al. [54] reported a higher incidence of HLA-B*4002 and HLA-A*0206 in 78 Japanese AA patients, suggesting a potential role of HLA class I genes even in Far East countries.

HLA genes revealing a protective role in developing AA have been identified too (see Table 2.2, b). Even if data refer mainly to a small series of patients, and may reflect natural polymorphism in the HLA system, again, a key role for HLA class II genes and their alleles is suggested. HLA-DRB1*13 appeared to be protective in a cohort of patients of Turkish origin [55], as well as HLA-DRB1*03:01, HLA-DRB1*11:01, and HLA-B1*51:01 alleles appear to be protective in a cohort of Chinese children [48]. In a small cohort of Pakistani patients [43], HLA-DRB1*03 had a higher frequency in healthy controls, suggesting a putative protective role, and a similar observation is available for allele DRB1*1302 in the Korean population [56].

Even if AA has a typical bimodal age of incidence, the majority of studies did not look specifically into HLA frequency and age differences, mostly due to their retrospective nature and the rarity of the disease. Therefore, a good assumption could be that data on HLA allele frequency could be inferred to the pediatric setting. However, Fuhrer et al. [57] in a recent study involving 181 Caucasian children observed a positive association between HLA-A26 and HLA-B14 alleles, but not a higher incidence of HLA-DR2. Similarly, Chen et al. [48] in a retrospective survey conducted on 80 Chinese children showed a higher than expected incidence of class I HLA-B48 alleles and class II HLA-DRB*09 alleles. Finally, a frequency of the HLA-DR2 B15 allele not different from the normal population has been reported by Kook et al. [58] in North Korean AA children and by Yoshida et al. [59] in Japanese AA children. These limited data suggest a potentially different HLA landscape in children with AA, even if further investigation involving a higher number of patients is needed to specifically address this question (see Table 2.2, c).

Association between agranulocytosis and HLA genes has been reported for drug exposure in specific ethnic groups, suggesting that certain alleles may facilitate the initiation of AA through direct presentation of drug-derived antigens to T-cells [37]. HLA class II haplotypes have been reported to be associated with clozapine-induced agranulocytosis in Ashkenazi Jewish [60, 61] individuals, and an association between HLA-DRB1*08 alleles and thionamide-induced AA has been described for Japanese patients [62]. A similar mechanism of disease can be suggested for post-hepatitis AA, too, where the association between HLA class I, specifically HLA-B8, and hematological disease has been documented [24] (see Table 2.2, d).

Finally, some groups have shown that response to immunosuppressive therapy can be related to specific HLA genes. HLA-DRB1*1501 is the most clearly associated allele with a better response to Cyclosporine[41], and the presence of HLA-DR2 and a PNH clone independently predicts response to therapy in patients under immunosuppression [45]. On the other hand, HLA-DRB1*1502 allele [63], which represents a different allele variant of HLA-DR2, does not seem to have the same influence on treatment, even if its incidence is increased among older Japanese patients with AA. High-resolution genotyping of HLA-DRB1 showed that the HLA-DRB1*04 allele coding for alanine position 74 (HLA-DR4-Ala74) [64] predisposes to AA independently from HLA-DRB1*15 and that HLA-DRB1*04 alleles are associated with worse response to cyclosporine and the poorest prognosis (see Table 2.2, e).

AA and Autoimmune Disorders

Although AA is idiopathic in most cases, associations with other autoimmune diseases (AID) have been shown in numerous single-case reports. In rheumatic diseases such as systemic lupus erythematosus (SLE), rheumatoid arthritis (RA), and eosinophilic fasciitis (Shulman disease), there is a recognized association with AA [65, 66]. However, in most cases of rheumatic disease, cytopenias are frequently observed as immune cytopenias (immune thrombocytopenia, autoimmune hemolytic disease) or the result of ongoing inflammation or therapy-related (e.g., methotrexate, gold salts, etanercept) causes, whereas the full picture of AA with a hypocellular marrow is only anecdotally described [67, 68].

Two large, different studies have specifically looked into the incidence of autoimmune conditions among AA patients. In a single-center series [69] of 253 individuals, 5.3% of patients with AA had a previous diagnosis of AID, and 4.5% developed an AID after AA was diagnosed. Similarly, 4% of patients recorded in the EBMT database [70] for AA have been found to be diagnosed with a previous AID in a retrospective analysis. Interestingly, in both studies, patients' age at diagnosis of AA seems to be higher (>50 years) than normal. The impact of immunosuppressive treatment for AA on concomitant AID and the effects on its natural history remain, at the moment, a controversial topic.

AA During Pregnancy

There are no prospective studies about the incidence of AA during pregnancy. Curiously, AA was first described in a pregnant woman by Ehrlich in 1888. Since then, there have been a few published reports of AA during pregnancy. Tichelli et al. [71] described a case series of 36 pregnancies in women with AA. Their study showed that a successful pregnancy with a normal outcome is possible in women with AA who have been previously treated with immunosuppression. Nineteen percent of women were found to have a relapse of AA, and a further 14% needed transfusion support at the time of delivery. Complications appear to be more likely in patients with low platelet counts and paroxysmal nocturnal hemoglobinuria-associated AA.

Similarly, Choudhry et al. [72] described 10 cases of AA and concomitant pregnancies, reporting successful delivery in 10 of 11 cases, with adverse outcomes related to fatal bleeding in only two patients.

Although pregnancy remains an immunomodulatory state, with a higher incidence of autoimmune disease reported, the causative relationship with AA remains controversial. However, the description of spontaneous improvement in blood count after delivery, as far as cases of multiple pregnancies and subsequent disease relapses in single women [73], suggests a potential immune trigger even for this phenomenon.

AA Post-vaccination

There have been several case reports of AA following vaccination (e.g., hepatitis B, anthrax, varicella zoster, H1N1 influenza) [74]. Most recently, also Aplastic Anemia cases have been reported to occur after SARS-CoV-2 mRNA vaccination. Systematic case-control studies for the incidence of AA following vaccination are not known. Although the mechanism of how vaccinations can induce AA is unclear, some speculate that it may trigger an autoimmune reaction leading to the destruction of hematopoietic stem cells. This should alert health care providers to vigilantly monitor patients for potential adverse events following vaccination. Also, patients with AA who have been treated with immunosuppressive treatment and, therefore, might still be at risk for a reemerging immune attack should also be cautiously monitored for the theoretical risk of disease relapse [1]. Nevertheless, this drawback has to be weighed against the benefits of vaccinations, as AA patients under immunosuppressive treatment are also prone to severe infections and therefore can also profit from vaccinations. With respect to COVID-19, a recent EBMT study of a large cohort of 361 non-transplanted AA patients reported that vaccination was overall well-tolerated, with low complication and relapse rates. There were no deaths from COVID-19 reported after vaccination. Against historical recommendations, advising generally against the vaccinations in AA patients due to a potential relapse risk, caregivers nowadays should carefully evaluate and discuss with the individual patients the benefits and drawbacks of each vaccination.

Problems with Epidemiological Studies in AA and Future Strategies

AA remains a rare disease with an annual incidence between 0.6 and 6 million per annum. It is innately difficult to conduct a population-based study in a rare disease such as AA. Reporting of cases with AA is likely to be only from areas and centers that have a high coverage of health services. It is likely that there had been underreporting of cases with AA in regions with poor access to tertiary health care services or facilities for diagnostic tests, including special tests for genomic and molecular analysis.

Drug recording and reporting to the medicines regulatory body for association is not uniformly practiced, leading to under- or overestimation of association and causality (Chloramphenicol remains a case in point for an example of the latter). Given the catastrophic event of SAA in a given patient and the need to find explanations, the diagnosis may cause overreporting of drug associations. The notion of an autoimmune cause of the disease has led to a fall in the proportion of cases attributed to specific drugs.

The distinction between acquired and inherited disease may also present a clinical challenge, especially among pediatric cases.

Multicenter clinical trials for newer therapeutic agents or treatment strategies in AA may provide in different countries a uniform panel of recording data, including family history for inherited bone marrow-failure syndromes and special tests, including T-cell subset repertoire analysis, and next-generation technique molecular analysis.

Following this theme, future epidemiological studies for AA are likely to better explain the association to causality in AA, precise diagnosis and staging prognostic information, and also unravel key molecular pathways for therapeutic exploitation.

References

1. Killick S, Brown N, Cavenagh J, et al. Guidelines for the diagnosis and management of adult aplastic anemia. Br J Haem. 2016;172:187–207.
2. Montané E, Ibanez L, Vidal X, et al. Epidemiology of aplastic anaemia: a prospective multicenter study. Haematologica. 2008;93:518–23.
3. Kaufman DW, Kelly JP, Levy M, et al. The drug etiology of agranulocytosis and aplastic anemia. New York: Oxford University Press; 1991.
4. Cartwright RA, McKinney PA, Williams L, et al. Aplastic anaemia incidence in parts of the United Kingdom in 1985. Leuk Res. 1988;12:459–63.
5. Mary JY, Baumelou M, Guiguet M, The French Cooperative Group for Epidemiological Study of Aplastic Anemia. Epidemiology of aplastic anemia in France: a prospective multi-centric study. Blood. 1990;75:1646–53.
6. Clausen N, Kreuger A, Salmi T, et al. Severe aplastic anaemia in the Nordic countries: a population based study of incidence, presentation, course, and outcome. Arch Dis Child. 1996;74:319–22.
7. Maluf EM, Pasquini R, Eluf JN, et al. Aplastic anemia in Brazil: incidence and risk factors. Am J Hematol. 2002;71:268–74.
8. Issaragrisil S, Sriratanasatavorn C, Piankijagum A, et al. Incidence of aplastic anemia in Bangkok. The Aplastic Anemia Study Group. Blood. 1991;77(10):2166–8.
9. Issaragrisil S, Kaufman DW, Anderson T, et al. The epidemiology of aplastic anemia in Thailand. Blood. 2006;107:1299–307.
10. Yang C, Zhang X. Incidence survey of aplastic anemia in China. Chin Med Sci J. 1991;6:203–7.
11. Szklo M, Sesenbrenner L, Markowitz J, at. Incidence of aplastic anemia in metropolitan Baltimore. A population based study. Blood. 1985;66:115–9.
12. Yong AS, Goh M, Rahman J, et al. Epidemiology of aplastic anemia in the state of Sabah, Malaysia. Cell Immunol. 1996;1284:S75.
13. McCahon E, Tang K, Rogers PC, McBride ML, et al. The impact of Asian descent on the incidence of acquired severe aplastic anaemia in children. Br J Haematol. 2003;121(1):170–2.
14. Ahamed M, Anand M, Kumar A, Siddiqui MK. Childhood aplastic anaemia in Lucknow, India: incidence, organochlorines in the blood and review of case reports following exposure to pesticides. Clin Biochem. 2006;39(7):762–6.
15. Qing L, Luoping Z, Guilan L, et al. Hematotoxicity in workers exposed to low levels of Benzene. Science. 2004;306(5702):1774–6.
16. Qing L, Luoping Z, Min S, et al. Polymorphisms in cytokine and cellular adhesion molecule genes and susceptibility to Hematotoxicity among workers exposed to benzene. Cancer Res. 2005;65:9574–81.
17. Maluf E, Hamerschlak N, Cavalcanti AB, et al. Incidence and risk factors of aplastic anemia in Latin American countries: the LATIN case-control study. Haematologica. 2009;94(9):1220–6.
18. Young N, Kaufman D. The epidemiology of acquired aplastic anemia. Haematologica. 2008;93:489–92.
19. Heimpel H. Epidemiology and aetiology of aplastic anaemia. In: Schrezenmeier H, Bacigalupo A, editors. Aplastic anaemia: pathophysiology and treatment. Cambridge, UK: Cambridge University Press; 2000. p. 97–116.
20. Mahapatra M, Singh PK, Agarwal M, et al. Epidemiology, clinico-haematological profile and management of aplastic anaemia: AIIMS experience. J Assoc Physicians India. 2015;63(3 Suppl):30–5.
21. Adil SN, Kakepoto GN, Khurshi M. Epidemiological features of aplastic anaemia in Pakistan. JPMA. 2001;51:443.
22. Young NS. Bone marrow failure syndromes. Philadelphia: W.B. Saunders; 2000.
23. Hao LY, Armanios M, Strong MA, et al. Short telomeres, even in the presence of telomerase, limit tissue renewal capacity. Cell. 2005;123:1121–31.

24. Brown KE, Tisdale J, Barrett AJ, et al. Hepatitis-associated aplastic anemia. N Engl J Med. 1997;336:1059–64.
25. Locasciulli A, Bacigalupo A, Bruno B. Hepatitis-associated aplastic anaemia: epidemiology and treatment results obtained in Europe. A report of the EBMT aplastic anaemia working party. Br J Haematol. 2010;6:890–5.
26. Gonzalez-Casas R, Garcia-Buey L, Jones EA, et al. Systematic review: hepatitis-associated aplastic anaemia – a syndrome associated with abnormal immunological function. Aliment PharmacolTher. 2009;30:436–43.
27. Adachi Y, Yasui H, Yuasa H, Ishi Y, Imai K, Kato Y. Hepatitis B virus-associated aplastic anemia followed by myelodysplastic syndrome. Am J Med. 2002;112:330–2.
28. Byrnes JJ, Banks AT, Piatack M Jr, Kim JP. Hepatitis G-associated aplastic anaemia. Lancet. 1996;348:472.
29. Pardi DS, Romero Y, Mertz LE, Douglas DD. Hepatitis-associated aplastic anemia and acute parvovirus B19 infection: a report of two cases and a review of the literature. Am J Gastroenterol. 1998;93:468–70.
30. Lau YL, Srivastava G, Lee CW, et al. Epstein-Barr virus associated aplastic anaemia and hepatitis. J Paediatr Child Health. 1994;30:74–6.
31. Poovorawan Y, Tangkijvanich P, Theamboonlers A, et al. Transfusion transmissible virus TTV and its putative role in the etiology of liver disease. Hepato-Gastroenterology. 2001;48:256–60.
32. Imai T, Itoh S, Okada H, et al. Aplastic anemia following hepatitis associated with echovirus 3. Pediatr Int. 2002;44:522–4.
33. Fu¨hrer M, Rampf U, Baumann I, et al. Immunosuppressive therapy for aplastic anemia in children: a more severe disease predicts better survival. Blood. 2005;106:2102–4.
34. Young NS, Brown KE. Mechanisms of disease: parvovirus B19. N Engl J Med. 2004;350:586–97.
35. Mishra B, Malhotra P, Ratho RK, et al. Human Parvovirus B19 in patients with aplastic anemia. Am J Hematol. 2005;79:166–7.
36. Pagliuca S, Gérard L, Kulasekararaj A, et al. Characteristics and outcomes of aplastic anemia in HIV patients: a brief report from the severe aplastic anemia working party of the European Society of Blood and Bone Marrow Transplantation. Bone Marrow Transpl. 2016;51:313–5.
37. Young NS, Alter BP, Young NS. In: Young NS, Alter BP, editors. Aplastic anemia, acquired and inherited, drugs and chemicals. Philadelphia: W.B. Saunders; 1994. p. 100–32.
38. Chapuis B, Von Fliedner VE, Jeannet M, et al. Increased frequency of DR2 in patients with aplastic anaemia and increased DR sharing in their parents. Br J Haem. 1986;63:51–7.
39. Nimer SD, Ireland P, Meshkinpour A, et al. An increased HLA DR2 frequency is seen in aplastic anemia patients. Blood. 1994;84:923–7.
40. Shao W, Tian D, Congyan L, et al. Aplastic anemia is associated with HLA-DRB1*1501 in northern Han Chinese. Int J Hemat. 2000;71:350–2.
41. Nakao S, Takamatsu H, Chuhjo T, et al. Identification of a specific HLA class II haplotype strongly associated with susceptibility to cyclosporine-dependent aplastic anemia. Blood. 1995;84:4257–61.
42. Ilhan O, Beksac M, Arslan O, Koc H, et al. HLA-DR frequency in Turkish aplastic anemia patients and the impact of HLA-DR2 positivity in response rate in patients receiving immunosuppressive therapy, vol. 86. Blood; 1995.
43. Rehman S, Saba N, Khalilullah, et al. The frequency of HLA class I and II alleles in Pakistani patients with aplastic anemia. Imm Investigations. 2009;38:251–4.
44. Dhaliwal JS, Wong L, Kamaluddin MA. Susceptibility to aplastic anemia is associated with HLA-DRB1* 1501 in an aboriginalpopulation in Sabah, Malaysia. Human Immunol. 2011;72:889–92.
45. Maciejewski JP, Follmann D, Nakamura R. Increased frequency of HLA-DR2 in patients with paroxysmal nocturnal hemoglobinuria and the PNH/aplastic anemia syndrome. Blood. 2001;98:3513–9.

46. Nakao S, Takami A, Takamatsu H. Isolation of a T-cell clone showing HLA-DRB1*0405-restricted cytotoxicity for hematopoietic cells in a patient with aplastic anemia. Blood. 1997;89:3691.
47. Yari F, Sobhani M, Vaziri MZ, et al. Association of Aplastic Anemia and Fanconi's disease with HLA-DRB1 alleles. Int J Imm. 2008;35:453–6.
48. Chen C, Lu S, Luo M, et al. Correlations between HLA-A, HLA-B and HLA-DRB1 allele polymorphism to acquired aplastic anemia. Acta Haematol. 2012;128:23–7.
49. Odum N, Platz P, Morling N, et al. Increased frequency of HLA-DPw3 in severe aplastic anemia. Tissue Antigens. 1987;29:184–5.
50. Albert E, et al. HLA antigens and haplotypes in 200 patients with aplastic anemia. Transplantation. 1976;22:528–31.
51. Dausset J, Gluckman E, et al. Excess of HLA-A2 and HLA-A2 homozygotes in patients with aplastic anemiaFanconi'sanemias. Nouv Rev Fr Hematol Blood Cells. 1977;18:315–24.
52. Gluckman E. HLA markers in patients suffering from aplastic anaemia. Haematologia. 1981;14:165–72.
53. D'Amaro J, et al. HLA associations in Italian and non-Italian Caucasoid aplastic anemia patients. Tissue Antigens. 1983;21:184–91.
54. Shichishima T, Noji H, Ikeda K, et al. The frequency of HLA class I alleles in Japanese patients with bone marrow failure. Haematologica. 2006;91:857.
55. Oguz FS, Yalman N, Diler S, et al. HLA-DR15 and pediatric Aplastic anemia patients. Haematologica. 2002;87:772–4.
56. Song EY, Park S, Lee DS, et al. Association of human leukocyte antigen-DRB1 alleles with disease susceptibility and severity of Aplastic anemia in Korean patients. Human Immun. 2008;69:354–9.
57. Fuhrer M, Durner J, Brunnler G, et al. HLA association is different in children and adults with severe acquired Aplastic anemia. Pediatr Blood Cancer. 2007;48:186–91.
58. Kook H, Hwang TJ, Seo JJ, et al. The frequency of HLA alleles in Korean children with aplastic anemia and the correlation with the response to immunosuppressive treatment. Korean J Pediatr Hematol Oncol. 2003;10:177–88.
59. Yoshida N, Yagasaki H, Takahashi Y, et al. Clinical impact of HLA-DR15, a minor population of paroxysmal nocturnal haemoglobinuria-type cells, and an aplastic anaemia-associated autoantibody in children with acquired Aplastic anemia. Br J Haematol. 2008;142:427–35.
60. Yunis JJ, Corzo D, Salazar M, et al. HLA associations with clozapine-induced agranulocytosis. Blood. 1995;86:1777.
61. Corzo D, Yunis JJ, Salazar M, et al. The major histocompatibility complex region marked by HSP70-1 and HSP70-2 varisnts is associated with clozapine induced agranulocytosis in two different ethnic groups. Blood. 1995;86:3835–40.
62. Tamai H, Sudo T, Kimura A, et al. Association between the DRB1*08032 histocompatibility antigen and methimazole-induced agranulocytosis in Japanese patients with graves disease. Ann Intern Med. 1996;124:490–4.
63. Sugimori C, Yamazaki H, Feng X, et al. Roles of DRB1*1501 and DRB1*1502 in the pathogenesis of Aplastic anemia. Exp Hematol. 2007;35:13–20.
64. Kapustin SI, Popova TI, Lyshchov AA, et al. HLA-DR4-Ala74 beta is associated with high risk and poor outcome of severe aplastic anemia. Ann Haem. 2001;80:66–71.
65. Bacigalupo A. Aetiology of severe aplastic anaemia and outcome after allogeneic bone marrow transplantation or immunosuppression. Eur J Haematol. 1996;57(Suppl):16–9.
66. De Masson A. Severe aplastic anemia associated with eosinophilic fasciitis: report of 4 cases and review of the literature. Medicine (Baltimore). 2013;2:69–81.
67. Bhatt AS, Berliner N. Hematologic manifestations of SLE. In: Schur P, Massarotti E, editors. Lupus erythematosus: clinical evaluation and treatment. New York: Springer; 2012. p. 127–40.
68. Alishiri GH, Saburi A, Bayat N, et al. The initial presentation of systemic lupus erythematosis with aplastic anemia successfully treated with rituximab. Clin Rheumatol. 2012;31(2):381.

69. Stalder MP, Rovó A, Halter J, et al. Aplastic anemia and concomitant autoimmune disease. Ann Hematol. 2009;88:659–65.
70. Cesaro S, Marsh JC, Tridelli G, et al. Retrospective survey on the prevalence and outcome of prior autoimmune diseases in patients with aplastic anemia reported to the Registry of the European Group for Blood and Marrow Transplantation. Acta Haematol. 2010;124:19–22.
71. Tichelli A, Socié G, Marsh J, et al. Outcome of pregnancy and disease course among women with aplastic anemia treated with immunosuppression. Ann Intern Med. 2002;137(3):164.
72. Choudhry VP, Gupta S, Gupta M, et al. Pregnancy associated aplastic anemia—a series of 10 cases with review of the literature. Haematology. 2002;7:233–8.
73. Bourantas K, Makrydinas G, Georgiou I, et al. Aplastic anemia: report of a case with recurrent episodes in consecutive pregnancies. J Reprod Med. 1997;42:672–4.
74. Shah C, Lemke S, Singh V, et al. Case reports of aplastic anemia after vaccine administration. Am J Hematol. 2004;77(2):204.

Open Access This chapter is licensed under the terms of the Creative Commons Attribution 4.0 International License (http://creativecommons.org/licenses/by/4.0/), which permits use, sharing, adaptation, distribution and reproduction in any medium or format, as long as you give appropriate credit to the original author(s) and the source, provide a link to the Creative Commons license and indicate if changes were made.

The images or other third party material in this chapter are included in the chapter's Creative Commons license, unless indicated otherwise in a credit line to the material. If material is not included in the chapter's Creative Commons license and your intended use is not permitted by statutory regulation or exceeds the permitted use, you will need to obtain permission directly from the copyright holder.

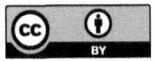

Chapter 3
Pathophysiology of Acquired Bone Marrow Failure

Nicholas C. Lee and Neal S. Young

Introduction: Evidence and Inferences from the Clinic

Acquired aplastic anemia (AA) is the prototypical bone marrow (BM) failure syndrome. AA is characterized by peripheral blood pancytopenia and BM hypoplasia. Low blood counts and "empty" marrow pathology imply the absence of stem and progenitor cells, which is consistent with the success of BM transplantation (BMT), where replacement of hematopoietic stem cells (HSCs) and immune cells is adequate to cure disease. Though if absent stem cells were the sole deficiency, twin donor or syngeneic transplants should be successful with BM infusion but a large proportion suffer graft failure. Conditioning eliminates graft failure, suggesting an immune pathophysiology [1]. Immunosuppressive regimens were developed in the context of graft failure and are widely employed when a stemcell transplant is not feasible. The efficacy of immunosuppressive therapy (IST) alone is strong evidence of an immune mechanism in most patients with AA: 60–70% respond to one course of horse antithymocyte globulin (hATG) and cyclosporine (CsA), and an additional 30% of primary nonresponders will respond to a second course of IST. Patients' blood counts often are dependent on continued administration of CsA, as would be expected of a T-cell-mediated disease. Eltrombopag, a thrombopoietin (TPO) mimetic, has activity in refractory SAA as a single agent and in increasing the complete response rate when combined with IST as first therapy. These results suggest there are residual HSCs that can repopulate the BM, even if they are not detectable. Genomic data applying whole-exome sequencing in AA shows that hematopoiesis can be sustained from a single or very few HSC clones. Clonal hematopoiesis has also been inferred from the frequent, unique association of paroxysmal nocturnal

N. C. Lee (✉) · N. S. Young
Hematology Branch, National Heart, Lung, and Blood Institutes, National Institutes of Health, Bethesda, MD, USA
e-mail: nicholas.lee3@nih.gov

hemoglobinuria (PNH), the origin of which is a somatic mutation in an X-linked gene, with acquired AA.

In vitro experiments with patients' cells are consistent with clinical observations in supporting an immune mechanism of AA. The presence of PNH or acquired copy-number neutral loss of heterozygosity of the 6p arms (6pLOH) clones supports clonal escape from immune-mediated BM destruction. Immune-mediated destruction of BM can be modeled in animals and animal experiments, employing myelotoxic drugs or myeloablative transplants, showing that very limited numbers of HSCs can support hematopoiesis for prolonged time periods. Clonal evolution, the development of myelodysplastic syndrome (MDS) and acute myeloid leukemia (AML) in a patient with typical AA, often after successful IST, demonstrates genomic instability in the setting of an immune or inflammatory disease environment (and occurs in other immune diseases, such as inflammatory bowel disease and chronic hepatitis). Short telomeres appear to predispose to genomic instability, with tissue culture and animal model experiments providing a mechanism of chromosome derangement. In some cases of clonal evolution, there is evidence of origin from a tiny clone of cells harboring a recurrent mutation in an MDS/AML candidate gene.

Pathophysiology

Hematopoiesis in AA

AA is a BM failure syndrome characterized by peripheral blood pancytopenia and BM hypoplasia [2–5]. Profound reduction in hematopoietic stem and progenitor cells (HSPCs) is a consistent finding [6–10]. Stem cells/early progenitor cells can be assayed by long-term culture-initiating cell assays (LTC-ICs) [8, 10] or cobblestone area-forming cells [11]; these cells are also markedly deficient in AA. The scant numbers of LTC-ICs per mononuclear cell suggest that only a small percentage of residual early hematopoietic cells remain at presentation in severely affected patients. There are few or no CD34+ cells on flow cytometry [9].

HSC fate-mapping analyses in mice have suggested that progenitors and not HSCs are fundamental for hematopoiesis under homeostatic conditions [12, 13]. Using a flow cytometric gating scheme to define MPPs (CD34+CD38–Thy1–CD45RA–CD49f–), CMPs (CD34+CD38+CD10–FLT3+CD45RA–), and MEPs (CD34+CD38+CD10–FLT3–CD45RA–), the progenitor hierarchy was examined in a few cases of AA [14]. Consistent with previous reports, the proportion of CD34+ cells within the overall mononuclear cell pool was much lower in AA compared with normal BM [7, 10]. The CD34+CD38– stem-cell compartment in AA was more significantly depleted compared with the CD34+CD38+ progenitor compartment. HSCs and MPPs were virtually undetectable in the residual CD34+CD38– compartment, confirming that HSCs are lost in AA, as determined by phenotype. Despite the loss of phenotypic HSCs, the CD34+CD38+ compartment was detectable in all cases. The percentage of myeloid progenitors was equivalent compared with normal BM. In contrast, erythroid progenitors were low, like HSCs, in all patients. These results suggest that ongoing erythropoiesis is more reliant on HSC input compared with myelopoiesis. Consistent with these findings, clinical data suggested that the baseline absolute reticulocyte count (ARC) and absolute lymphocyte count (ALC) together serve as a simple predictor of response to IST and a greater rate of 5-year survival [15].

While physiological studies of hematopoiesis and immunity in human subjects were once thought to be impossible, single-cell genomics is advancing our understanding of the complex interplay in bone marrow failure syndromes [16]. Single-cell studies have demonstrated that CD8+ T cells accumulate JAK-STAT and MAPK pathway somatic mutations [17], Th-17 polarized CD4+ CAMK4+ T cells have activated IL-6/JAK3/STAT3 pathways [18], CD38+CD8+ T cells directly infiltrate the bone marrow with evidence of inflammation [19], and cell-type-specific ligand-receptor interactions exist between HSPC and CD4+/CD8+ T cells, particularly FAS/FASL and TNF receptors/TNF-α [20]. A comprehensive study of AA patients compared to autoimmune diseases and healthy individuals revealed that highly expanded, individual-specific (private) clonotypes were not targeted toward viral antigens. Comparison of AA patients' private clonotypes seems to converge on a common epitope. Additionally, these private clonotypes in the bone marrow were most commonly the CD8+ effector phenotype, and the amount of clonotype correlated with IST response [21]. These initial studies have elucidated the nuanced interactions between hematopoiesis and the immune system, providing further evidence for possible therapeutic targets.

In AA, BM is not truly empty but replaced by fat cells [22]. BM adipocytes were reported to be possible negative regulators in the hematopoietic microenvironment [23]. To examine the role of adipocytes in BM failure, a recent study investigated peroxisomal proliferator-activated receptor gamma (PPARγ), a key transcription factor in adipogenesis, utilizing an antagonist of this factor [24]. While PPARγ antagonists inhibited adipogenesis as expected, they also suppressed T-cell infiltration of BM, reduced plasma inflammatory cytokines, decreased expression of multiple inflammasome genes, and ameliorated marrow failure. These results suggested that PPARγ antagonists acted as negative regulators of T cells in addition to their inhibition of BM adipogenesis. In murine models of fatty bone marrow and clonal hematopoiesis, IL-6 was found to be elevated, which provided a selective advantage to preleukemic HSPCs with *DNMT3A* mutations, which was negated by the administration of IL-6 neutralizing antibodies [25]. This provides further support that an "empty" bone marrow replaced with adipocytes may exert selective pressure on the residual stem cells.

AA is strongly associated with PNH [26]. PNH is a rare acquired disorder of HSCs characterized by hemolytic anemia, BM failure, and venous thrombosis. The etiology of PNH is a somatic mutation in the X-linked phosphatidylinositol glycan class A gene (*PIGA*), resulting in global deficiency of glycosyl phosphatidylinositol–anchored proteins (GPI–APs) [27]. Clinically, AA may coexist with or appear to evolve into other hematologic diseases that are characterized by proliferation of distinctive cell clones, as in PNH or MDS [2]. Nearly half of AA patients have clonal populations of cells lacking GPI–APs, PNH clones, because of somatic mutations in the *PIGA* gene [28, 29]. Most clones are small and do not lead to clinical manifestations of hemolysis or thrombosis [30], but classic PNH can be dominated by marrow failure (the "AA/PNH syndrome"). *PIGA* mutant cells can support hematopoiesis for the long term [31–33].

Recent studies have demonstrated clonal hematopoiesis in the majority of AA [34–38]. To clarify the origin, importance, and dynamics over time of clonal hematopoiesis in AA, and its relationship to the development of MDS, AML, or both, targeted deep-sequencing, SNP array karyotyping, and whole-exome sequencing were performed to identify genetic alterations in AA and describe their dynamics over long clinical courses [35]. Somatic mutations in myeloid cancer candidate genes were present in one-third of the AA patients, in a limited number of genes, and at low initial variant allele frequency [35]. Clonal hematopoiesis was detected in 47% of the AA, most frequently as acquired mutations. The prevalence of the mutations increased with age. *DNMT3A*-mutated and *ASXL1*-mutated clones tended to increase in size over time; the size of *BCOR/L1*-mutated and *PIGA*-mutated clones decreased or remained stable [35]. Specific mutations that were found to be associated with clonal evolution 6 months after IST were *RUNX1*, splicing factor mutations, and *ASXL1*, while *BCOR/L1* and *DNMT3A* were not associated [39]. Patients with *BCOR/L1* and *PIGA* mutations have improved IST response rates and overall survival.

These results show parallels between BM failure and normal aging of the hematopoietic compartment. The characteristic mutation signature and correlation of mutations with patient age suggested age-related, spontaneous conversion of methylated cytosine to thymidine at CpG sites as a major source of nucleotide alterations in AA [40]. Similar C-to-T conversion mutations accumulate in hematopoietic progenitors in healthy persons [41–43]. Mutations generally appeared at a low variant allele frequency and involved common mutational targets in myeloid cancers, which suggests that the origin and clonal selection of these mutations are similar to those in AA.

However, the exact mechanism of the selection of mutated cells in AA is unclear. DNMT3A is essential for hematopoietic stem-cell differentiation [43]. DNMT3A loss predisposes murine HSCs to malignant transformation [44]. Deletion of *ASXL1* results in myelodysplasia in vivo [45, 46]. Cells containing *DNMT3A* or *ASXL1* mutations may preferentially self-renew rather than differentiate in response to extrinsic signals. While *BCOR* and *BCORL1* mutations are overrepresented, the teleologic mechanism remains unclear, although *BCOR* is implicated in lymphoid malignancies [47] and myeloid neoplasms [48, 49], and can enhance granulopoiesis via *HoxA* regulation [50]. In contrast, overrepresentation of *PIGA* mutations, as well as frequent 6pUPD involving the specific human leukocyte antigens (HLA) classes, suggests a mechanism of immune evasion from pathogenic T cells [51, 52].

Immune Mechanisms in AA

Clinical Data

An immune mechanism was inferred decades ago from the recovery of autologous hematopoiesis in patients conditioned with ATG who failed to engraft after allogeneic stem-cell transplantation, demonstrating the utility of lymphocyte-depletion with ATG [53]. Also, the majority of syngeneic transplantations where BM was infused without conditioning failed due to rejection, implying an immune mechanism [54]. The responsiveness of AA to IST in most patients is the best evidence of an underlying immune pathophysiology: the majority of patients show hematologic improvement after only transient T-cell depletion by ATGs, relapse usually responds to ATG, and dependence of adequate blood counts on low-dose CsA administration is not infrequent [2].

T Cells and Cytokines

In early laboratory experiments, removal of lymphocytes from aplastic BMs improved colony numbers in tissue culture, and their addition to normal marrow inhibited hematopoiesis in vitro [55]. Immunity to HSCs by activated T cells has been considered to be responsible for the pathogenesis of AA [56, 57]. Laboratory in vitro data have further reinforced the immune pathogenesis in AA, with the principal findings including:

1. An increased cytokine (IFN-γ) of activated T cells is identified both in the blood and BM [58–64]; CD8+ CTLs are expanded in AA, leading to the production of proinflammatory cytokines (e.g., IFN-γ) that induce apoptosis of CD34+ cells [62, 63].
2. In a murine model of AA, JAK1/2 inhibition with ruxolitinib demonstrated profound efficacy in the treatment of bone marrow failure, suppressing the immune response (decreased IFN-γ, TNF-α) [65]. Ruxolitinib improved blood counts, preserved hematopoietic stem cells, and improved survival of the mice.
3. Oligoclonal skewing of the T-cell repertoire indicating expansion of pathogenic CD8+ T cells [66–68]. In general, patients at presentation demonstrate oligoclonal expansions of a few Vβ subfamilies, which diminish or disappear with successful IST; original clones reemerge with relapse, sometimes accompanied by new clones, consistent with spreading of the immune response. Occasionally, a large clone persists in remission, perhaps evidence of T-cell tolerance.
4. A reduction of regulatory T cells (Treg) and an increase in Th17-related T cells resulting in a high Th17/Treg ratio at diagnosis, which tends to normalize in patients responding to IST [69, 70]; a reduction in Treg numbers correlates with disease severity, and the defect is most prominent in severe and very severe AA [71]. Treg depletion is dependent on FASL-mediated apoptosis, which can be overcome with high concentrations of IL-2 in vitro [72].

5. Increased transcription of Th1-related genes in activated T cells of AA patients [73, 74]. In BM failure mouse models, NOTCH signaling is a primary driver of Th1-mediated pathogenesis in AA and may represent a novel target for therapeutic intervention.
6. Confirmation in murine models on the role of Th1 and Th17 cells and related cytokines in producing destruction of marrow progenitor cells, and the positive effects of Th17 blocking antibodies and infusion of regulatory T cells in reversing BM failure in these models [70, 75–79].
7. At the single-cell level, in patients with SAA, CD8+ memory and effector T cells highly express genes associated with activation, exhaustion, and cytokines. The number of cell-type-specific ligand-receptor pairs between HSPCs and CD4+/CD8+ T cells is significantly increased in patients with SAA, including known pathways of FAS/FASL and TNF receptors/TNF-α. These interactions are inactivated with immunosuppressive treatment, though an abnormal transcription state remains in remission [20].

The impact of the T-cell attack on the BM can be modeled in vitro and in vivo. IFN-γ (and tumor necrosis factor-α) in increasing doses reduces the number of human hematopoietic progenitors assayed in vitro. The cytokines efficiently induce apoptosis in CD34+ target cells, at least partially through the Fas-dependent pathway of cell death [56, 80], which can be overcome by IL-2 in vitro [72]. In long-term culture of human BM, in which stromal cells were engineered to constitutively express IFN-γ, the output of long-term culture-initiating cells (LTCI-ICs) was markedly diminished, despite low concentrations of the cytokine in the media, consistent with local amplification of toxicity in the marrow milieu [61]. Measurements of soluble circulating mediating factors in BM failure were limited largely to one or two cytokines in AA [81–84]. High TPO levels have been observed in patients with AA, and these abnormal levels correlate with disease severity [81, 82]. Comprehensive analysis of 31 cytokines identified that high levels of TPO and granulocyte colony-stimulating factor were part of a signature profile for AA [85]. An increase in IL-17-producing Th17 cells in the peripheral blood and BM of patients with AA has also been reported [70, 86, 87]. A recent study showed that TPO and IL-17 levels are useful for differentiating hypocellular refractory cytopenia of childhood (RCC) from pediatric AA [88].

HLA and Cytokine Gene Polymorphisms

There have been a number of studies on the human leukocyte antigens (HLA) and their association with AA. In patients treated with ATG+IST, class I MHC loss was somatically mutated in 13% of individuals, and 7% had somatic mutations and 6pLOH, leading to MHC I loss. *HLA-A*02:01*, *HLA-B*40:02*, *HLA-B*08:01*, and *HLA-B*07:02* were most frequently affected [89]. Olson et al. analyzed the pathogenicity, structural characteristics, and impact of HLA class I and found these same alleles to be overrepresented, but only *HLA-B*40:02* was classified as a higher-pathogenicity allele [90]. While higher-pathogenicity alleles increased the risk of developing AA, they did not affect response to IST or HSCT.

HLA-DR2 is overrepresented among patients [91], suggesting a role for antigen recognition, and its presence is predictive of a better response to CsA [92]. Further research showed *HLA-DRB1*1501* was associated with a good response to IST in Japanese cohorts [93, 94]. Polymorphisms in cytokine genes, associated with an increased immune response, also may be more prevalent: a nucleotide polymorphism in the TNF-α (TNF2) promoter at −308 [95], homozygosity for a variable number of dinucleotide repeats in the gene encoding IFN-γ [96], and polymorphisms in the CTLA4 [97].

Immune Escape Clones (PNH, 6pLOH)

Certain clones may escape the immune attack within the BM environment, proliferate, and attain a survival advantage over normal HSCs. The global absence of a large number of cell-surface proteins in PNH has been hypothesized to allow escape and survival of a preexisting mutant clone. Association of PNH clones with IST response suggests that the escape is from immune attack [29, 98–102]. Small PNH clones present at diagnosis usually remain stable over time but may expand sufficiently to produce symptomatic hemolysis [103]. Comparison by microarray shows that residual cells of normal phenotype in the PNH BM upregulate the same apoptosis and cell-death genes as do CD34+ cells in aplastic marrow, while the *PIGA* mutant clone appears transcriptionally similar to CD34+ cells from healthy donors [104]. Alternatively, NK-cell-mediated cytotoxicity may play a role: immunoglobulin-like receptors (KIR) may be differentially expressed in PNH compared to normal, resulting in cytotoxicity of normal HSCs [105]. Recent work has suggested expansion of autoreactive, CD1d-restricted, GPI-specific T cells in PNH [51]. Cell-extrinsic factors are important in PNH cell clonal expansion.

AA patients possessing clonal/oligoclonal hematopoiesis with copy-number neutral loss of heterozygosity (CNN-LOH) of the 6p arms (6pLOH) specifically lost either HLA haplotype containing the *HLA-B*40:02, HLA-A*31:01, HLA-A*02:01*, and *HLA-A*02:06* [106]. Approximately 10% of AA have acquired CNN-LOH in 6pLOH, postulated to emerge by immune selection against specific HLA alleles [106–108]. This clonal hematopoiesis may represent a signature of an escape from cytotoxic T cells targeting autoantigens and strengthen the hypothesis of the immune-mediated pathogenesis of AA, although the exact mechanism is still unclear. Isolation of HLA-B*40:02-restricted CTLs specific for HSCs that were present in AA patient peripheral blood or BM further supports the immune hypothesis [109]. Reports show that acquired CN-6pLOH occurs in GPI-AP+ granulocytes, but not in GPI-AP⁻ granulocytes, suggesting that a hostile immune environment drives selection of immune evasive hematopoietic cell clones [110]. Comprehensive sequencing re-demonstrates that while patients can have HLA loss and PNH clones, they do not coexist in the same cells [89], emphasizing there is likely no natural selection advantage to concomitantly possessing HLA loss and GPI-AP⁻ in the same cell.

STAT3 Mutant Clones

Large granular lymphocyte leukemia (LGL) is often associated with immune cytopenias and can occur in BM failure, such as AA and MDS [111, 112]. *STAT3* mutations in LGL clonal expansions are detected [113, 114]. *STAT3* clones can be found not only in known LGL concomitant cases but in a small population of other BM failure cases (7% AA and 2.5% MDS) [88]. *STAT3*-mutated AA patients trend toward better IST responses, and an association with the presence of HLA-DR15 was found. In patients with AA, CD8+ T cells are enriched for mutations in JAK-STAT and MAPK pathways, with STAT3 p.Y640F mutated cells forming a unique phenotype cluster, higher expression of *STAT3* target genes, and changes in clone size with successful IST [17]. Similarly, in pediatric SAA patients, Th17-polarized CD4+ naïve T cells with JAK3/STAT3 pathway activation [18], although somatic mutations were not evaluated. *STAT3* mutant clones may facilitate a persistently dysregulated autoimmune activation responsible for the primary induction of BM failure in a subset of AA and MDS, as they can in other disorders [115].

Innate Immunity

Transcriptional analysis of T cells from AA has implicated some components of innate immunity in AA, including toll-like receptors and natural killer cells [116]. There are some experimental results that support the natural killer cells' involvement in AA [117, 118]. KIR and KIR ligand (KIR-L) genotype study showed that AA and PNH showed decreased frequency of KIR-2DS1 and KIR-2DS5 genes [117]. The reduced frequency of these KIRs in AA and PNH may indicate an immunogenetic relationship between these diseases.

microRNA

There is emerging evidence that microRNA (miRNA) controls and modulates immunity. Dysregulation of miRNA can lead to autoimmune diseases, such as rheumatoid arthritis, multiple sclerosis, and inflammatory bowel disease. Based on exosomal miRNA screening and validation, miR-126-5p was identified as being specific to SAA and was the only miR that demonstrated a strong association with response to IST (AUC 0.79). Of note, higher relative expression of miR-126-5p at diagnosis had the shortest progression-free survival and levels of miR-126-5p decreased with response to IST [119]. There are potential regulatory roles of miR-145-5p and miR-126-3p in T-cell activation in AA, in which MYC and PIK3R2 are the respective targets of these miRNAs [120]. Dysregulated miR-145-5p and miR-126-3p promote T-cell proliferation and increase GZMB and IFN-γ production. Targeting or employing miRNA mimics might be a novel therapeutic approach in AA.

Autoantibodies

Autoantibodies are frequently detected in patients with AA [121–124]. Antimoesin [121], diazepam-binding inhibitor-related protein 1 [122], kinectin [123], postmeiotic segregation increased 1 [123], and HNRNPK antibodies [124] were reported to be expressed in AA. A recent study using SEREX identified autoantibodies that are expressed in AA, accompanied by an immune abnormality [125]. Eight candidates were identified: CLIC1, SLIRP, HSPB11, NHP2L1, SLC50A1, RPL41, RPS27, and SNRPF. Most recently, in a microarray screen of >9000 proteins, a novel anti-COX2 autoantibody (aCOX-2 Ab) that binds to the C-terminal end was identified in 37% of all adult patients with AA [126], demonstrating a sensitivity of 83% in patients >40 years old with *HLA-DRB1*15:01*.

Immune-Mediated BM Failure Mouse Models

Mouse models of AA, produced by the destruction of BM cells using radiation, cytotoxic drugs, and immune cells, have been useful in defining the hematopoietic stem cell and illustrating the potency of small numbers of lymphocytes in specifically inducing apoptosis of BM targets and their cytokines (e.g., IFN-γ-) as negative effector molecules [127–130]. Murine models mimicking AA have used exposure to agents that result in marrow destruction through a direct toxic effect, but models that explore antigenic disparities between strains have resulted in immune-mediated destruction of the marrow, more closely modeling human AA [131]. Infusion of parental lymph node cells into F1 hybrid donors caused pancytopenia, profound marrow aplasia, and death [79]. Not only a murine version of ATG and CsA, but also monoclonal antibodies to IFN-γ and tumor necrosis factor abrogated hematologic disease, rescuing animals. A powerful "innocent bystander" effect, in which activated cytotoxic T cells kill genetically identical targets, was present in secondary transplantation experiments [78]. In a minor histocompatibility antigen-discordant model, marrow destruction resulted from activity of an expanded H60 antigen-specific T-cell clone [77]. Treatment with the CsA abolished H60-specific T-cell expansion and rescued animals from fatal pancytopenia. The development of BM failure was associated with a significant increase in activated CD4+CD25+ T cells that did not express intracellular FoxP3, whereas inclusion of normal CD4+CD25+ regulatory T cells in combination with C57BL/6 LN cells aborted H60-specific T-cell expansion and prevented BM destruction. Trafficking of T cells to the marrow has also been shown to be important in AA pathogenesis in murine models [132].

Mouse Models of Chemical and Drug Hematopoietic Toxicity

In a few instances, mouse models have been utilized to examine chemical and drug toxicity for hematopoiesis. Industrial exposure to benzene has numerous deleterious hematologic effects in human workers. When benzene was subcutaneously injected into CD1 mice, they showed lethargy, irritability, and weight loss, with decreased hemoglobin, erythrocytes, leukocytes, and BM cells indicative of BM failure [133].

Chronic, delayed hematotoxicity of the chemotherapy drug busulfan was recapitulated in a mouse model: following a course of therapy, animals maintained normal blood and BM cell counts for 1 year before developing pancytopenia and frank marrow aplasia, with a significant decline in splenic colony-forming units (CFU) [134]. BALB/c mice were treated eight times with busulfan over 23 days and found reductions in nucleated marrow cells, granulocyte-macrophage (CFU-GM), CFU-erythroid, erythrocytes, leukocytes, platelets, and reticulocytes on day 1, which continued until days 91 and 112 posttreatment [135].

Genetic Risk Factors in AA

Telomeres are DNA sequences with a structure that protects chromosomes from erosion, and a specific enzyme, telomerase, is involved in their repair after mitosis [136, 137]. Telomeres are repeated nucleotide sequences that cap the ends of chromosomes and protect them from damage. Acquired and congenital AA have been linked molecularly and pathophysiologically by abnormal telomere maintenance [138, 139]. Telomeres are eroded with cell division, but in HSCs, maintenance of their length is mediated by telomerase. Accelerated telomere shortening is virtually universal in dyskeratosis congenita due to mutations in genes encoding components of telomerase, the telomerase-dedicated shelterin complex, or accessory factors (*TERT*, *TERC*, *DKC1*, *NOP10*, *TINF2*, *NHP2*, *WRAP53*, *CTC1*, *RTEL1*, *PARN*, *RPA1*, and *DCLRE1B*) [140–145]. These mutations can cause low telomerase activity, accelerated telomere shortening, and diminished proliferative capacity of hematopoietic progenitors. Sex hormones increase telomerase activity by upregulating the *TERT* gene [146]. Blood count improvement can be obtained with androgen therapy in patients with a mutation in telomere-repair complex genes [147]. Short telomeres were found in leukocytes from approximately one-third of patients with AA, especially those who do not have a response to IST [148, 149]. Systematic screening of patients with apparently AA showed a few patients with *TERT* or *TERC* mutations [150, 151]. Patients with SAA undergoing transplant with pretransplant relative telomere length <10th percentile-for-age was increased with an increased risk of post-HCT mortality [152]. For more information about telomeres, please refer to Chap. 15.

Mutation of *SBDS* underlies Shwachman-Diamond syndrome (SDS), an inherited syndrome featuring BM failure, which clinically presents with skeletal abnormalities, exocrine pancreatic insufficiency, and fat malabsorption with the hematologic hallmark of neutropenia and risk for myeloid malignancy in homozygotes or compound heterozygotes [151]. *SBDS* encodes the SBDS protein, which promotes the creation of the mature, translationally active 80S ribosome. Heterozygosis for the 258 + 2 T > C *SBDS* gene was associated with AA (4 of 91 AA) and leukocyte telomere shortening—three of these patients did not respond to IST and another relapsed shortly after IST [153]. A pediatric patient with a concomitant *TERT* 1062A>T gene variant rapidly evolved to monosomy 7, highlighting that these mutations may be able to cooperate to alter malignant predispositions.

Germline *GATA2* gene mutations, leading to haploinsufficiency, have been identified in patients with familial MDS/AML [154], monocytopenia and mycobacterial infections [155, 156], Emberger syndrome [157], and dendritic cell, monocyte, B-, and NK-cell deficiency [158, 159]. *GATA2* mutations have also been identified in a subset of patients presenting with chronic neutropenia [160] and young adults with AA [161], highlighting the clinical heterogeneity and variable hematologic phenotypes associated with a single genetic defect. The BM from patients with GATA2 deficiency is typically hypocellular, with varying degrees of dysplasia. The marrow had severely reduced monocytes, B cells, and NK cells; absent hematogones; and inverted CD4:CD8 ratios. Atypical megakaryocytes and abnormal cytogenetics were more common in GATA2 marrows. Routine BM flow cytometry, morphology, and cytogenetics in patients who present with cytopenias can identify patients for whom GATA2 sequencing is indicated [161]. If GATA2 mutations are identified, it is important to screen family members who may be potential donors, as HSCT is the only definitive therapy for GATA2 deficiency [162, 163], and there have been reports of donor-derived myeloid malignancy due to donor GATA2 deficiency [164].

Familial AA is an extremely rare inherited subtype affecting multiple individuals in a family. Patients typically only have features of AA; the absence of any somatic features makes it distinct from other inherited AA. By exome sequencing, the causative homozygous *MPL* mutation in a family with familial AA is reported [165]. Biallelic constitutional mutations in *MPL* have been described in congenital amegakaryocytic thrombocytopenia (CAMT) [166]. *MPL* mutations can be found in children with familial AA in whom CAMT was not diagnosed or suspected. Additional studies will be needed to further clarify the relationship between CAMT, AA, and *MPL*.

While there is interplay between isolated mutations in IBMFS genes, for acquired bone marrow failure, the focus is on excluding an inherited syndrome through clinical history, genetic screening, and focused laboratory testing [167]. It is crucial to promptly test for IBMFS with genetic sequencing, chromosomal breakage, and telomere length, as it will determine whether immunosuppressive therapy or hematopoietic stemcell transplant will be pursued (including whether conditioning should include radiation in the latter scenario). Unrecognized IBMFS undergoing transplant for presumed SAA is associated with worse survival [168]. For centers without a bone marrow failure specialist, distinguishing between inherited and immune-mediated marrow failure syndromes can be aided with an algorithm developed with machine learning (https://dir.nhlbi.nih.gov/DDxAA/) [169].

Clonality and Clonal Evolution in AA

Distinguishing between clonality, which is poorly defined, and clonal evolution is essential [170]. All hematopoiesis is clonal, arising from a finite number of stem cells, which is more pronounced in marrow failure disorders. The selection of clones, defined as an identical cell population, is complex in immune aplastic anemia and related to the existing populations at the initial immune destruction (e.g., preexisting age-related clonal hematopoiesis), natural selection due to cell-intrinsic factors and microenvironment (e.g., monosomy 7), and the target of immune attack itself (e.g., *PIGA* mutations, HLA loss). While acquired adaptations can be beneficial for stem-cell fitness in a marrow under immune attack, the concern remains whether these clones—with mutations often found in myeloid malignancy genes—will sustain functioning hematopoiesis or evolve into myeloid malignancy.

Clonal evolution occurs in approximately 15% of patients with AA treated with IST when defined as any chromosomal abnormality [39, 171]. Importantly, high-risk clonal evolution, defined as overt myeloid neoplasia, monosomy 7, or complex karyotype, arises in 9% of patients [39]. Monosomy 7 and/or complex karyotype have been associated with inferior survival primarily due to malignant transformation [172]. At the time of monosomy 7 identification, 64% of patients met criteria for MDS/AML, and this was strongly associated with progression to high-risk MDS or AML, even if no morphologic dysplasia was present [39]. In contrast, +8 and del13q may appear in AA that is responsive to IST and associated with a good prognosis [172–174]. 13q deletion is the most common chromosomal abnormality to progress to overt myeloid neoplasm, monosomy 7, or complex karyotype [39]. In AA patients with PNH clones, cytogenetic abnormalities usually occur in hematopoietic cells that are of normal phenotype (GPI-AP positive), suggesting these cells have a different origin [33, 174].

Telomere dynamics play a role in the development of myeloid cancers in patients with AA not associated with a telomere biology disorder (TBD). In adult patients with severe AA undergoing IST (without a known TBD), pretreatment telomere length in the bottom quartile for age (by qPCR) was a significant risk factor for evolution to MDS [175]. Patients with the shortest telomeres had more uncapped telomere-free chromosome ends as compared to the patients with the longest telomeres [176]. More recently, with flow-FISH, TL <10th percentile in lymphocytes was not predictive of clonal evolution [39, 177], though this requires further study given the difference in assays. Analysis of patients without TBDs and with normal telomere length at the time of diagnosis who developed monosomy 7 found these patients had dramatically accelerated telomere attrition before developing MDS [178]. Rapid telomere loss led to an accumulation of individual chromosomes bearing extremely short telomeres prior to the development of monosomy 7. Dependence on a limited stemcell pool to support hematopoiesis would require an increased rate of cell division and accelerate telomere attrition.

The evaluation of HLA class I has revealed contradictory associations with clonal evolution. *HLA-B*14:02* has been associated with increased rates of clonal evolution in a number of studies [89, 90, 179]. Additionally, HLA loss was also associated with increased risk for clonal evolution [89], although longer follow-up in the NIH cohort did not demonstrate this association and did not assess HLA genotype [39]. Interestingly, while clonal evolution does not originate in GPI-AP negative clones, it can originate in clones with HLA loss, hinting at possible differences between immune escape mechanisms related to *PIGA* mutations and HLA loss.

Advances in sequencing have allowed visualization of clonality in AA via somatic mutations [34–38]. The most frequently mutated genes are *BCOR*, *BCORL1*, *PIGA*, *DNMT3A*, and *ASXL1* [35]. *BCOR/L1* and *PIGA* clones remained stable over time, and patients with these clones had a better response to IST [35]. Clonal evolution to overt myeloid neoplasm, monosomy 7, or complex karyotype had more frequent somatic mutations, particularly in *RUNX1*, splicing factors, and *ASXL1*, 6 months after IST [39], suggesting these patients should be monitored more frequently. Despite the association of specific somatic mutations with increased rates of high-risk clonal evolution, there have been no prospective trials regarding intervention based on these data, so the standard of care remains active observation.

Treatments for AA

BMT with Matched Sibling Donors

HSCT is the treatment of choice in newly diagnosed patients up to 40 years of age eligible for HSCT with an HLA-matched sibling donor (MSD) [180]. For all other patients, IST with horse ATG/CsA is the preferred treatment modality. The long-term survival for either therapy is about 80% for patients of all ages, with younger patients (<20) faring better in general [181]. Standard treatment for patients who have a matched sibling donor is HSCT, which provides a cure in about 80–90% of patients [180]. Although randomized trials did not achieve adequate power to detect a difference [182], cyclophosphamide (CY) with ATG as a conditioning regimen results in improved overall survival in retrospective analyses [182, 183]. Survival in adults older than 40 years of age remains consistent at 50% [184, 185].

BM source, conditioning with CY+ATG, and GVHD prophylaxis by CsA + MTX represent the gold standard in MSD transplantation for AA. Given the excellent overall survival, prevention and early detection of late HSCT complications is the main objective [186]. Thus, the use of peripheral blood stem cells is discouraged because they increase the incidence of chronic GVHD compared to the use of BM as a stem cell source, leading to an unacceptably higher risk of treatment-related mortality [187, 188].

BMT from Alternative Donors

For patients who lack an HLA-identical sibling donor, IST remains first-line treatment. However, 30–40% of patients will be refractory or relapse to IST and will thus be considered for transplantation using an alternative donor. HSCT is indicated if refractory AA patients are fit and have a suitably matched donor, typically a matched unrelated donor (MUD) [189]. This strategy is based on the relatively high risk of complications for MUD transplant recipients, such as graft rejection, GvHD, and infections [190, 191]. However, the outcome of unrelated donor transplants has significantly improved [192, 193]. Current outcomes of UD transplants for AA are non-inferior compared to sibling transplants, although patients are at greater risk of acute and chronic GVHD [194]. The risk of death with UD grafts was higher, but not significantly higher, compared to a sibling donor. Outcomes are better when marrow is the graft source rather than peripheral blood, ATG is utilized in the conditioning regimen, donors are young, and time to transplantation is short.

Haploidentical and Cord Blood HSCT

Other alternative sources of stem cells include umbilical cord blood and a haploidentical family donor [195]. A difficult situation is when a patient with refractory AA has no suitably matched UD, which is not uncommon. The options for these individuals include a second course of IST, an alternative immunosuppressive drug or novel agent, or transplantation using an alternative donor source, namely cord blood or a haploidentical family donor. HSCT offers possibilities of a cure but risks of alternative donor HSCT remain graft rejection and GVHD, especially chronic GVHD, which affects mortality and quality of life.

The key features of a haploidentical graft are short graft procurement time, low cost, and widespread availability for most patients, as a half-matched donor should be present in nearly every family. Historically, haploidentical HSCT was invariably unsuccessful with high rates of graft rejection and GVHD. A recent review of 73 patients receiving HSCT between 1976 and 2011 and mostly using nonmyeloablative regimens showed a 3-year OS of 37% [196]. An updated approach is nonmyeloablative conditioning with high-dose posttransplantation CY given on days +3 and +4 (PTCy) to prevent GVHD by depleting dividing donor-alloreactive T cells while sparing quiescent, non-alloreactive T cells.

In a prospective, multicenter, single-arm Phase 2 trial (BMT CTN 1502) for haploidentical HSCT with PTCy in 31 relapsed or refractory SAA patients, the 1-year OS was 81%, aGVHD was 16%, and cGVHD was 26% [197]. In the treatment-naïve setting, 27 patients with acquired or inherited AA underwent haploidentical HSCT PTCy with a 3-year OS of 92%, 1-year engraftment of 89%, aGVHD of 7%, and 2-year cGVHD of 4% [198]. After the initial 7 patients were treated, the protocol was amended to increase the TBI dose from 200 cGy to 400 cGy—both deaths occurred in patients who received 200 cGy TBI. Similarly, in a report from the EBMT reviewing all patients undergoing haploidentical transplant with PTCy, most of whom had received IST, the 2-year overall survival was similar at 78% [199].

The largest retrospective study of unrelated cord blood transplantation comprised 71 AA patients (9 with PNH) [200]. The main problem was engraftment failure, with a cumulative incidence of neutrophil recovery of only 51% at 2 months and a 3-year OS of 38%. All those patients receiving total body irradiation of 12 Gy as part of the conditioning regimen died, indicating that an RIC rather than a myeloablative regimen is preferable. Significantly improved OS was seen in recipients of >3.9 × 10^7 TNCs/kg pre-freezing [200]. Data for cord blood transplantation (CBT) from MSD is predominantly retrospective from the Eurocord dataset. Most recently described in 2017, 117 patients (median age 6.7 years) underwent transplantation from 1988 to 2014, with 97 IBMFS patients and 20 acquired BMFS patients in the cohort. With a median follow-up of 86.7 months, overall survival at 7 years was 88% (95% CI 91–93%), D+100 aGVHD was 15.2%, and cGVHD was 14.5% [201]. In 2018, de Latour et al. reported a Phase 2 study on unrelated CBT for patients with idiopathic refractory aplastic anemia [202]. Over a median follow-up of 39 months, 26 patients with a median age of 16 years who underwent FLU-CY-ATG-2-Gy TBI conditioning had a 1-year overall survival of 88.5%, D+100 aGVHD of 45.8%, and 1-year cGVD of 36% [202]. A Phase 2 clinical trial showed that haplocord HSCT is an effective treatment option for severe AA patients (including those evolving to MDS) who lack an HLA-matched donor, with an overall survival of 83% at a median of 7.5 years through haploidentical myeloid engraftment, reducing infection risk, followed by long-term umbilical graft hematopoiesis [203].

Immunosuppressive Therapy

The possibility that the pathophysiology of AA could be immune-mediated was initially proposed by Barnes and Mole and later reinforced by autologous hematologic recovery after ATG exposure [131, 204]. The combination of ATG/CsA was shown to be superior to ATG alone and became the standard IST option in patients not eligible for HSCT [205]. Extensive experience with this regimen showed that 60–70% of patients responded to the combination of horse ATG/CsA, making it the standard IST regimen. Across these studies, hematologic response correlated with excellent long-term survival [205–208].

Mounting evidence that AA had an immune-mediated pathogenesis led to the exploration of more immunosuppressive agents in clinical protocols. This development was conducted in two manners: [1] adding a third immunosuppressive agent to horse ATG/CsA and [2] using more potent lymphocyte-depleting agents than horse ATG. Neither strategy improved the outcomes. Adding mycophenolate mofetil or sirolimus to horse ATG/CsA did not improve outcomes in SAA and the use of more lymphocyte-depleting agents (cyclophosphamide, alemtuzumab, rabbit ATG) was equally ineffective [209, 210]. Cyclophosphamide, despite being an active agent in SAA, is associated with prohibitive toxicity impeding its use [211, 212]. Toxicity was considerable, mainly due to prolonged absolute neutropenia, which occurred regardless of pretherapy blood counts and persisted an average of 2 months [212]. Alemtuzumab is associated with a low response rate (about 20%) when given as first therapy [213]. Noteworthy are the disappointing results with rabbit ATG/CsA when compared directly to horse ATG/CsA in a randomized study [214]. The anticipation was for a higher response rate with rabbit ATG/CsA, given its more lymphocyte-depleting properties, Treg-inducing property, activity in horse ATG/

CsA refractory cases, and superiority to horse ATG in solid organ transplant [215–218]. However, results showed a lower response rate of about 35–40% compared to the expected 60–70% seen with horse ATG/CsA [214]. This difference resulted in superior survival outcomes with horse ATG/CsA compared to rabbit ATG/CsA. Other observations from prospective studies confirmed this observation [219]. Therefore, horse ATG/CsA remains the optimal, first-line immunosuppressive regimen in SAA.

The options for patients who fail initial horse ATG/CsA include HSCT from a related (in older patients) or unrelated (in younger patients) HLA-matched donor or a repeat course of IST [194, 220]. Rabbit ATG/CsA or alemtuzumab in this refractory setting can salvage about 30–40% of patients who can achieve a hematologic response [213, 216]. The ability to salvage a proportion of patients with transplant and nontransplant modalities, along with advances in supportive care, has resulted in improved survival outcomes in IST-refractory patients [221]. Even among very refractory patients to IST who do not undergo HSCT, long-term survival can be achieved with supportive care measures, such as transfusions, antimicrobials, growth factors, androgens, and iron chelation. Neutrophil count is the principal determinant of survival [221]. A longer, tapering course of CsA following horse ATG up to 24 months as initial therapy delayed but did not ultimately prevent relapses [222]. Therefore, efforts to improve beyond the outcomes achieved with horse ATG/CsA were ineffective until recently.

StemCell Stimulation

TPO mimetics, such as romiplostim and eltrombopag, were developed to treat patients with refractory immune thrombocytopenia but have been investigated for the treatment of BM failure syndromes [223]. TPO is the main regulator for platelet production, and its receptor (c-MPL) is present on megakaryocytes and HSCs [224, 225]. Historically, the use of G-CSF and erythropoietin has not been effective in systematic AA studies and did not change the natural history of the disease [226]. The use of a TPO agonist was of particular interest given the expression of the TPO agonist receptor in marrow progenitor cells and the reduced numbers of HSCs in murine TPO receptor knockout models [227]. However, the very high endogenous TPO levels in SAA could render this approach ineffective [228]. In a pilot study ($n = 26$), eltrombopag was investigated at an initial dose of 50 mg/day titrated up to 150 mg in an IST-refractory SAA cohort [229]. The overall response rate was 44%, with some bi- and trilineage hematologic improvements observed. The degree and quality of improvement in blood counts with eltrombopag in patients with refractory AA was unanticipated. Responses were striking in several respects: they were not restricted to platelets and were robust, resulting in transfusion independence. In an extended experience ($n = 43$), the response rate was confirmed at 40% and multilineage increments in blood counts continued to be observed [230]. Discontinuation of eltrombopag was possible in a few patients who had achieved a robust hematologic recovery without worsening of the counts. Eight of 43 patients developed new cytogenetic abnormalities. The most common chromosomal changes were chromosome 7 abnormalities, which developed in five of the eight evolvers. This clonal transformation is associated with a poor outcome, but all patients who developed chromosome 7 changes were successfully transplanted. An increase in bone marrow cellularity was observed in some responding patients, suggesting that eltrombopag was stimulating a more primitive progenitor population, leading to improvement in marrow function and an increase in blood counts.

Eltrombopag was evaluated in a Phase 1/2, prospective study in treatment-naïve patients with SAA, which demonstrated an increase in overall response to 74% at 3 months and 80% at 6 months, which is 20–30% higher than historical overall response rates of hATG with CsA [231]. Long-term follow-up with a median of 4 years re-demonstrated the benefit of EPAG-IST, though the relapse rate was 43% [177]. While clonal evolution was identified at earlier timepoints, there was no increase in events, suggesting that HSC stimulation by EPAG promotes existing clone growth to a detectable level. A European Phase 3 trial, The Randomized, Multicenter Trial Comparing Horse ATG Plus Cyclosporine with or without eltrombopag as first-line (RACE), met its primary endpoint of hematologic response at 3 months (IST: 10% versus EPAG-IST 22%) [232], cementing the role of eltrombopag in addition to IST as upfront treatment for SAA and VSAA.

Investigations into alternative TPO agonists, romiplostim and avatrombopag, are underway. A dose-finding study of romiplostim identified a target dose of 10 µg/kg [233], but the single-lineage benefit in refractory AA has been contradictory, from 7% in a French nationwide survey to 84% in a Phase 2/3 Japanese and Korean study [234, 235]. In eltrombopag-refractory patients, increasing the dose up to 20 µg/kg has resulted in transfusion independence [236]. Trials of avatrombopag are ongoing in treatment-naïve and refractory settings in China and Australia. While there is extensive investigation into a class effect of TPO mimetics, eltrombopag remains the evidence-based choice in both treatment-naïve and refractory SAA [229–232].

Supportive Care

Management of AA has been dramatically improved since the late 1970s with the introduction of allogeneic stem-cell transplantation (alloSCT) and IST, as well as optimized supportive care [221]. Supportive care has positively impacted these different treatment modalities. The advent of oral antifungals with activity against *Aspergillus* sp. (voriconazole, posaconazole, isavuconazole) has allowed for continued outpatient therapy against these pathogens that represent the deadliest infectious culprit in SAA [221, 237]. The use of granulocyte transfusion in selected cases has allowed for better control of fungal infections when neutropenia is severe and persistent and antifungals are not resolutive alone [238–240]. Oral iron chelators have allowed for continued long-term transfusion programs in refractory patients, minimizing the risks associated with iron accumulation in the long term [241], and the management of iron status is aided by the iron-chelating effects of eltrombopag [242]. In aggregate, these advances have allowed for patients who failed IST and are not HSCT eligible to be supported for long periods of time.

Conclusions

Investigations into the pathophysiology of aplastic anemia have yielded insights into genetics, the immune system, and stem cell biology. Our understanding of these concepts has improved recognition of immune marrow failure and informed treatment of this once lethal disease with stemcell transplant, immunosuppression, and/or stemcell stimulation. Ongoing research efforts continue to produce results that are being translated into the clinic to provide therapeutic benefit to our patients.

References

1. Gerull S, Stern M, Apperley J, Beelen D, Brinch L, Bunjes D, et al. Syngeneic transplantation in aplastic anemia: pre-transplant conditioning and peripheral blood are associated with improved engraftment: an observational study on behalf of the Severe Aplastic Anemia and Pediatric Diseases Working Parties of the European Group for Blood and Marrow Transplantation. Haematologica. 2013;98(11):1804–9.
2. Young NS, Calado RT, Scheinberg P. Current concepts in the pathophysiology and treatment of aplastic anemia. Blood. 2006;108(8):2509–19.
3. Young NS, Bacigalupo A, Marsh JCW. Aplastic anemia: pathophysiology and treatment. Biol Blood Marrow Transplant. 2010;16(1):S119–S25.
4. Killick SB, Bown N, Cavenagh J, Dokal I, Foukaneli T, Hill A, et al. Guidelines for the diagnosis and management of adult aplastic anaemia. Br J Haematol. 2016;172(2):187–207.
5. Young NS. Aplastic anemia. N Engl J Med. 2018;379(17):1643–56.
6. Scopes J, Bagnara M, Gordon-Smith EC, Ball SE, Gibson FM. Haemopoietic progenitor cells are reduced in aplastic anaemia. Br J Haematol. 1994;86(2):427–30.
7. Marsh JC, Chang J, Testa NG, Hows JM, Dexter TM. The hematopoietic defect in aplastic anemia assessed by long-term marrow culture. Blood. 1990;76(9):1748–57.
8. Maciejewski JP, Selleri C, Sato T, Anderson S, Young NS. A severe and consistent deficit in marrow and circulating primitive hematopoietic cells (long-term culture-initiating cells) in acquired aplastic anemia. Blood. 1996;88(6):1983–91.
9. Matsui WH, Brodsky RA, Smith BD, Borowitz MJ, Jones RJ. Quantitative analysis of bone marrow CD34 cells in aplastic anemia and hypoplastic myelodysplastic syndromes. Leukemia. 2006;20(3):458–62.
10. Rizzo S, Scopes J, Elebute M, Papadaki H, Gordon-Smith E, Gibson F. Stem cell defect in aplastic anemia: reduced long term culture-initiating cells (LTC-IC) in CD34+ cells isolated from aplastic anemia patient bone marrow. Hematol J. 2002;3(5):230–6.
11. Schrezenmeier H, Jenal M, Herrmann F, Heimpel H, Raghavachar A. Quantitative analysis of cobblestone area-forming cells in bone marrow of patients with aplastic anemia by limiting dilution assay. Blood. 1996;88(12):4474–80.
12. Sun J, Ramos A, Chapman B, Johnnidis JB, Le L, Ho Y-J, et al. Clonal dynamics of native haematopoiesis. Nature. 2014;514(7522):322–7.

13. Busch K, Klapproth K, Barile M, Flossdorf M, Holland-Letz T, Schlenner SM, et al. Fundamental properties of unperturbed haematopoiesis from stem cells in vivo. Nature. 2015;518(7540):542–6.
14. Notta F, Zandi S, Takayama N, Dobson S, Gan OI, Wilson G, et al. Distinct routes of lineage development reshape the human blood hierarchy across ontogeny. Science. 2016;351(6269):aab2116.
15. Scheinberg P, Wu CO, Nunez O, Young NS. Predicting response to immunosuppressive therapy and survival in severe aplastic anaemia. Br J Haematol. 2009;144(2):206–16.
16. Wu Z, Young NS. Single-cell genomics in acquired bone marrow failure syndromes. Blood. 2023;142(14):1193–207.
17. Lundgren S, Keränen MAI, Kankainen M, Huuhtanen J, Walldin G, Kerr CM, et al. Somatic mutations in lymphocytes in patients with immune-mediated aplastic anemia. Leukemia. 2021;35(5):1365–79.
18. Zhang J, Liu T, Duan Y, Chang Y, Chang L, Liu C, et al. Single-cell analysis highlights a population of Th17-polarized CD4+ naïve T cells showing IL6/JAK3/STAT3 activation in pediatric severe aplastic anemia. J Autoimmun. 2023;136:103026.
19. You X, Yang Q, Yan K, Wang S-R, Huang R-R, Wang S-Q, et al. Multi-omics profiling identifies pathways associated with CD8+ T-cell activation in severe aplastic anemia. Front Genet. 2022;12:790990.
20. Zhu C, Lian Y, Wang C, Wu P, Li X, Gao Y, et al. Single-cell transcriptomics dissects hematopoietic cell destruction and T-cell engagement in aplastic anemia. Blood. 2021;138(1):23–33.
21. Huuhtanen J, Lundgren S, Keränen MA, Feng X, Kerr CM, Jokinen E, et al. T cell landscape of immune aplastic anemia reveals a convergent antigen-specific signature. Blood. 2019;134(Supplement_1):108.
22. Takaku T, Malide D, Chen J, Calado RT, Kajigaya S, Young NS. Hematopoiesis in 3 dimensions: human and murine bone marrow architecture visualized by confocal microscopy. Blood. 2010;116(15):e41–55.
23. Naveiras O, Nardi V, Wenzel PL, Hauschka PV, Fahey F, Daley GQ. Bone-marrow adipocytes as negative regulators of the haematopoietic microenvironment. Nature. 2009;460(7252):259–63.
24. Sato K, Feng X, Chen J, Li J, Muranski P, Desierto MJ, et al. PPARγ antagonist attenuates mouse immune-mediated bone marrow failure by inhibition of T cell function. Haematologica. 2016;101(1):57–67.
25. Zioni N, Bercovich AA, Chapal-Ilani N, Bacharach T, Rappoport N, Solomon A, et al. Inflammatory signals from fatty bone marrow support DNMT3A driven clonal hematopoiesis. Nat Commun. 2023;14(1):2070.
26. Young NS, Maciejewski JP, Sloand E, Chen G, Zeng W, Risitano A, et al. The relationship of aplastic anemia and PNH. Int J Hematol. 2002;76(Suppl 2):168–72.
27. Takeda J, Miyata T, Kawagoe K, Iida Y, Endo Y, Fujita T, et al. Deficiency of the GPI anchor caused by a somatic mutation of the PIG-A gene in paroxysmal nocturnal hemoglobinuria. Cell. 1993;73(4):703–11.
28. Scheinberg P, Marte M, Nunez O, Young NS. Paroxysmal nocturnal hemoglobinuria clones in severe aplastic anemia patients treated with horse anti-thymocyte globulin plus cyclosporine. Haematologica. 2010;95(7):1075–80.
29. Dunn DE, Tanawattanacharoen P, Boccuni P, Nagakura S, Green SW, Kirby MR, et al. Paroxysmal nocturnal hemoglobinuria cells in patients with bone marrow failure syndromes. Ann Intern Med. 1999;131(6):401–8.
30. Wang H, Chuhjo T, Yasue S, Omine M, Nakao S. Clinical significance of a minor population of paroxysmal nocturnal hemoglobinuria–type cells in bone marrow failure syndrome. Blood. 2002;100(12):3897–902.
31. Shen W, Clemente MJ, Hosono N, Yoshida K, Przychodzen B, Yoshizato T, et al. Deep sequencing reveals stepwise mutation acquisition in paroxysmal nocturnal hemoglobinuria. J Clin Invest. 2014;124(10):4529–38.

32. Katagiri T, Kawamoto H, Nakakuki T, Ishiyama K, Okada-Hatakeyama M, Ohtake S, et al. Individual hematopoietic stem cells in human bone marrow of patients with aplastic anemia or myelodysplastic syndrome stably give rise to limited cell lineages. Stem Cells. 2013;31(3):536–46.
33. Sloand EM, Fuhrer M, Keyvanfar K, Mainwaring L, Maciejewski J, Wang Y, et al. Cytogenetic abnormalities in paroxysmal nocturnal haemoglobinuria usually occur in haematopoietic cells that are glycosylphosphatidylinositol-anchored protein (GPI-AP) positive. Br J Haematol. 2003;123(1):173–6.
34. Babushok DV, Perdigones N, Perin JC, Olson TS, Ye W, Roth JJ, et al. Emergence of clonal hematopoiesis in the majority of patients with acquired aplastic anemia. Cancer Genet. 2015;208(4):115–28.
35. Yoshizato T, Dumitriu B, Hosokawa K, Makishima H, Yoshida K, Townsley D, et al. Somatic mutations and clonal hematopoiesis in aplastic anemia. N Engl J Med. 2015;373(1):35–47.
36. Kulasekararaj AG, Jiang J, Smith AE, Mohamedali AM, Mian S, Gandhi S, et al. Somatic mutations identify a subgroup of aplastic anemia patients who progress to myelodysplastic syndrome. Blood. 2014;124(17):2698–704.
37. Lane AA, Odejide O, Kopp N, Kim S, Yoda A, Erlich R, et al. Low frequency clonal mutations recoverable by deep sequencing in patients with aplastic anemia. Leukemia. 2013;27(4):968–71.
38. Heuser M, Schlarmann C, Dobbernack V, Panagiota V, Wiehlmann L, Walter C, et al. Genetic characterization of acquired aplastic anemia by targeted sequencing. Haematologica. 2014;99(9):e165–e7.
39. Groarke EM, Patel BA, Shalhoub R, Gutierrez-Rodrigues F, Desai P, Leuva H, et al. Predictors of clonal evolution and myeloid neoplasia following immunosuppressive therapy in severe aplastic anemia. Leukemia. 2022;36(9):2328–37.
40. Alexandrov LB, Nik-Zainal S, Wedge DC, Aparicio SAJR, Behjati S, Biankin AV, et al. Signatures of mutational processes in human cancer. Nature. 2013;500(7463):415–21.
41. Welch John S, Ley Timothy J, Link Daniel C, Miller Christopher A, Larson David E, Koboldt Daniel C, et al. The origin and evolution of mutations in acute myeloid leukemia. Cell. 2012;150(2):264–78.
42. Jaiswal S, Fontanillas P, Flannick J, Manning A, Grauman PV, Mar BG, Lindsley RC, Mermel CH, Burtt N, Chavez A, Higgins JM. Age-related clonal hematopoiesis associated with adverse outcomes. N Engl J Med. 2014;371(26):2488–98.
43. Challen GA, Sun D, Jeong M, Luo M, Jelinek J, Berg JS, et al. Dnmt3a is essential for hematopoietic stem cell differentiation. Nat Genet. 2012;44(1):23–31.
44. Mayle A, Yang L, Rodriguez B, Zhou T, Chang E, Curry CV, et al. Dnmt3a loss predisposes murine hematopoietic stem cells to malignant transformation. Blood. 2015;125(4):629–38.
45. Abdel-Wahab O, Gao J, Adli M, Dey A, Trimarchi T, Chung YR, et al. Deletion of Asxl1 results in myelodysplasia and severe developmental defects in vivo. J Exp Med. 2013;210(12):2641–59.
46. Wang J, Li Z, He Y, Pan F, Chen S, Rhodes S, et al. Loss of Asxl1 leads to myelodysplastic syndrome–like disease in mice. Blood. 2014;123(4):541–53.
47. Sportoletti P, Sorcini D, Falini B. BCOR gene alterations in hematologic diseases. Blood. 2021;138(24):2455–68.
48. Tara S, Isshiki Y, Nakajima-Takagi Y, Oshima M, Aoyama K, Tanaka T, et al. Bcor insufficiency promotes initiation and progression of myelodysplastic syndrome. Blood. 2018;132(23):2470–83.
49. Sportoletti P, Sorcini D, Guzman AG, Reyes JM, Stella A, Marra A, et al. Bcor deficiency perturbs erythro-megakaryopoiesis and cooperates with Dnmt3a loss in acute erythroid leukemia onset in mice. Leukemia. 2021;35(7):1949–63.
50. Cao Q, Gearhart MD, Gery S, Shojaee S, Yang H, Sun H, et al. BCOR regulates myeloid cell proliferation and differentiation. Leukemia. 2016;30(5):1155–65.

51. Gargiulo L, Papaioannou M, Sica M, Talini G, Chaidos A, Richichi B, et al. Glycosylphosphatidylinositol-specific, CD1d-restricted T cells in paroxysmal nocturnal hemoglobinuria. Blood. 2013;121(14):2753–61.
52. Murakami Y, Kosaka H, Maeda Y, Nishimura J-I, Inoue N, Ohishi K, et al. Inefficient response of T lymphocytes to glycosylphosphatidylinositol anchor–negative cells: implications for paroxysmal nocturnal hemoglobinuria. Blood. 2002;100(12):4116–22.
53. Speck B, Gluckman E, Hark HL, Rood JJV. Treatment of aplastic anaemia by antilymphocyte globulin with and without allogeneic bone-marrow infusions. Lancet. 1977;310(8049):1145–8.
54. Hinterberger W, Rowlings PA, Hinterberger-Fischer M, Gibson J, Jacobsen N, Klein JP, et al. Results of transplanting bone marrow from genetically identical twins into patients with aplastic anemia. Ann Intern Med. 1997;126(2):116.
55. Young NS. Hematopoietic cell destruction by immune mechanisms in acquired aplastic anemia. Semin Hematol. 2000;37(1):3–14.
56. Maciejewski J, Selleri C, Anderson S, Young NS. Fas antigen expression on CD34+ human marrow cells is induced by interferon γ and tumor necrosis factor α and potentiates cytokine-mediated hematopoietic suppression in vitro. Blood. 1995;85(11):3183–90.
57. Nakao S, Takami A, Takamatsu H, Zeng W, Sugimori N, Yamazaki H, et al. Isolation of a T-cell clone showing HLA-DRB1*0405-restricted cytotoxicity for hematopoietic cells in a patient with aplastic anemia. Blood. 1997;89(10):3691–9.
58. Zoumbos NC, Gascon P, Djeu JY, Young NS. Interferon is a mediator of hematopoietic suppression in aplastic anemia in vitro and possibly in vivo. Proc Natl Acad Sci. 1985;82(1):188–92.
59. Gascon P, Zoumbos NC, Scala G, Djeu JY, Moore JG, Young NS. Lymphokine abnormalities in aplastic anemia: implications for the mechanism of action of antithymocyte globulin. Blood. 1985;65(2):407–13.
60. Zoumbos NC, Gascón P, Djeu JY, Trost SR, Young NS. Circulating activated suppressor T lymphocytes in aplastic anemia. N Engl J Med. 1985;312(5):257–65.
61. Selleri C, Maciejewski JP, Sato T, Young NS. Interferon-gamma constitutively expressed in the stromal microenvironment of human marrow cultures mediates potent hematopoietic inhibition. Blood. 1996;87(10):4149–57.
62. Hosokawa K, Muranski P, Feng X, Townsley DM, Liu B, Knickelbein J, et al. Memory stem T cells in autoimmune disease: high frequency of circulating CD8+ memory stem cells in acquired aplastic anemia. J Immunol. 2016;196(4):1568–78.
63. Sloand E, Kim S, Maciejewski JP, Tisdale J, Follmann D, Young NS. Intracellular interferon-γ in circulating and marrow T cells detected by flow cytometry and the response to immunosuppressive therapy in patients with aplastic anemia. Blood. 2002;100(4):1185–91.
64. Sato T, Selleri C, Young NS, Maciejewski JP. Inhibition of interferon regulatory Factor-1 expression results in predominance of cell growth stimulatory effects of interferon-γ due to phosphorylation of Stat1 and Stat3. Blood. 1997;90(12):4749–58.
65. Groarke EM, Feng X, Aggarwal N, Manley AL, Wu Z, Gao S, et al. Efficacy of JAK1/2 inhibition in murine immune bone marrow failure. Blood. 2023;141(1):72–89.
66. Risitano AM, Maciejewski JP, Green S, Plasilova M, Zeng W, Young NS. In-vivo dominant immune responses in aplastic anaemia: molecular tracking of putatively pathogenetic T-cell clones by TCR β-CDR3 sequencing. Lancet. 2004;364(9431):355–64.
67. Kook H, Risitano AM, Zeng W, Wlodarski M, Lottemann C, Nakamura R, et al. Changes in T-cell receptor VB repertoire in aplastic anemia: effects of different immunosuppressive regimens. Blood. 2002;99(10):3668–75.
68. Zeng W, Maciejewski JP, Chen G, Young NS. Limited heterogeneity of T cell receptor BV usage in aplastic anemia. J Clin Invest. 2001;108(5):765–73.
69. Solomou EE, Rezvani K, Mielke S, Malide D, Keyvanfar K, Visconte V, et al. Deficient CD4+ CD25+ FOXP3+ T regulatory cells in acquired aplastic anemia. Blood. 2007;110(5):1603–6.
70. Latour RPD, Visconte V, Takaku T, Wu C, Erie AJ, Sarcon AK, et al. Th17 immune responses contribute to the pathophysiology of aplastic anemia. Blood. 2010;116(20):4175–84.

71. Kordasti S, Marsh J, Al-Khan S, Jiang J, Smith A, Mohamedali A, et al. Functional characterization of CD4+ T cells in aplastic anemia. Blood. 2012;119(9):2033–43.
72. Lim SP, Costantini B, Mian SA, Abellan PP, Gandhi S, Llordella MM, et al. Treg sensitivity to FasL and relative IL-2 deprivation drive idiopathic aplastic anemia immune dysfunction. Blood. 2020;136(7):885–97.
73. Solomou EE, Keyvanfar K, Young NS. T-bet, a Th1 transcription factor, is up-regulated in T cells from patients with aplastic anemia. Blood. 2006;107(10):3983–91.
74. Roderick JE, Gonzalez-Perez G, Kuksin CA, Dongre A, Roberts ER, Srinivasan J, et al. Therapeutic targeting of NOTCH signaling ameliorates immune-mediated bone marrow failure of aplastic anemia. J Exp Med. 2013;210(7):1311–29.
75. Tang Y, Desierto MJ, Chen J, Young NS. The role of the Th1 transcription factor T-bet in a mouse model of immune-mediated bone-marrow failure. Blood. 2010;115(3):541–8.
76. Omokaro SO, Desierto MJ, Eckhaus MA, Ellison FM, Chen J, Young NS. Lymphocytes with aberrant expression of Fas or Fas ligand attenuate immune bone marrow failure in a mouse model. J Immunol. 2009;182(6):3414–22.
77. Chen J, Ellison FM, Eckhaus MA, Smith AL, Keyvanfar K, Calado RT, et al. Minor antigen H60-mediated aplastic anemia is ameliorated by immunosuppression and the infusion of regulatory T cells. J Immunol. 2007;178(7):4159–68.
78. Chen J, Lipovsky K, Ellison FM, Calado RT, Young NS. Bystander destruction of hematopoietic progenitor and stem cells in a mouse model of infusion-induced bone marrow failure. Blood. 2004;104(6):1671–8.
79. Bloom ML, Wolk AG, Simon-Stoos KL, Bard JS, Chen J, Young NS. A mouse model of lymphocyte infusion-induced bone marrow failure. Exp Hematol. 2004;32(12):1163–72.
80. Maciejewski JP, Selleri C, Sato T, Anderson S, Young NS. Increased expression of Fas antigen on bone marrow CD34+ cells of patients with aplastic anaemia. Br J Haematol. 1995;91(1):245–52.
81. Marsh JCW, Gibson FM, Prue RL, Bowen A, Dunn VT, Hornkohl AC, et al. Serum thrombopoietin levels in patients with aplastic anaemia. Br J Haematol. 1996;95(4):605–10.
82. Kojima S, Matsuyama T, Kodera Y, Tahara T, Kato T. Measurement of endogenous plasma thrombopoietin in patients with acquired aplastic anaemia by a sensitive enzyme-linked immunosorbent assay. Br J Haematol. 1997;97(3):538–43.
83. Kojima S, Matsuyama T, Kodera Y, Nishihira H, Ueda K, Shimbo T, et al. Measurement of endogenous plasma granulocyte colony-stimulating factor in patients with acquired aplastic anemia by a sensitive chemiluminescent immunoassay. Blood. 1996;87(4):1303–8.
84. Hirayama Y, Sakamaki S, Matsunaga T, Kuga T, Kuroda H, Kusakabe T, et al. Concentrations of thrombopoietin in bone marrow in Normal subjects and in patients with idiopathic thrombocytopenic purpura, aplastic anemia, and essential thrombocythemia correlate with its mRNA expression of bone marrow stromal cells. Blood. 1998;92(1):46–52.
85. Feng X, Scheinberg P, Wu CO, Samsel L, Nunez O, Prince C, et al. Cytokine signature profiles in acquired aplastic anemia and myelodysplastic syndromes. Haematologica. 2011;96(4):602–6.
86. Du H-Z, Wang Q, Ji J, Shen B-M, Wei S-C, Liu L-J, et al. Expression of IL-27, Th1 and Th17 in patients with aplastic anemia. J Clin Immunol. 2013;33(2):436–45.
87. Gu Y, Hu X, Liu C, Qv X, Xu C. Interleukin (IL)-17 promotes macrophages to produce IL-8, IL-6 and tumour necrosis factor-α in aplastic anaemia. Br J Haematol. 2008;142(1):109–14.
88. Elmahdi S, Hama A, Manabe A, Hasegawa D, Muramatsu H, Narita A, et al. A cytokine-based diagnostic program in pediatric aplastic anemia and hypocellular refractory cytopenia of childhood. Pediatr Blood Cancer. 2016;63(4):652–8.
89. Zaimoku Y, Patel BA, Adams SD, Shalhoub R, Groarke EM, Lee AAC, et al. HLA associations, somatic loss of HLA expression, and clinical outcomes in immune aplastic anemia. Blood. 2021;138(26):2799–809.
90. Olson TS, Frost BF, Duke JL, Dribus M, Xie HM, Prudowsky ZD, et al. Pathogenicity and impact of HLA class I alleles in aplastic anemia patients of different ethnicities. JCI Insight. 2022;7(22):e163040.

91. Chapuis B, Fliedner VEV, Jeannet M, Merica H, Vuagnat P, Gratwohl A, et al. Increased frequency of DR2 in patients with aplastic anaemia and increased DR sharing in their parents. Br J Haematol. 1986;63(1):51–7.
92. Maciejewski JP, Follmann D, Nakamura R, Saunthararajah Y, Rivera CE, Simonis T, et al. Increased frequency of HLA-DR2 in patients with paroxysmal nocturnal hemoglobinuria and the PNH/aplastic anemia syndrome. Blood. 2001;98(13):3513–9.
93. Sugimori C, Yamazaki H, Feng X, Mochizuki K, Kondo Y, Takami A, et al. Roles of DRB1∗1501 and DRB1∗1502 in the pathogenesis of aplastic anemia. Exp Hematol. 2007;35(1):13–20.
94. Nakao S, Takamatsu H, Chuhjo T, Ueda M, Shiobara S, Matsuda T, et al. Identification of a specific HLA class II haplotype strongly associated with susceptibility to cyclosporine-dependent aplastic anemia. Blood. 1994;84(12):4257–61.
95. Babushok DV, Duke JL, Xie HM, Stanley N, Atienza J, Perdigones N, et al. Somatic HLA mutations expose the role of class I–mediated autoimmunity in aplastic anemia and its clonal complications. Blood Adv. 2017;1(22):1900–10.
96. Demeter J, Messer G, Schrezenmeier H. Clinical relevance of the TNF-alpha promoter/enhancer polymorphism in patients with aplastic anemia. Ann Hematol. 2002;81(10):566–9.
97. Dufour C, Capasso M, Svahn J, Marrone A, Haupt R, Bacigalupo A, et al. Homozygosis for (12) CA repeats in the first intron of the human IFN-γ gene is significantly associated with the risk of aplastic anaemia in Caucasian population. Br J Haematol. 2004;126(5):682–5.
98. Svahn J, Capasso M, Lanciotti M, Marrone A, Haupt R, Bacigalupo A, et al. The polymorphisms −318C>T in the promoter and 49A>G in exon 1 of CTLA4 and the risk of aplastic anemia in a Caucasian population. Bone Marrow Transplant. 2005;35(Suppl 1):S89–92.
99. Nakao S, Sugimori C, Yamazaki H. Clinical significance of a small population of paroxysmal nocturnal hemoglobinuria—type cells in the management of bone marrow failure. Int J Hematol. 2006;84(2):118–22.
100. Sugimori C, Chuhjo T, Feng X, Yamazaki H, Takami A, Teramura M, et al. Minor population of CD55-CD59- blood cells predicts response to immunosuppressive therapy and prognosis in patients with aplastic anemia. Blood. 2006;107(4):1308–14.
101. Hosokawa K, Sugimori N, Katagiri T, Sasaki Y, Saito C, Seiki Y, et al. Increased glycosylphosphatidylinositol-anchored protein-deficient granulocytes define a benign subset of bone marrow failures in patients with trisomy 8. Eur J Haematol. 2015;95(3):230–8.
102. Kulagin A, Lisukov I, Ivanova M, Golubovskaya I, Kruchkova I, Bondarenko S, et al. Prognostic value of paroxysmal nocturnal haemoglobinuria clone presence in aplastic anaemia patients treated with combined immunosuppression: results of two-centre prospective study. Br J Haematol. 2014;164(4):546–54.
103. Shah YB, Priore SF, Li Y, Tang CN, Nicholas P, Kurre P, et al. The predictive value of PNH clones, 6p CN-LOH, and clonal TCR gene rearrangement for aplastic anemia diagnosis. Blood Adv. 2021;5(16):3216–26.
104. Sugimori C, Mochizuki K, Qi Z, Sugimori N, Ishiyama K, Kondo Y, et al. Origin and fate of blood cells deficient in glycosylphosphatidylinositol-anchored protein among patients with bone marrow failure. Br J Haematol. 2009;147(1):102–12.
105. Chen G, Zeng W, Maciejewski JP, Kcyvanfar K, Billings EM, Young NS. Differential gene expression in hematopoietic progenitors from paroxysmal nocturnal hemoglobinuria patients reveals an apoptosis/immune response in 'normal' phenotype cells. Leukemia. 2005;19(5):862–8.
106. van Bijnen ST, Withaar M, Preijers F, van der Meer A, de Witte T, Muus P, et al. T cells expressing the activating NK-cell receptors KIR2DS4, NKG2C and NKG2D are elevated in paroxysmal nocturnal hemoglobinuria and cytotoxic toward hematopoietic progenitor cell lines. Exp Hematol. 2011;39(7):751–62.e3.
107. Katagiri T, Sato-Otsubo A, Kashiwase K, Morishima S, Sato Y, Mori Y, et al. Frequent loss of HLA alleles associated with copy number-neutral 6pLOH in acquired aplastic anemia. Blood. 2011;118(25):6601–9.

108. Babushok DV, Xie HM, Roth JJ, Perdigones N, Olson TS, Cockroft JD, et al. Single nucleotide polymorphism array analysis of bone marrow failure patients reveals characteristic patterns of genetic changes. Br J Haematol. 2014;164(1):73–82.
109. Afable MG, Wlodarski M, Makishima H, Shaik M, Sekeres MA, Tiu RV, et al. SNP array-based karyotyping: differences and similarities between aplastic anemia and hypocellular myelodysplastic syndromes. Blood. 2011;117(25):6876–84.
110. Inaguma Y, Akatsuka Y, Hosokawa K, Maruyama H, Okamoto A, Katagiri T, et al. Induction of HLA-B*40:02-restricted T cells possessing cytotoxic and suppressive functions against haematopoietic progenitor cells from a patient with severe aplastic anaemia. Br J Haematol. 2016;172(1):131–4.
111. Ueda Y, Ji N, Murakami Y, Kajigaya S, Kinoshita T, Kanakura Y, et al. Paroxysmal nocturnal hemoglobinuria with copy number-neutral 6pLOH in GPI (+) but not in GPI (−) granulocytes. Eur J Haematol. 2014;92(5):450–3.
112. Loughran TP. Clonal diseases of large granular lymphocytes. Blood. 1993;82(1):1–14.
113. Saunthararajah Y, Molldrem JJ, Rivera M, Williams A, Stetler-Stevenson M, Sorbara L, et al. Coincident myelodysplastic syndrome and T-cell large granular lymphocytic disease: clinical and pathophysiological features. Br J Haematol. 2001;112(1):195–200.
114. Koskela HL, Eldfors S, Ellonen P, van Adrichem AJ, Kuusanmäki H, Andersson EI, Lagström S, Clemente MJ, Olson T, Jalkanen SE, Majumder MM, et al. Somatic STAT3 mutations in large granular lymphocytic leukemia. N Engl J Med. 2012;366(20):1905–13.
115. Jerez A, Clemente MJ, Makishima H, Koskela H, LeBlanc F, Ng KP, et al. STAT3 mutations unify the pathogenesis of chronic lymphoproliferative disorders of NK cells and T-cell large granular lymphocyte leukemia. Blood. 2012;120(15):3048–57.
116. Mustjoki S, Young NS. Somatic mutations in "benign" disease. N Engl J Med. 2021;384(21):2039–52.
117. Zeng W, Kajigaya S, Chen G, Risitano AM, Nunez O, Young NS. Transcript profile of CD4+ and CD8+ T cells from the bone marrow of acquired aplastic anemia patients. Exp Hematol. 2004;32(9):806–14.
118. Howe EC, Wlodarski M, Ball EJ, Rybicki L, Maciejewski JP. Killer immunoglobulin-like receptor genotype in immune-mediated bone marrow failure syndromes. Exp Hematol. 2005;33(11):1357–62.
119. Poggi A, Negrini S, Zocchi MR, Massaro A-M, Garbarino L, Lastraioli S, et al. Patients with paroxysmal nocturnal hemoglobinuria have a high frequency of peripheral-blood T cells expressing activating isoforms of inhibiting superfamily receptors. Blood. 2005;106(7):2399–408.
120. Giudice V, Banaszak LG, Gutierrez-Rodrigues F, Kajigaya S, Panjwani R, Ibanez MPF, et al. Circulating exosomal microRNAs in acquired aplastic anemia and myelodysplastic syndromes. Haematologica. 2018;103(7):1150–9.
121. Hosokawa K, Muranski P, Feng X, Keyvanfar K, Townsley DM, Dumitriu B, et al. Identification of novel microRNA signatures linked to acquired aplastic anemia. Haematologica. 2015;100(12):1534–45.
122. Takamatsu H, Feng X, Chuhjo T, Lu X, Sugimori C, Okawa K, et al. Specific antibodies to moesin, a membrane-cytoskeleton linker protein, are frequently detected in patients with acquired aplastic anemia. Blood. 2007;109(6):2514–20.
123. Feng X, Chuhjo T, Sugimori C, Kotani T, Lu X, Takami A, et al. Diazepam-binding inhibitor-related protein 1: a candidate autoantigen in acquired aplastic anemia patients harboring a minor population of paroxysmal nocturnal hemoglobinuria–type cells. Blood. 2004;104(8):2425–31.
124. Hirano N, Butler MO, Guinan EC, Nadler LM, Kojima S. Presence of anti-kinectin and anti-PMS1 antibodies in Japanese aplastic anaemia patients. Br J Haematol. 2005;128(2):221–3.
125. Qi Z, Takamatsu H, Espinoza JL, Lu X, Sugimori N, Yamazaki H, et al. Autoantibodies specific to hnRNP K: a new diagnostic marker for immune pathophysiology in aplastic anemia. Ann Hematol. 2010;89(12):1255–63.

126. Goto M, Kuribayashi K, Takahashi Y, Kondoh T, Tanaka M, Kobayashi D, et al. Identification of autoantibodies expressed in acquired aplastic anaemia. Br J Haematol. 2013;160(3):359–62.
127. Kelkka T, Tyster M, Lundgren S, Feng X, Kerr C, Hosokawa K, et al. Anti-COX-2 autoantibody is a novel biomarker of immune aplastic anemia. Leukemia. 2022;36(9):2317–27.
128. Bruin AMD, Voermans C, Nolte MA. Impact of interferon-γ on hematopoiesis. Blood. 2014;124(16):2479–86.
129. Bruin AMD, Demirel Ö, Hooibrink B, Brandts CH, Nolte MA. Interferon-γ impairs proliferation of hematopoietic stem cells in mice. Blood. 2013;121(18):3578–85.
130. Chen J, Feng X, Desierto MJ, Keyvanfar K, Young NS. IFN-γ-mediated hematopoietic cell destruction in murine models of immune-mediated bone marrow failure. Blood. 2015;126(24):2621–31.
131. Lin F-C, Karwan M, Saleh B, Hodge DL, Chan T, Boelte KC, et al. IFN-γ causes aplastic anemia by altering hematopoietic stem/progenitor cell composition and disrupting lineage differentiation. Blood. 2014;124(25):3699–708.
132. Scheinberg P, Chen J. Aplastic anemia: what have we learned from animal models and from the clinic. Semin Hematol. 2013;50(2):156–64.
133. Kuksin CA, Gonzalez-Perez G, Minter LM. CXCR4 expression on pathogenic T cells facilitates their bone marrow infiltration in a mouse model of aplastic anemia. Blood. 2015;125(13):2087–94.
134. Lezama RV, Escorcia EB, Torres AM, Aguilar RT, Ramírez CG, Lorenzana MG, et al. A model for the induction of aplastic anemia by subcutaneous administration of benzene in mice. Toxicology. 2001;162(3):179–91.
135. Morley A, Blake J. An animal model of chronic aplastic marrow failure. I. Late marrow failure after Busulfan. Blood. 1974;44(1):49–56.
136. Gibson FM, Andrews CM, Diamanti P, Rizzo S, Macharia G, Gordon-Smith EC, et al. A new model of busulphan-induced chronic bone marrow aplasia in the female BALB/c mouse. Int J Exp Pathol. 2003;84(1):31–48.
137. Szostak JW, Blackburn EH. Cloning yeast telomeres on linear plasmid vectors. Cell. 1982;29(1):245–55.
138. Greider CW, Blackburn EH. Identification of a specific telomere terminal transferase activity in tetrahymena extracts. Cell. 1985;43(2):405–13.
139. Calado RT, Young NS. Telomere maintenance and human bone marrow failure. Blood. 2008;111(9):4446–55.
140. Calado RT, Young NS. Telomere diseases. N Engl J Med. 2009;361(24):2353–65.
141. Heiss NS, Knight SW, Vulliamy TJ, Klauck SM, Wiemann S, Mason PJ, et al. X-linked dyskeratosis congenita is caused by mutations in a highly conserved gene with putative nucleolar functions. Nat Genet. 1998;19(1):32–8.
142. Armanios M, Chen J-L, Chang Y-PC, Brodsky RA, Hawkins A, Griffin CA, et al. Haploinsufficiency of telomerase reverse transcriptase leads to anticipation in autosomal dominant dyskeratosis congenita. Proc Natl Acad Sci. 2005;102(44):15960–4.
143. Vulliamy T, Marrone A, Goldman F, Dearlove A, Bessler M, Mason PJ, et al. The RNA component of telomerase is mutated in autosomal dominant dyskeratosis congenita. Nature. 2001;413(6854):432–5.
144. Walne AJ, Vulliamy T, Marrone A, Beswick R, Kirwan M, Masunari Y, et al. Genetic heterogeneity in autosomal recessive dyskeratosis congenita with one subtype due to mutations in the telomerase-associated protein NOP10. Hum Mol Genet. 2007;16(13):1619–29.
145. Savage SA, Giri N, Baerlocher GM, Orr N, Lansdorp PM, Alter BP. TINF2, a component of the shelterin telomere protection complex, is mutated in dyskeratosis congenita. Am J Hum Genet. 2008;82(2):501–9.
146. Revy P, Kannengiesser C, Bertuch AA. Genetics of human telomere biology disorders. Nat Rev Genet. 2023;24(2):86–108.

147. Calado RT, Yewdell WT, Wilkerson KL, Regal JA, Kajigaya S, Stratakis CA, et al. Sex hormones, acting on the TERT gene, increase telomerase activity in human primary hematopoietic cells. Blood. 2009;114(11):2236–43.
148. Ziegler P, Schrezenmeier H, Akkad J, Brassat U, Vankann L, Panse J, et al. Telomere elongation and clinical response to androgen treatment in a patient with aplastic anemia and a heterozygous hTERT gene mutation. Ann Hematol. 2012;91(7):1115–20.
149. Ball SE, Gibson FM, Sn R, Tooze JA, Marsh JCW, Gordon-Smith EC. Progressive telomere shortening in aplastic anemia. Blood. 1998;91(10):3582–92.
150. Brümmendorf TH, Maciejewski JP, Mak J, Young NS, Lansdorp PM. Telomere length in leukocyte subpopulations of patients with aplastic anemia. Blood. 2001;97(4):895–900.
151. Yamaguchi H, Baerlocher GM, Lansdorp PM, Chanock SJ, Nunez O, Sloand E, et al. Mutations of the human telomerase RNA gene (TERC) in aplastic anemia and myelodysplastic syndrome. Blood. 2003;102(3):916–8.
152. Dror Y. Shwachman-diamond syndrome. Pediatr Blood Cancer. 2005;45(7):892–901.
153. Wang Y, McReynolds LJ, Dagnall C, Katki HA, Spellman SR, Wang T, et al. Pre-transplant short telomeres are associated with high mortality risk after unrelated donor haematopoietic cell transplant for severe aplastic anaemia. Br J Haematol. 2020;188(2):309–16.
154. Calado RT, Graf SA, Wilkerson KL, Kajigaya S, Ancliff PJ, Dror Y, et al. Mutations in the SBDS gene in acquired aplastic anemia. Blood. 2007;110(4):1141–6.
155. Hahn CN, Chong C-E, Carmichael CL, Wilkins EJ, Brautigan PJ, Li X-C, et al. Heritable GATA2 mutations associated with familial myelodysplastic syndrome and acute myeloid leukemia. Nat Genet. 2011;43(10):1012–7.
156. Vinh DC, Patel SY, Uzel G, Anderson VL, Freeman AF, Olivier KN, et al. Autosomal dominant and sporadic monocytopenia with susceptibility to mycobacteria, fungi, papillomaviruses, and myelodysplasia. Blood. 2010;115(8):1519–29.
157. Hsu AP, Sampaio EP, Khan J, Calvo KR, Lemieux JE, Patel SY, et al. Mutations in GATA2 are associated with the autosomal dominant and sporadic monocytopenia and mycobacterial infection (MonoMAC) syndrome. Blood. 2011;118(10):2653–5.
158. Ostergaard P, Simpson MA, Connell FC, Steward CG, Brice G, Woollard WJ, et al. Mutations in GATA2 cause primary lymphedema associated with a predisposition to acute myeloid leukemia (Emberger syndrome). Nat Genet. 2011;43(10):929–31.
159. Dickinson RE, Griffin H, Bigley V, Reynard LN, Hussain R, Haniffa M, et al. Exome sequencing identifies GATA-2 mutation as the cause of dendritic cell, monocyte, B and NK lymphoid deficiency. Blood. 2011;118(10):2656–8.
160. Bigley V, Haniffa M, Doulatov S, Wang X-N, Dickinson R, McGovern N, et al. The human syndrome of dendritic cell, monocyte, B and NK lymphoid deficiency. J Exp Med. 2011;208(2):227–34.
161. Pasquet M, Bellanné-Chantelot C, Tavitian S, Prade N, Beaupain B, LaRochelle O, et al. High frequency of GATA2 mutations in patients with mild chronic neutropenia evolving to MonoMac syndrome, myelodysplasia, and acute myeloid leukemia. Blood. 2013;121(5):822–9.
162. Ganapathi KA, Townsley DM, Hsu AP, Arthur DC, Zerbe CS, Cuellar-Rodriguez J, et al. GATA2 deficiency-associated bone marrow disorder differs from idiopathic aplastic anemia. Blood. 2015;125(1):56–70.
163. Grossman J, Cuellar-Rodriguez J, Gea-Banacloche J, Zerbe C, Calvo K, Hughes T, et al. Nonmyeloablative allogeneic hematopoietic stem cell transplantation for GATA2 deficiency. Biol Blood Marrow Transplant. 2014;20(12):1940–8.
164. Cuellar-Rodriguez J, Gea-Banacloche J, Freeman AF, Hsu AP, Zerbe CS, Calvo KR, et al. Successful allogeneic hematopoietic stem cell transplantation for GATA2 deficiency. Blood. 2011;118(13):3715–20.
165. Galera P, Hsu AP, Wang W, Droll S, Chen R, Schwartz JR, et al. Donor-derived MDS/AML in families with germline GATA2 mutation. Blood. 2018;132(18):1994–8.

166. Walne AJ, Dokal A, Plagnol V, Beswick R, Kirwan M, Fuente JDL, et al. Exome sequencing identifies MPL as a causative gene in familial aplastic anemia. Haematologica. 2012;97(4):524–8.
167. Ballmaier M, Germeshausen M, Schulze H, Cherkaoui K, Lang S, Gaudig A, et al. c-mpl mutations are the cause of congenital amegakaryocytic thrombocytopenia. Blood. 2001;97(1):139–46.
168. Gutierrez-Rodrigues F, Patel BA, Groarke EM. When to consider inherited marrow failure syndromes in adults. Hematology. 2023;2023(1):548–55.
169. McReynolds LJ, Rafati M, Wang Y, Ballew BJ, Kim J, Williams VV, et al. Genetic testing in severe aplastic anemia is required for optimal hematopoietic cell transplant outcomes. Blood. 2022;140(8):909–21.
170. Gutierrez-Rodrigues F, Munger E, Ma X, Groarke EM, Tang Y, Patel BA, et al. Differential diagnosis of bone marrow failure syndromes guided by machine learning. Blood. 2023;141(17):2100–13.
171. Khincha PP, Savage SA. Genomic characterization of the inherited bone marrow failure syndromes. Semin Hematol. 2013;50(4):333–47.
172. Cooper JN, Young NS. Clonality in context: hematopoietic clones in their marrow environment. Blood. 2017;130(22):2363–72.
173. Socié G, Rosenfeld S, Frickhofen N, Gluckman E, Tichelli A. Late clonal diseases of treated aplastic anemia. Semin Hematol. 2000;37(1):91–101.
174. Maciejewski JP, Risitano A, Sloand EM, Nunez O, Young NS. Distinct clinical outcomes for cytogenetic abnormalities evolving from aplastic anemia. Blood. 2002;99(9):3129–35.
175. Ishiyama K, Karasawa M, Miyawaki S, Ueda Y, Noda M, Wakita A, et al. Aplastic anaemia with 13q–: a benign subset of bone marrow failure responsive to immunosuppressive therapy. Br J Haematol. 2002;117(3):747–50.
176. Hosokawa K, Katagiri T, Sugimori N, Ishiyama K, Sasaki Y, Seiki Y, et al. Favorable outcome of patients WHO have 13q deletion: a suggestion for revision of the WHO 'MDS-U' designation. Haematologica. 2012;97(12):1845–9.
177. Scheinberg P, Cooper JN, Sloand EM, Wu CO, Calado RT, Young NS. Association of telomere length of peripheral blood leukocytes with hematopoietic relapse, malignant transformation, and survival in severe aplastic anemia. JAMA. 2010;304(12):1358–64.
178. Calado RT, Cooper JN, Padilla-Nash HM, Sloand EM, Wu CO, Scheinberg P, et al. Short telomeres result in chromosomal instability in hematopoietic cells and precede malignant evolution in human aplastic anemia. Leukemia. 2012;26(4):700–7.
179. Patel BA, Groarke EM, Lotter J, Shalhoub R, Gutierrez-Rodrigues F, Rios O, et al. Long-term outcomes in patients with severe aplastic anemia treated with immunosuppression and eltrombopag: a phase 2 study. Blood. 2022;139(1):34–43.
180. Dumitriu B, Feng X, Townsley DM, Ueda Y, Yoshizato T, Calado RT, et al. Telomere attrition and candidate gene mutations preceding monosomy 7 in aplastic anemia. Blood. 2015;125(4):706–9.
181. Marsh JCW, Mufti GJ. Clinical significance of acquired somatic mutations in aplastic anaemia. Int J Hematol. 2016;104(2):159–67.
182. Ogawa S. Clonal hematopoiesis in acquired aplastic anemia. Blood. 2016;128(3):337–47.
183. Betensky M, Babushok D, Roth JJ, Mason PJ, Biegel JA, Busse TM, et al. Clonal evolution and clinical significance of copy number neutral loss of heterozygosity of chromosome arm 6p in acquired aplastic anemia. Cancer Genet. 2016;209(1–2):1–10.
184. Scheinberg P, Young NS. How I treat acquired aplastic anemia. Blood. 2012;120(6):1185–96.
185. Scheinberg P, Wu CO, Nunez O, Young NS. Long-term outcome of pediatric patients with severe aplastic anemia treated with antithymocyte globulin and cyclosporine. J Pediatr. 2008;153(6):814–9.e1.
186. Champlin RE, Perez WS, Passweg JR, Klein JP, Camitta BM, Gluckman E, et al. Bone marrow transplantation for severe aplastic anemia: a randomized controlled study of conditioning regimens. Blood. 2007;109(10):4582–5.

187. Bejanyan N, Kim S, Hebert KM, Kekre N, Abdel-Azim H, Ahmed I, et al. Choice of conditioning regimens for bone marrow transplantation in severe aplastic anemia. Blood Adv. 2019;3(20):3123–31.
188. Gupta V, Eapen M, Brazauskas R, Carreras J, Aljurf M, Gale RP, et al. Impact of age on outcomes after bone marrow transplantation for acquired aplastic anemia using HLA-matched sibling donors. Haematologica. 2010;95(12):2119–25.
189. Giammarco S, Latour RPD, Sica S, Dufour C, Socie G, Passweg J, et al. Transplant outcome for patients with acquired aplastic anemia over the age of 40: has the outcome improved? Blood. 2018;131(17):1989–92.
190. Socié G. Allogeneic BM transplantation for the treatment of aplastic anemia: current results and expanding donor possibilities. Hematology. 2013;2013(1):82–6.
191. Bacigalupo A, Socié G, Schrezenmeier H, Tichelli A, Locasciulli A, Fuehrer M, et al. Bone marrow versus peripheral blood as the stem cell source for sibling transplants in acquired aplastic anemia: survival advantage for bone marrow in all age groups. Haematologica. 2012;97(8):1142–8.
192. Schrezenmeier H, Passweg JR, Marsh JCW, Bacigalupo A, Bredeson CN, Bullorsky E, et al. Worse outcome and more chronic GVHD with peripheral blood progenitor cells than bone marrow in HLA-matched sibling donor transplants for young patients with severe acquired aplastic anemia. Blood. 2007;110(4):1397–400.
193. Bacigalupo A, Marsh JCW. Unrelated donor search and unrelated donor transplantation in the adult aplastic anaemia patient aged 18–40 years without an HLA-identical sibling and failing immunosuppression. Bone Marrow Transplant. 2013;48(2):198–200.
194. Deeg HJ, Amylon MD, Harris RE, Collins R, Beatty PG, Feig S, et al. Marrow transplants from unrelated donors for patients with aplastic anemia: minimum effective dose of total body irradiation. Biol Blood Marrow Transplant. 2001;7(4):208–15.
195. Kojima S, Matsuyama T, Kato S, Kigasawa H, Kobayashi R, Kikuta A, et al. Outcome of 154 patients with severe aplastic anemia who received transplants from unrelated donors: the Japan Marrow Donor Program. Blood. 2002;100(3):799–803.
196. Viollier R, Socié G, Tichelli A, Bacigalupo A, Korthof ET, Marsh J, et al. Recent improvement in outcome of unrelated donor transplantation for aplastic anemia. Bone Marrow Transplant. 2008;41(1):45–50.
197. Maury S, Balère-Appert M-L, Chir Z, Boiron J-M, Galambrun C, Yakouben K, et al. Unrelated stem cell transplantation for severe acquired aplastic anemia: improved outcome in the era of high-resolution HLA matching between donor and recipient. Haematologica. 2007;92(5):589–96.
198. Bacigalupo A, Socié G, Hamladji RM, Aljurf M, Maschan A, Kyrcz-Krzemien S, et al. Current outcome of HLA identical sibling versus unrelated donor transplants in severe aplastic anemia: an EBMT analysis. Haematologica. 2015;100(5):696–702.
199. Marsh JCW, Kulasekararaj AG. Management of the refractory aplastic anemia patient: what are the options? Blood. 2013;122(22):3561–7.
200. Ciceri F, Lupo-Stanghellini MT, Korthof ET. Haploidentical transplantation in patients with acquired aplastic anemia. Bone Marrow Transplant. 2013;48(2):183–5.
201. DeZern AE, Eapen M, Wu J, Talano J-A, Solh M, Saldaña BJD, et al. Haploidentical bone marrow transplantation in patients with relapsed or refractory severe aplastic anaemia in the USA (BMT CTN 1502): a multicentre, single-arm, phase 2 trial. Lancet Haematol. 2022;9(9):e660–e9.
202. DeZern AE, Zahurak M, Symons HJ, Cooke KR, Huff CA, Jain T, et al. Alternative donor BMT with posttransplant cyclophosphamide as initial therapy for acquired severe aplastic anemia. Blood. 2023;141(25):3031–8.
203. Prata PH, Eikema D-J, Afansyev B, Bosman P, Smiers F, Diez-Martin JL, et al. Haploidentical transplantation and posttransplant cyclophosphamide for treating aplastic anemia patients: a report from the EBMT Severe Aplastic Anemia Working Party. Bone Marrow Transplant. 2020;55(6):1050–8.

204. Latour RPD, Purtill D, Ruggeri A, Sanz G, Michel G, Gandemer V, et al. Influence of nucleated cell dose on overall survival of unrelated cord blood transplantation for patients with severe acquired aplastic anemia: a study by eurocord and the aplastic anemia working party of the European group for blood and marrow transplantation. Biol Blood Marrow Transplant. 2011;17(1):78–85.
205. Childs RW, Tian X, Vo P, Purev E, Kotecha RR, Carlsten M, et al. Combined haploidentical and cord blood transplantation for refractory severe aplastic anaemia and hypoplastic myelodysplastic syndrome. Br J Haematol. 2021;193(5):951–60.
206. Pagliuca S, Latour RPD, Volt F, Locatelli F, Zecca M, Dalle J-H, et al. Long-term outcomes of cord blood transplantation from an HLA-identical sibling for patients with bone marrow failure syndromes: a report from Eurocord, Cord Blood Committee and Severe Aplastic Anemia Working Party of the European Society for Blood and Marrow Transplantation. Biol Blood Marrow Transplant. 2017;23(11):1939–48.
207. Latour RPD, Chevret S, Jubert C, Sirvent A, Galambrun C, Ruggeri A, et al. Unrelated cord blood transplantation in patients with idiopathic refractory severe aplastic anemia: a nationwide phase 2 study. Blood. 2018;132(7):750–4.
208. Barnes DWH, Mole RH. Aplastic anaemia in sublethally irradiated mice given allogeneic lymph node cells. Br J Haematol. 1967;13(s1):482–91.
209. Frickhofen N, Kaltwasser JP, Schrezenmeier H, Raghavachar A, Vogt HG, Herrmann F, et al. Treatment of aplastic anemia with antilymphocyte globulin and methylprednisolone with or without cyclosporine. N Engl J Med. 1991;324(19):1297–304.
210. Bacigalupo A, Bruno B, Saracco P, Bona ED, Locasciulli A, Locatelli F, et al. Antilymphocyte globulin, cyclosporine, prednisolone, and granulocyte colony-stimulating factor for severe aplastic anemia: an update of the GITMO/EBMT study on 100 patients. Blood. 2000;95(6):1931–4.
211. Kojima S, Hibi S, Kosaka Y, Yamamoto M, Tsuchida M, Mugishima H, et al. Immunosuppressive therapy using antithymocyte globulin, cyclosporine, and danazol with or without human granulocyte colony-stimulating factor in children with acquired aplastic anemia. Blood. 2000;96(6):2049–54.
212. Rosenfeld SJ, Kimball J, Vining D, Young NS. Intensive immunosuppression with antithymocyte globulin and cyclosporine as treatment for severe acquired aplastic anemia. Blood. 1995;85(11):3058–65.
213. Scheinberg P, Nunez O, Wu C, Young NS. Treatment of severe aplastic anaemia with combined immunosuppression: anti-thymocyte globulin, ciclosporin and mycophenolate mofetil. Br J Haematol. 2006;133(6):606–11.
214. Scheinberg P, Wu CO, Nunez O, Scheinberg P, Boss C, Sloand EM, et al. Treatment of severe aplastic anemia with a combination of horse antithymocyte globulin and cyclosporine, with or without sirolimus: a prospective randomized study. Haematologica. 2009;94(3):348–54.
215. Tisdale JF, Dunn DE, Maciejewski J. Cyclophosphamide and other new agents for the treatment of severe aplastic anemia. Semin Hematol. 2000;37(1):102–9.
216. Scheinberg P, Townsley D, Dumitriu B, Scheinberg P, Weinstein B, Daphtary M, et al. Moderate-dose cyclophosphamide for severe aplastic anemia has significant toxicity and does not prevent relapse and clonal evolution. Blood. 2014;124(18):2820–3.
217. Scheinberg P, Nunez O, Weinstein B, Scheinberg P, Wu CO, Young NS. Activity of alemtuzumab monotherapy in treatment-naive, relapsed, and refractory severe acquired aplastic anemia. Blood. 2012;119(2):345–54.
218. Scheinberg P, Nunez O, Weinstein B, Scheinberg P, Biancotto A, Wu CO, et al. Horse versus rabbit antithymocyte globulin in acquired aplastic anemia. N Engl J Med. 2011;365(5):430–8.
219. Feng X, Kajigaya S, Solomou EE, Keyvanfar K, Xu X, Raghavachari N, et al. Rabbit ATG but not horse ATG promotes expansion of functional CD4+CD25highFOXP3+ regulatory T cells in vitro. Blood. 2008;111(7):3675–83.

220. Scheinberg P, Nunez O, Young NS. Retreatment with rabbit anti-thymocyte globulin and ciclosporin for patients with relapsed or refractory severe aplastic anaemia. Br J Haematol. 2006;133(6):622–7.
221. Scheinberg P, Fischer SH, Li L, Nunez O, Wu CO, Sloand EM, et al. Distinct EBV and CMV reactivation patterns following antibody-based immunosuppressive regimens in patients with severe aplastic anemia. Blood. 2007;109(8):3219–24.
222. Gaber AO, First MR, Tesi RJ, Gaston RS, Mendez R, Mulloy LL, et al. Results of the double-blind, randomized, multicenter, phase iii clinical trial of thymoglobulin versus atgam in the treatment of acute graft rejection episodes after renal transplantation1, 2. Transplantation. 1998;66(1):29–37.
223. Marsh JC, Bacigalupo A, Schrezenmeier H, Tichelli A, Risitano AM, Passweg JR, et al. Prospective study of rabbit antithymocyte globulin and cyclosporine for aplastic anemia from the EBMT Severe Aplastic Anaemia Working Party. Blood. 2012;119(23):5391–6.
224. Marsh JC, Pearce RM, Koh MBC, Lim Z, Pagliuca A, Mufti GJ, et al. Retrospective study of alemtuzumab vs ATG-based conditioning without irradiation for unrelated and matched sibling donor transplants in acquired severe aplastic anemia: a study from the British Society for Blood and Marrow Transplantation. Bone Marrow Transplant. 2014;49(1):42–8.
225. Valdez JM, Scheinberg P, Nunez O, Wu CO, Young NS, Walsh TJ. Decreased infection-related mortality and improved survival in severe aplastic anemia in the past two decades. Clin Infect Dis. 2011;52(6):726–35.
226. Scheinberg P, Rios O, Scheinberg P, Weinstein B, Wu CO, Young NS. Prolonged cyclosporine administration after antithymocyte globulin delays but does not prevent relapse in severe aplastic anemia. Am J Hematol. 2014;89(6):571–4.
227. Townsley DM, Desmond R, Dunbar CE, Young NS. Pathophysiology and management of thrombocytopenia in bone marrow failure: possible clinical applications of TPO receptor agonists in aplastic anemia and myelodysplastic syndromes. Int J Hematol. 2013;98(1):48–55.
228. Kaushansky K. The molecular mechanisms that control thrombopoiesis. J Clin Invest. 2005;115(12):3339–47.
229. Zeigler FC, Sauvage FD, Widmer HR, Keller GA, Donahue C, Schreiber RD, et al. In vitro megakaryocytopoietic and thrombopoietic activity of c-mpl ligand (TPO) on purified murine hematopoietic stem cells. Blood. 1994;84(12):4045–52.
230. Marsh JCW, Ganser A, Stadler M. Hematopoietic growth factors in the treatment of acquired bone marrow failure states. Semin Hematol. 2007;44(3):138–47.
231. Kuter DJ. Biology and chemistry of thrombopoietic agents. Semin Hematol. 2010;47(3):243–8.
232. Feng X, Scheinberg P, Samsel L, Rios O, Chen J, McCoy JP, et al. Decreased plasma cytokines are associated with low platelet counts in aplastic anemia and immune thrombocytopenic purpura. J Thromb Haemost. 2012;10(8):1616–23.
233. Olnes MJ, Scheinberg P, Calvo KR, Desmond R, Tang Y, Dumitriu B, et al. Eltrombopag and improved hematopoiesis in refractory aplastic anemia. N Engl J Med. 2012;367(1):11–9.
234. Desmond R, Townsley DM, Dumitriu B, Olnes MJ, Scheinberg P, Bevans M, et al. Eltrombopag restores trilineage hematopoiesis in refractory severe aplastic anemia that can be sustained on discontinuation of drug. Blood. 2014;123(12):1818–25.
235. Townsley DM, Scheinberg P, Winkler T, Desmond R, Dumitriu B, Rios O, et al. Eltrombopag added to standard immunosuppression for aplastic anemia. N Engl J Med. 2017;376(16):1540–50.
236. Latour RP, Kulasekararaj A, Iacobelli S, Terwel SR, Cook R, Griffin M, et al. Eltrombopag added to immunosuppression in severe aplastic anemia. N Engl J Med. 2022;386(1):11–23.
237. Lee JW, Lee S-E, Jung CW, Park S, Keta H, Park SK, et al. Romiplostim in patients with refractory aplastic anaemia previously treated with immunosuppressive therapy: a dose-finding and long-term treatment phase 2 trial. Lancet Haematol. 2019;6(11):e562–e72.
238. Zhao L-P, Fontbrune FSD, Contejean A, Abraham J, Terriou L, Chabrot C, et al. Nationwide survey in France on the use of romiplostim in patients with refractory severe aplastic anemia. Bone Marrow Transplant. 2019;54(7):1161–3.

239. Jang JH, Tomiyama Y, Miyazaki K, Nagafuji K, Usuki K, Uoshima N, et al. Efficacy and safety of romiplostim in refractory aplastic anaemia: a phase II/III, multicentre, open-label study. Br J Haematol. 2021;192(1):190–9.
240. Hosokawa K, Yamazaki H, Tanabe M, Imi T, Sugimori N, Nakao S. High-dose romiplostim accelerates hematologic recovery in patients with aplastic anemia refractory to eltrombopag. Leukemia. 2021;35(3):906–9.
241. Valdez JM, Scheinberg P, Young NS, Walsh TJ. Infections in patients with aplastic anemia. Semin Hematol. 2009;46(3):269–76.
242. O'Donghaile D, Childs RW, Leitman SF. Blood consult: granulocyte transfusions to treat invasive aspergillosis in a patient with severe aplastic anemia awaiting mismatched hematopoietic progenitor cell transplantation. Blood. 2012;119(6):1353–5.

Open Access This chapter is licensed under the terms of the Creative Commons Attribution 4.0 International License (http://creativecommons.org/licenses/by/4.0/), which permits use, sharing, adaptation, distribution and reproduction in any medium or format, as long as you give appropriate credit to the original author(s) and the source, provide a link to the Creative Commons license and indicate if changes were made.

The images or other third party material in this chapter are included in the chapter's Creative Commons license, unless indicated otherwise in a credit line to the material. If material is not included in the chapter's Creative Commons license and your intended use is not permitted by statutory regulation or exceeds the permitted use, you will need to obtain permission directly from the copyright holder.

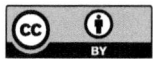

Part II
Diagnosis and Classification

Chapter 4
Diagnosis of Acquired Aplastic Anemia with Figures

Alicia Rovó, Carlo Dufour, André Tichelli, and On behalf of the SAA-WP EBMT

Introduction

Aplastic anemia (AA) is a rare, potentially life-threatening, nonmalignant disease caused by autoimmune destruction of early hematopoietic cells. AA presents with geographic rate variability, with a global incidence rate range of 0.7–5 cases per million inhabitants per year, with two- to three-fold higher rates in Asia than in Europe and the United States [1, 2]. The low incidence of its occurrence makes its diagnosis a challenge. The lack of experience in approaching such a patient can lead to misdiagnosis or unnecessary delay for diagnosis and treatment initiation. During the last years, the continuous increase of new information has contributed to a better understanding of the current landscape of bone marrow failure syndrome (BMFs) [3].

AA is defined by persistent pancytopenia with an empty bone marrow with fat replacement (Figs. 4.1 and 4.2) [4] and has no specific disease markers. A

A. Rovó (✉)
Department of Hematology and Central Hematology Laboratory, Inselspital, Bern University Hospital, University of Bern, Bern, Switzerland
e-mail: Alicia.Rovo@insel.ch

C. Dufour
Hematology Unit, IRCCS Istituto Giannina Gaslini, Genoa, Italy

A. Tichelli
Division of Hematology, University Hospital Basel, Basel, Switzerland

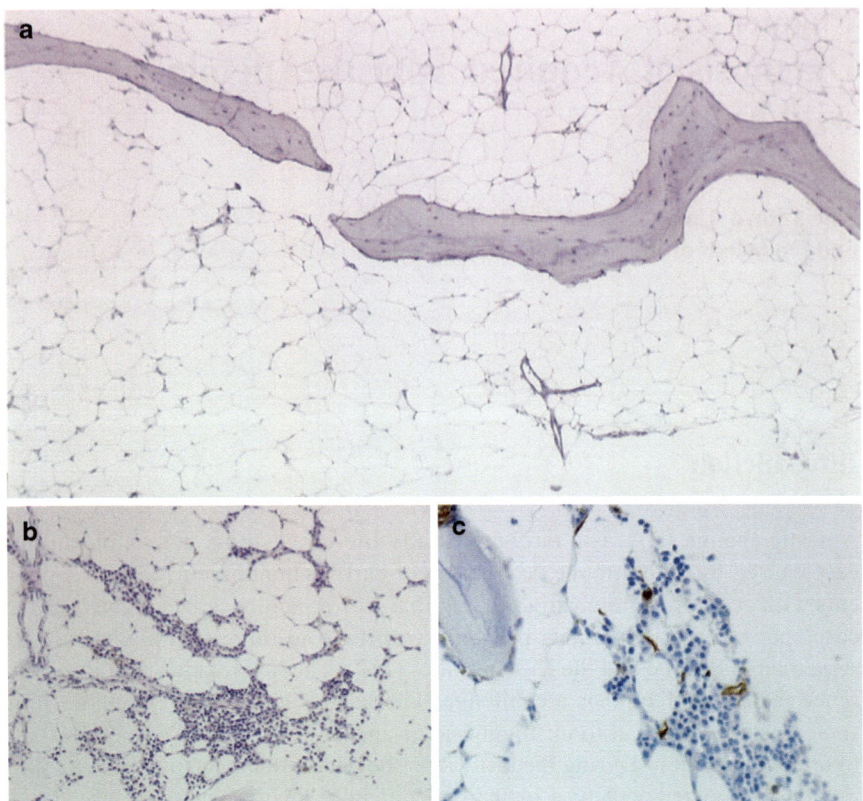

Fig. 4.1 Histology and immunohistology of bone marrow from a patient with SAA. (**a**) PAS staining of a patients with SAA; (**b**) HE staining, hotspot of erythropoiesis of a patient with SAA; (**c**) immunostaining with CD34 of the hotspot, showing absence of CD34 positive cells. (Picture courtesy of Professor Stephan Dirnhofer and Professor Alexandar Tzankov, Institute of Pathology, University Hospital of Basel, Basel, Switzerland)

number of BMFs have a similar presentation that makes the diagnosis difficult. Additional information on accelerated telomere attrition [5, 6], cytogenetic changes [7], somatic [8, 9] and germline mutations [10–12], and flow cytometry [13, 14] are nowadays the main contributors in the diagnosis of AA. In this chapter, we will focus on the diagnostic approach of AA in adults and its differential diagnosis.

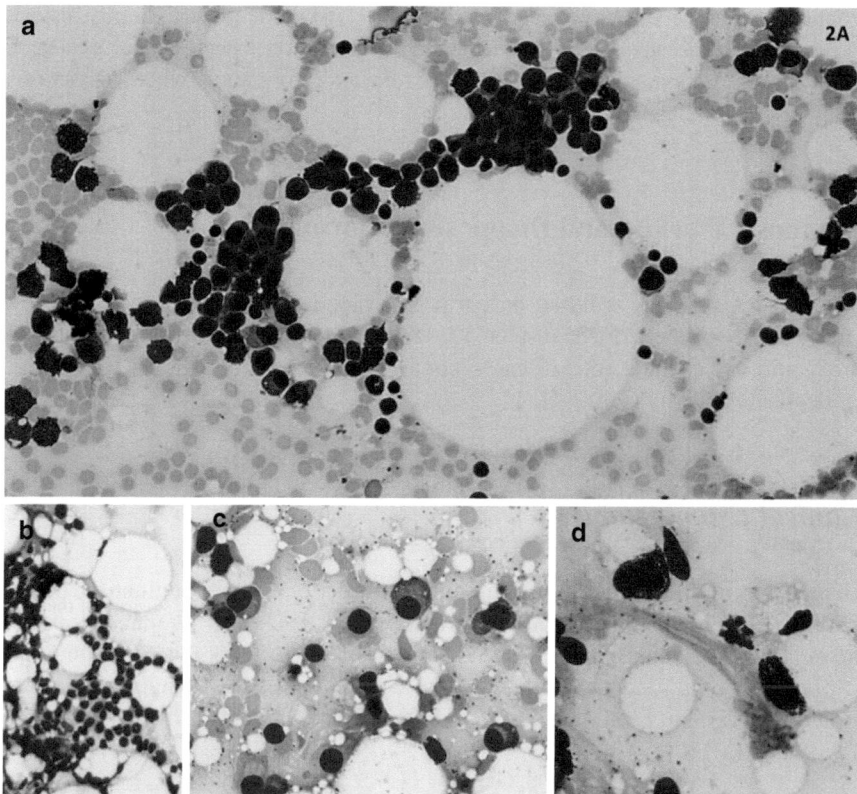

Fig. 4.2 Cytomorphology of an aspiration of bone marrow from patients with aplastic anemia. (**a**) Hotspot with a nest of erythroid cells; (**b**) reactive lymphoid infiltrate; (**c**) reactive plasma cells; (**d**) mast cells

Diagnosis Approach of Aplastic Anemia

Different pathogenic mechanisms may be involved in the development of AA. Identifying the underlying mechanism has therapeutic implications, since although every patient with AA could benefit from an allogeneic hematopoietic transplant (allo-HCT), only autoimmune forms will respond to immunosuppression (IST) [15]. AA lacks specific markers and therefore the differential diagnosis is part of the diagnostic process, for which much experience is required. Thus, a number of diseases like paroxysmal nocturnal hemoglobinuria (PNH), hypoplastic myelodysplastic syndromes (hMDS), hypoplastic acute leukemia, large granular lymphocyte (LGL) leukemia, and autoimmune diseases, including primary immune dysregulation disorders (PIRD), should be considered systematically. An inherited marrow failure syndrome (IBMFS), such as Fanconi anemia (FA) and telomere biology disease (TBD), as a cause for the aplasia is more likely, although not exclusively, in younger adults, generally younger than 50 years [16]. Patient's age, family history, exposure to toxic substances or medicaments, infections, professional exposure, clinical presentation, and comorbidities are relevant information, which helps to set priorities in the diagnostic process.

Diagnosis Workup and Diagnosis Confirmation

The diagnosis of AA is based on peripheral blood investigations, bone marrow (BM), and cytogenetic/FISH results [17, 18] (Fig. 4.3). A number of investigations are required to exclude other diseases, confirm and characterize the AA, and define its degree of severity (Fig. 4.4).

Clinical Examination

Except for findings related to bleeding or infections, the examination in AA patients presents mainly negative characteristics: absence of lymphadenopathy, no enlarged spleen or liver, and no infiltration of any other organ. Such findings, if present, would render the diagnosis of AA most unlikely. Somatic malformations and liver, lung, and bone disease abnormalities should alert to the possibility of an IBMFS [3, 19].

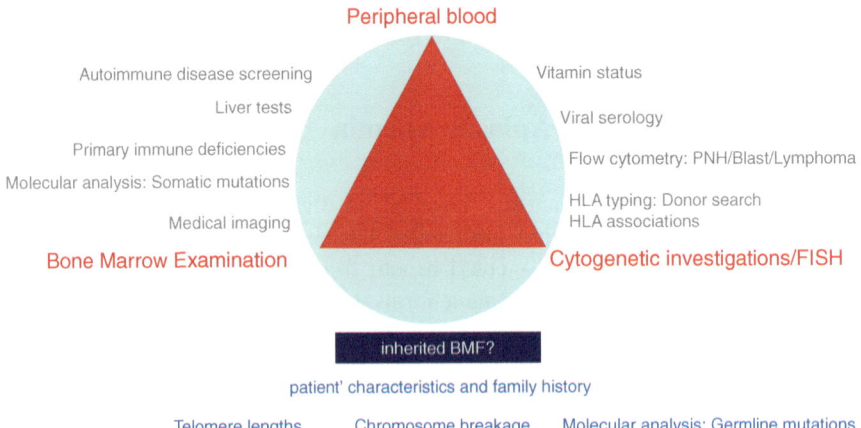

Fig. 4.3 Aplastic anemia—workup. Abbreviations: PNH paroxysmal nocturnal hemoglobinuria, HLA human leukocyte antigens, BMF bone marrow failure, FISH Fluorescence in situ hybridization

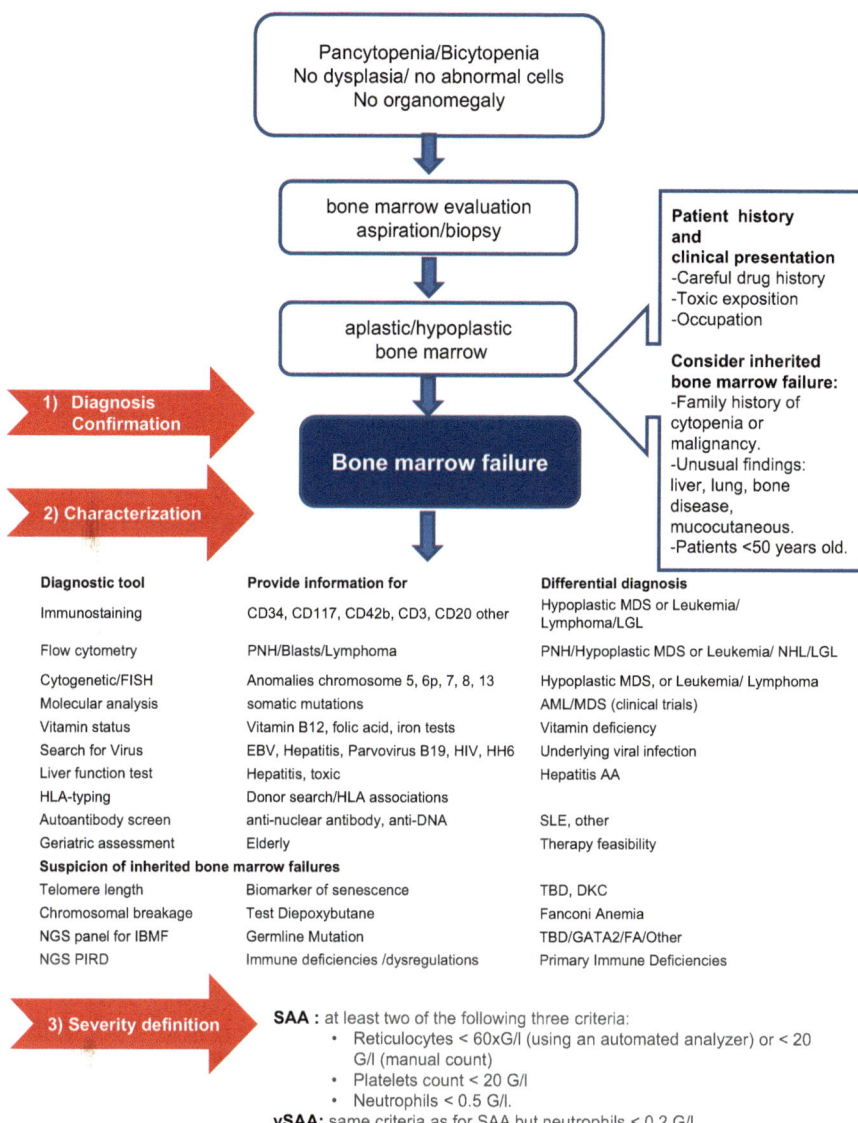

Fig. 4.4 Stepwise diagnostic phases of aplastic anemia. Abbreviations: AA aplastic anemia, BMF bone marrow failure, DKC dyskeratosis congenita, EBV Epstein-Barr-Virus, FISH fluorescence in situ hybridization, GATA2 GATA binding protein 2, HHV6 human herpesvirus 6, HLA human leukocyte antigens, IBMF inherited marrow failure syndrome, LGL large granular lymphocytic leukemia, MDS myelodysplastic syndrome, NHL non-Hodgkin lymphoma, NGS next-generation sequencing, PIRD primary immune dysregulation disorders, PNH paroxysmal nocturnal hemoglobinuria, SAA severe aplastic anemia, SLE systemic lupus erythematosus, TBD telomere biology disease, vSAA very SAA

Complete Blood Count

Pancytopenia is the main manifestation in the peripheral blood, but at least two cell lines should be decreased for the diagnosis. In early stages, isolated cytopenia, particularly thrombocytopenia and non-regenerative anemia, is common. Red blood cells (RBCs) classically do not show anisocytosis or poikilocytosis; macrocytosis is a common feature. RBC changes due to underlying iron deficiency can confuse the diagnosis. Iron deficiency is rare in AA. In such cases, an association with PNH should be investigated. For the evaluation of white blood cell (WBC) differentiation, absolute numbers and not relative percentages should be considered. Neutropenia is frequent with varying degrees of severity. Lymphocyte count is usually preserved. Monocytopenia can be present and imposes the differential diagnosis of hairy cell leukemia. A careful examination of blood film is indicated, this allow to assess morphology of RBCs and dysplastic changes of all hematopoietic lines, including the presence of abnormal cells like blasts, hairy cells, and abnormal platelets morphology. Any of these findings would be a strong argument against the diagnosis of AA. Fetal hemoglobin (Hb) can be increased in AA [20] and in other pathologies, particularly in children [21, 22]. Pancytopenia, despite being typical in AA, may be the first presentation of many other diseases. Therefore, strategies with a straightforward algorithm are useful to guide the diagnosis [23].

Bone Marrow Examination

Bone marrow (BM) aspiration and trephine biopsy are of paramount relevance for the diagnosis of AA. Both evaluations are complementary; aspiration allows a better assessment of cellular morphology and dysplasia. Trephine biopsy is crucial to assess overall cellularity, topography of hematopoietic cells, abnormal infiltrates, and fibrosis. A BM biopsy containing at least five to six intertrabecular spaces, with a core of 20–30 mm length, is considered as representative [24]. Dry tap is unusual and suggests diagnoses other than AA. Overall, cellularity is more often reduced rather than completely absent. Aplastic and hypocellular BM based on trephine biopsy is defined by <10% (empty marrow) and <30% of hematopoietic cells, respectively. This cutoff has been established mainly for children and young adults. Besides the variable amounts of residual hematopoietic cells, there are prominent fat spaces and an increase in stromal cells, such as plasma cells, lymphocytes forming follicles, and mast cells, which can be a confounding finding. The increment of stromal cells can mimic the picture of a marrow with normal cellularity, stromal cells have to be excluded in the global estimation for cellularity. The presence of nests of erythropoiesis [20], conforming to the so-called "hot spots," is frequent in AA marrow; they may show a certain degree of dyserythropoiesis, mainly with macro/megaloblastic changes (Fig. 4.2), which can be misinterpreted as MDS. Megakaryopoiesis is usually decreased or absent. Immunostaining allows the identification and assessment of the topographical distribution of blasts, megakaryocytes, abnormal cells, and infiltrates in the BM histology (Fig. 4.1). It might occasionally identify the unusual association with lymphoma [25–27]. Fibrosis is not present in AA. Repeat BM biopsy may be necessary and is recommended in any unclear case, particularly in the case of subcortical trephine biopsy, which may be hypocellular in adult patients, leading to wrong interpretation. Flow cytometry of BM aspiration may contribute to identifying abnormal populations. Furthermore, immunostained BM tissues can be successfully mapped by multicolour immunofluorescence using confocal reflection microscopy but its use is not incorporated into the diagnostic routine [28].

Cytogenetic

Cytogenetic abnormalities can be present in up to 12–15% of otherwise typical AA patients; therefore, cytogenetic investigations should be systematically performed [7]. Due to the scarcity of hematopoietic cells, insufficient metaphases for an adequate analysis are common. FISH targeting specific anomalies should therefore be considered. Most frequent chromosome anomalies in AA include trisomy 8, uniparental disomy of the 6p (6pUPD) [29], and 13. Abnormal cytogenetic clones often are small at diagnosis, may arise during the course of the disease, or may be transient and disappear after IST [30, 31]. While abnormalities of chromosomes 7 and 5, even in the absence of dysplasia, make the diagnosis more likely in MDS, other cytogenetic findings are less categorical. An abnormal cytogenetic clone does, however, not necessarily imply the diagnosis of MDS or AML. Del(13q) has been reported in patients with MDS and other hematologic malignancy cases [32]. The presence of del(13q) in AA was reported with a good response to IST [33, 34]. Patients with AA are at risk of developing MDS or AML, so monitoring over time is recommended [35, 36].

Molecular Genetics

Molecular analysis, including next-generation sequencing (NGS), is increasingly used to understand disease pathophysiology. Somatic mutations are present in 20–30% of cases of idiopathic AA, especially during the disease course [18, 37]. The prevalence of the mutations increased with age, and mutations had an age-related signature. Common mutations in AA patients are PIGA, BCOR, and BCORL1, which correlate with a better response to IST and a longer and higher rate of overall and progression-free survival. In contrast, mutations such as DNMT3A and ASXL1 are associated with worse outcomes. The pattern of somatic clones is, however, variable, and the outcome frequently unpredictable [9, 38]. It also seems that between pediatric patients and older adults, there are potential differences in the mutational spectrum since adults are more likely to carry age-related somatic mutations associated with malignancy [39]. In clinical practice, the finding of somatic mutations tends to be interpreted as a signature for malignancy; this belief may be true for certain mutations, but not necessarily for all of them.

Telomere Length Measurement

Telomere attrition offers an interesting prognostic tool in acquired AA. Telomere shortening in AA patients was associated with both numerical and structural chromosome abnormalities. Patients with shorter telomeres were at higher risk of malignant transformation. Average telomere lengths were inversely correlated with monosomy 7 at diagnosis [5]. Patients who evolved to MDS and AML showed marked progressive telomere attrition before the emergence of −7 [6]. Due to constraints on health care budgets, telomere length measurements might not be systematically covered by insurance. Inclusion of patients in clinical trials addressing this aspect is strongly recommended [3, 18].

HLA-Typing

Human leukocyte antigen (HLA)-typing of the patient and his family belongs to the diagnostics of patients with BMFs. Early knowledge of the HLA-type of the patient and identification of a possible sibling donor allows including early transplantation in the treatment decision process. Matched unrelated donor transplantation looks like a consistent front-line option in children [40]. Wider applicability of alternative-donor transplantation for AA is under investigation and will be discussed in several chapters of the book [41, 42].

Characterization of Aplastic Anemia

Exclusion of Inherited Bone Marrow Failures (IBMFS)

Unusual clinical features like somatic malformations and liver, lung, and bone abnormalities, as well as a positive family history of cytopenia, somatic malformations, or malignancy, suggest an IBMFS. However, a normal clinical examination does not definitively rule out "cryptic" TBD [43, 44] or a nonclassical Fanconi anemia [45]. BM morphology cannot differentiate such diseases from acquired AA. Cytogenetic abnormalities have a particular value in this setting [16]. To exclude FA, tests to demonstrate increased sensitivity to chromosomal breakage with mitomycin C or diepoxybutane should be performed. This test should also be done in all patients with any suspected IBMF before transplantation because of the eventual need for conditioning adaptation. Screening should also include sibling donors of FA patients. Awareness about an underlying cryptic form of FA is needed, particularly due to the higher risk of secondary cancers in these patients and the lack of response to standard IST. Telomere shortening is a consistent and typical finding of TBD [10]. TERC and TERT gene mutations cause telomeropathies in both children and adults [11, 12]. In adult patients, symptoms and clinical signs are often milder than in children; mucocutaneous findings and other physical anomalies are infrequent. The pattern of organ abnormalities is extremely variable among affected individuals. The misdiagnosis of IBMFS can expose patients to ineffective and expensive therapies, toxic transplant conditioning regimens, and inappropriate use of an affected family member as a stem cell donor. In this complex diagnosis constellation, machine learning models integrating clinical and laboratory tests demonstrated a potential contribution in this field [46]. Given the higher frequency of IBMFS in children, an age-tailored diagnostic workup for AA in pediatric age is included in the Chap. 8 of this textbook.

Differential Diagnosis of AA from the Hypocellular Variant of MDS

The distinction between AA and hMDS is certainly the most difficult diagnostic task in elderly adult patients. Both diseases present with markedly hypocellular BM and increased fat cells [47–49]. Dysplasia of erythropoiesis may be present in both entities and therefore may not help for diagnosis differentiation. The absence of dysplasia in the megakaryopoiesis and myelopoiesis, as well as the lack of blast cells confirmed by immunostaining with CD34 and/or CD117 and/or flow cytometry, are the most conspicuous arguments supporting the diagnosis of AA. Findings like BM fibrosis or splenomegaly favor the diagnosis of MDS (Table 4.1). PNH clones are present in 50% of AA patients [4, 50] and less frequently in MDS. The presence of abnormal cytogenetic clones seen in around 12–15% of patients with AA may not necessarily indicate a diagnosis of MDS [32]. Some clones like +8 or del13q [33, 34] are associated with a good response to IST and consequently linked more closely to AA. Cases presenting with isolated monosomy 7, even lacking dysplastic changes, will be frequently classified as hMDS, even if the cytogenetic abnormality is the only criterion to support this diagnosis. The poor prognosis of monosomy 7 [51] is the strongest argument to avoid classifying it as a benign disease. Moreover, despite similar clinical presentations, distinct cytokine profiles were observed between AA and hMDS [52]. Mutational profiles can contribute to defining disease diagnosis [8, 38]. Among 5–52% of AA patients, MDS-associated mutations will be present, typically with a low allele burden, below 10%, while the presence of mutations with an allele burden greater than 10%, particularly those

Table 4.1 Distinction between AA and hypoplastic MDS

Parameters	Aplastic anemia	Hypoplastic MDS
Cytopenia	Present	Present
Bone marrow investigation		
BM cellularity	Aplastic (<10% cellularity or significantly hypocellular)	Hypocellular
Erythropoiesis	Present in nests, "hot spots"	Present
Granulopoiesis	Typically decreased	Present
Megakaryopoiesis	Decreased or absent	Present
BM fat replacement	Typical	Possible
Dysplasia		
Dyserythropoesis	Possible	Frequent
Granulocytic dysplasia	Normal morphology	Frequent
Megakaryocytic dysplasia	Normal morphology	Frequent
Ring sideroblasts	Absent	Possible
Blasts	Absent	Variable
CD34+ or CD117+ immunohistochemistry	No increase	Normal or increased
Marrow fibrosis	Absent	Possible
Additional information		
PNH clone	Frequent	Less frequent
Splenomegaly at diagnosis	Absent	Possible
Karyotype	Clonal abnormality possible (~12%)	Abnormal ~50%
Recurrent cytogenetic abnormalities	At diagnosis: del(13q), +8 Evolution: −7, −5/del(5q), del(20q)	−Y, del(11q), −5/del(5q), del(12p), del(20q), −i7/del(7q), +8, +19, i(17q), inv(3)/t(3q)/del(3q)
Complex cytogenetics (≥3 abnormalities)	Absent	Possible
Acquired CN-LOH	Possible (<20%)	Possible
Somatic mutated genes	Particularly PIGA, ASXL1, BCOR, BCORL1; 5–52% of patients will present MDS-associated mutations *(lower allele burden)*	SF3B1, SRSF2, U2AF1, ZRSR2, TET2, DNMT3A, IDH1, IDH2, ASXL1, EZH2, RUNX1, NRAS, BCOR, TP53, STAG2 *(allele burden > 10%)*
Germline mutations	Investigate if underlying inherited BMF is suspected	Investigate if underlying germline predisposition is suspected

Modified from Refs. [49, 129]

AA aplastic anemia, *hMDS* hypoplastic myelodysplastic syndrome, *BM* bone marrow, *PNH* paroxysmal nocturnal hemoglobinuria, *CN-LOH* copy number-neutral loss of heterozygosity associated with an unfavorable prognosis, is more likely associated with an hMDS [38]. In vitro cultures of colony-forming cells show different growing patterns for AA and MDS [53, 54] but they are no longer used in daily practice.

AA and PNH

There is a close correlation between AA and PNH [4]. PNH is a clonal, nonmalignant hematopoietic stem cell disorder with features including hemolytic anemia, marrow failure, and thrombosis. This disease will be discussed in detail in the chapter "Bone Marrow Failure in Paroxysmal Nocturnal Hemoglobinuria." Patients with typical PNH can develop AA during the course of their disease [50] and patients with AA often present a PNH clone [13]. Even the presence of a very small PNH clone is a strong argument for AA. Flow cytometry is the gold standard method for screening and diagnosis of PNH. This is currently best achieved by analysis of glycophosphatidylinositol (GPI)-linked antigen using monoclonal antibodies and fluorescent aerolysin [14]. About 40–50% of patients with acquired AA have a detectable PNH clone [55]; they are small, and normally, patients do not have PNH-related symptoms. According to the British guidelines, AA patients should be screened for PNH at the time of diagnosis. If the test is persistently negative, PNH tests should be done every 6 months for 2 years before moving to annual testing until symptoms/signs develop. If the PNH screen is, or becomes, positive, the test should be done every 3 months for the first 2 years, with reduced frequency only if the proportion of PNH cells remains stable [17, 18]. In some patients, the PNH clone can increase after IST; some of them will develop a clinical form of PNH.

AA and Viral Infections

Viruses can affect various cell lineages in the BM, causing uncommon aplasia. Epstein-Barr virus, dengue, parvovirus B19, human herpes virus 6, HIV, and disseminated adenovirus infections have been reported to cause marrow suppression mainly in patients with chronic hemolytic anemia, immunocompromised patients, and transplant recipients [56–61]; most will have transient aplasia with recovery. Hemophagocytic lymphohistiocytosis (HLH) is a rare life-threatening hyperinflammatory syndrome, occurring either as a familial disorder or a sporadic condition often triggered by viral infections. Pancytopenia is observed in the majority of these patients who present with febrile illness. An extremely high ferritin level might help to differentiate this entity from AA [62]. Association between AA and HLH, despite being rare, might occur [63]. Recently, the SARS-CoV-2 virus was added to the viral infections implicated in the pathogenesis of AA in children [64, 65] and adults [66–68].

AA and Hepatitis

The association with seronegative hepatitis has been described in approximately 5–10% of patients with acquired AA [69–71]. This association mainly affects young, healthy males with severe but self-limited liver inflammation. Therefore, liver function tests and viral hepatitis studies (serological and DNA/RNA) looking for HCV, HDV, HEV, HGV, parvovirus B19, EBV, and CMV should be performed. Patients with post-hepatitis AA were reported as having a similar response to IST compared to patients with idiopathic acquired AA [70]. In a Chinese cohort, some findings suggest that patients with hepatitis-associated AA have a more severe T cell imbalance and a poorer prognosis [72]. Compared to other countries, in the Pakistani population, the etiology of hepatitis-associated AA has been predominantly viral, and the idiopathic form is less common [73]. Severe hepatitis-associated AA following COVID-19 mRNA vaccination has also been reported [74]. Candidates for allo-HCT will particularly benefit from early transplantation (<75 days), careful donor selection, and improving post-transplant liver events, which were considered crucial to optimize outcomes [75].

Drug-Induced AA

For years, a number of drugs, particularly some nonsteroidal anti-inflammatories, chloramphenicol, gold, antiepileptics, nifedipine, and sulphonamides, have been associated with AA. Most are commonly used, and the cause for the rare association with BMF remains unclear. A report of a new drug-induced AA described it as associated with levamisole-contaminated cocaine [76], methimazole [77], leflunomide [78], and mesalazine [79]. Some anecdotal reports about drug-induced AA without recovery using first- and second-generation tyrosine kinase inhibitors in the treatment of chronic myeloid leukemia were also communicated without a clear underlying mechanism [80, 81]. Despite most cases of AA being idiopathic, a careful drug history must be taken, and any putative causative drug should be discontinued. Novel treatment modalities for other diseases have been associated with the occurrence of AA. Thus, hematological toxicity is an emerging complication observed after chimeric antigen receptor (CAR)-T cell therapy. Severe cytopenia after CAR-T cell therapy can last for weeks and, in some cases, become irreversible, thus constituting an emerging cause of BMF [82–85]. AA is also a rare immune-related adverse event after immune checkpoint inhibitor administration, with poorly understood incidence and outcomes [86, 87].

AA Associated with Chemicals

There is some evidence that AA risk is increased by certain industrial chemicals [88, 89]. Results from occupational epidemiology studies have shown increased risk of AA associated with pesticide and benzene exposures [2, 90]. The higher incidence among working-age adults suggests that environmental or occupational factors may play a role in the development of AA [2, 91, 92]. A large-scale case-control study reported a higher proportion of AA patients exposed to pesticides, solvents, glues, paints, and fuel. However, due to the diversity of compounds, a clear relationship was not conclusive [92, 93].

AA and Association with Autoimmune Diseases

The association between AA and other autoimmune diseases is not surprising. AA is a very rare complication of systemic lupus erythematosus (SLE) or its immunosuppression treatment. The underlying mechanism for the occurrence of aplasia is postulated as immune-mediated through autoantibodies against BM precursors [94–96]. Autoantibody screen panel according to clinical presentation, including antinuclear antibody and anti-DNA antibody, should be investigated when SLE is suspected as the underlying disease. Autoimmune myelofibrosis is an extremely uncommon cause of cytopenia in patients with SLE. It can be diagnosed with a BM biopsy, responds well to immunosuppression, and has a favorable prognosis compared to primary myelofibrosis, which is a myeloproliferative neoplasm [97, 98]. Associations of AA with other autoimmune diseases have been shown in single-case reports [99–101]. In a single-center report, 5.3% of the patients had an autoimmune disease before the diagnosis of AA, and 4.5% after diagnosis and treatment of AA [102]. Autoimmune diseases affected older AA patients (> 50 years) more frequently. In a large multicenter study, 50 of 1251 AA patients had an autoimmune disease [103]. Whether or not the IST applied to treat the AA has an influence on the outcome of the autoimmune disease still remains controversial.

AA and HLA-DR

HLA-DR typing might be useful for predicting a response to IST in AA patients. HLA-DR15, and more specifically DRB1(*)1502, was markedly more frequent in AA patients 40 years of age and older (52.4%) than in those below 40 years [104]. Ethnicity seems to play a role in the relationship between HLA-related factors and AA. In Japanese patients, DRB1*1501 seems to be associated with the presence of a small population of PNH-type cells and a good response to the IST [105]. In a study on 37 Korean patients with severe AA, responders to IST had a significantly higher HLA-DR15 and a lower DR4 frequency compared with nonresponders [106]. A study in which HLA-A, B, C, DRB1, and DQB1 alleles were compared between 96 Chinese severe AA patients and 600 healthy people showed a different gene profile in both groups. Comparison among AA patients with various severity also exhibited significant differences of specific alleles, identifying thus several risk and protective HLA alleles among Chinese AA patients [107]. An analysis of gene frequencies of HLA-DRB1 alleles in Mexican mestizo patients with AA showed, in coincidence with previously reported data, a positive association of the DRB1(*)15 allele and AA [108]. A comprehensive meta-analysis of 16 studies with 4428 AA patients suggests that HLA-DRB1 polymorphisms could play roles in the occurrence of AA [109]. Also, HLA-DQ expression levels were closely related to disease severity and immune status of AA patients, thus stressing the potential role of HLA-DQ in the immunopathogenesis of AA [110].

AA and LGL

LGL is a clonal lymphoid disorder characterized by cytopenia and clonal expansion of either CD3-positive cytotoxic T lymphocytes or CD3-negative natural killer (NK) cells. Although LGL can be associated with other entities such as AA or MDS, it is a distinct clinical entity with a specific diagnostic pathway [111, 112]. Abnormal T-cell populations expressing NK markers and downregulation of normal T-cell markers (i.e., CD5, CD7) suggest this diagnosis [113]. STAT3 mutations may distinguish truly malignant lymphoproliferations involving T and NK cells from reactive expansions [114]. Since LGL clones can accompany a number of diseases, additional investigations are necessary to confirm the LGL as the etiology of the BMFS [115, 116].

Diagnosis of AA in the Elderly

The diagnostic procedure of AA does not differ essentially in elderly patients. There are, however, aspects that need to be considered. BM cellularity changes with age, is highest at birth, and declines progressively with age. There is approximately a 10% decrease in cellularity by decade, although with huge variations. Overall, it is 40–70% in adults and declines below 30% in healthy elderly [117]. Therefore, the definition of hypocellular BM is particularly difficult in elderly patients. Furthermore, subcortical BM, even in a healthy elderly person, is likely to be of low cellularity [118]. Moreover, a relevant point in the elderly is the difficult distinction between AA and hMDS, particularly because of the high frequency of MDS in this population (Table 4.1). AA patients are more likely to carry age-related somatic mutations associated with malignancy, and it does not mean that they necessarily have MDS [38, 39]. Misdiagnosis can lead to unnecessary treatments with harmful consequences, particularly in elderly patients. Furthermore, a comprehensive geriatric assessment should be integrated into the diagnosis to formulate appropriate therapeutic decisions. This aspect is discussed in the Chap. 9.

Defining Severity of AA

Once the diagnosis of AA is confirmed and the AA characterized, the severity has to be defined. The severity definition of the disease is *crucial* for therapy decisions. The severity is based exclusively on values of the peripheral blood. Hence, three groups of AA are defined. Severe AA (SAA) [119], when at least two of the following three criteria are fulfilled: (1) reticulocytes <60 × 10^9/L (using an automated analyzer) or <20 × 10^9/L (using manual count), (2) platelets <20 × 10^9/L, (3) neutrophils <0.5 × 10^9/L. Very severe SAA (vSAA) [120], when SAA criteria are fulfilled but the neutrophil count is <0.2 × 10^9/L. Non-severe AA, when the criteria for SAA and vSAA are not fulfilled.

Defining Response After Treatment

The definition of the response criteria for IST treatment belongs to the diagnostic tasks. The normalization of blood values is considered a complete response (CR). For the definition of CR, several criteria are used worldwide [121, 122]; however, they have minor impact on the clinical outcome. Partial remission (PR) covers a wide range of blood values; it includes all patients who do not meet criteria for SAA any longer and are independent of transfusions but are not in CR.

Future Challenges in the Diagnostics of AA

There is a current better understanding of the underlying mechanisms involved in BMFs; however, diagnostic delimitation between the different entities still needs improvement. New advances in diagnostic technology provide additional fascinating information, which might solve unmet diagnostic problems in the future. In the diagnosis of AA, it should be considered that health insurance will only cover validated diagnostic methods; therefore, innovative diagnostic methods may be limited to their use in clinical trials until their validation is available.

We still lack markers to identify AA patients who will not respond to IST. A number of parameters have been postulated as possible predictors of response to IST, including reticulocytes and lymphocytes [123], WBC in children [124], and response to G-CSF [121], but a robust parameter in this regard is not yet available. Currently, molecular methods allow a more accurate differentiation between AA and myeloid diseases with hypoplastic presentation, an important aspect due to the worse prognosis of the latter [35, 36], which has constituted a clear progress. Early identification of true IST refractoriness would be crucial, as these patients could benefit from early transplantation or be considered for new therapeutic options [125, 126].

Artificial intelligence might improve and lead to faster diagnosis of rare diseases. Reports on deep learning models for automatic recognition of AA, MDS, and AML based on a BM smear [127], or using machine learning with magnetic resonance imaging for the quantitative analysis of pelvic bone fat to distinguish AA from MDS [128], showed interesting results. Differential diagnosis of bone BMFs guided by machine learning integrating clinical and laboratory variables in the initial evaluation, including telomere length and mutation profile, could potentially be used to help hematologists and health care providers not specialized in BMFs in the diagnosis, avoiding significant diagnostic delays [46].

Conflict of Interest Alicia Rovó (AR); Carlo Dufour (CD); André Tichelli (AT).

AR: Research grants: Novartis, CSL Behring, Alexion Pharmaceuticals. Expert consultant/speaker: Novartis, Alexion Pharmaceuticals, Swedish Orphan Biovitrum GmbH, OrPha Swiss GmbH. Advisory boards: Novartis, Alexion Pharmaceuticals, Swedish Orphan Biovitrum GmbH, Bristol Myers Squibb, OrPha Swiss GmbH, GlaxoSmithKline AG, Blueprint Medicines GmbH.

CD: Advisory Board: Novartis, Pfizer, Sobi, Biocryst, Rocket, Consultations: Gilead, ONO.

AT: No conflict of interest.

References

1. Young NS, Kaufman DW. The epidemiology of acquired aplastic anemia. Haematologica. 2008;93(4):489–92.
2. Issaragrisil S, Kaufman DW, Anderson T, Chansung K, Leaverton PE, Shapiro S, et al. The epidemiology of aplastic anemia in Thailand. Blood. 2006;107(4):1299–307.
3. Townsley DM, Dumitriu B, Young NS. Bone marrow failure and the telomeropathies. Blood. 2014;124(18):2775–83.
4. Young NS. Acquired aplastic anemia. Ann Intern Med. 2002;136(7):534–46.
5. Calado RT, Cooper JN, Padilla-Nash HM, Sloand EM, Wu CO, Scheinberg P, et al. Short telomeres result in chromosomal instability in hematopoietic cells and precede malignant evolution in human aplastic anemia. Leukemia. 2012;26(4):700–7.
6. Dumitriu B, Feng X, Townsley DM, Ueda Y, Yoshizato T, Calado RT, et al. Telomere attrition and candidate gene mutations preceding monosomy 7 in aplastic anemia. Blood. 2015;125(4):706–9.
7. Gupta V, Brooker C, Tooze JA, Yi QL, Sage D, Turner D, et al. Clinical relevance of cytogenetic abnormalities at diagnosis of acquired aplastic anaemia in adults. Br J Haematol. 2006;134(1):95–9.
8. Kulasekararaj AG, Jiang J, Smith AE, Mohamedali AM, Mian S, Gandhi S, et al. Somatic mutations identify a subgroup of aplastic anemia patients who progress to myelodysplastic syndrome. Blood. 2014;124(17):2698–704.
9. Peffault de Latour R, Kulasekararaj A, Iacobelli S, Terwel SR, Cook R, Griffin M, et al. Eltrombopag added to immunosuppression in severe aplastic anemia. N Engl J Med. 2022;386(1):11–23.
10. Shimamura A. Clinical approach to marrow failure. Hematology Am Soc Hematol Educ Program. 2009:329–37.
11. Yamaguchi H, Baerlocher GM, Lansdorp PM, Chanock SJ, Nunez O, Sloand E, et al. Mutations of the human telomerase RNA gene (TERC) in aplastic anemia and myelodysplastic syndrome. Blood. 2003;102(3):916–8.
12. Yamaguchi H, Calado RT, Ly H, Kajigaya S, Baerlocher GM, Chanock SJ, et al. Mutations in TERT, the gene for telomerase reverse transcriptase, in aplastic anemia. N Engl J Med. 2005;352(14):1413–24.

13. Pu JJ, Brodsky RA. Paroxysmal nocturnal hemoglobinuria from bench to bedside. Clin Transl Sci. 2011;4(3):219–24.
14. Brodsky RA, Mukhina GL, Li S, Nelson KL, Chiurazzi PL, Buckley JT, et al. Improved detection and characterization of paroxysmal nocturnal hemoglobinuria using fluorescent aerolysin. Am J Clin Pathol. 2000;114(3):459–66.
15. Young NS. Aplastic Anemia. N Engl J Med. 2018;379(17):1643–56.
16. Cuccuini W, Collonge-Rame MA, Auger N, Douet-Guilbert N, Coster L, Lafage-Pochitaloff M. Cytogenetics in the management of bone marrow failure syndromes: guidelines from the Groupe Francophone de Cytogenetique Hematologique (GFCH). Curr Res Transl Med. 2023;71(4):103423.
17. Killick SB, Bown N, Cavenagh J, Dokal I, Foukaneli T, Hill A, et al. Guidelines for the diagnosis and management of adult aplastic anaemia. Br J Haematol. 2016;172(2):187–207.
18. Kulasekararaj A, Cavenagh J, Dokal I, Foukaneli T, Gandhi S, Garg M, et al. Guidelines for the diagnosis and management of adult aplastic anaemia: a British Society for Haematology guideline. Br J Haematol. 2024;204(3):784–804.
19. Triemstra J, Pham A, Rhodes L, Waggoner DJ, Onel K. A review of Fanconi anemia for the practicing pediatrician. Pediatr Ann. 2015;44(10):444–5, 8, 50 passim.
20. Tichelli A, Gratwohl A, Nissen C, Signer E, Stebler Gysi C, Speck B. Morphology in patients with severe aplastic anemia treated with antilymphocyte globulin. Blood. 1992;80(2):337–45.
21. Hasle H, Baumann I, Bergstrasser E, Fenu S, Fischer A, Kardos G, et al. The International Prognostic Scoring System (IPSS) for childhood myelodysplastic syndrome (MDS) and juvenile myelomonocytic leukemia (JMML). Leukemia. 2004;18(12):2008–14.
22. Hasle H, Niemeyer CM. Advances in the prognostication and management of advanced MDS in children. Br J Haematol. 2011;154(2):185–95.
23. Gnanaraj J, Parnes A, Francis CW, Go RS, Takemoto CM, Hashmi SK. Approach to pancytopenia: diagnostic algorithm for clinical hematologists. Blood Rev. 2018;32(5):361–7.
24. Bain BJ, Clark DM, Wilkins BS. Bone Marrow pathology. 4th ed. Wiley; 2009.
25. Medinger M, Buser A, Stern M, Heim D, Halter J, Rovo A, et al. Aplastic anemia in association with a lymphoproliferative neoplasm: coincidence or causality? Leuk Res. 2012;36(2):250–1.
26. Zonder JA, Keating M, Schiffer CA. Chronic lymphocytic leukemia presenting in association with aplastic anemia. Am J Hematol. 2002;71(4):323–7.
27. Rovo A, Kulasekararaj A, Medinger M, Chevallier P, Ribera JM, Peffault de Latour R, et al. Association of aplastic anaemia and lymphoma: a report from the severe aplastic anaemia working party of the European Society of Blood and Bone Marrow Transplantation. Br J Haematol. 2019;184(2):294–8.
28. Takaku T, Malide D, Chen J, Calado RT, Kajigaya S, Young NS. Hematopoiesis in 3 dimensions: human and murine bone marrow architecture visualized by confocal microscopy. Blood. 2010;116(15):e41–55.
29. Katagiri T, Sato-Otsubo A, Kashiwase K, Morishima S, Sato Y, Mori Y, et al. Frequent loss of HLA alleles associated with copy number-neutral 6pLOH in acquired aplastic anemia. Blood. 2011;118(25):6601–9.
30. Tichelli A, Gratwohl A, Nissen C, Speck B. Late clonal complications in severe aplastic anemia. Leuk Lymphoma. 1994;12(3–4):167–75.
31. Socie G, Rosenfeld S, Frickhofen N, Gluckman E, Tichelli A. Late clonal diseases of treated aplastic anemia. Semin Hematol. 2000;37(1):91–101.
32. Steensma DP, Dewald GW, Hodnefield JM, Tefferi A, Hanson CA. Clonal cytogenetic abnormalities in bone marrow specimens without clear morphologic evidence of dysplasia: a form fruste of myelodysplasia? Leuk Res. 2003;27(3):235–42.
33. Hosokawa K, Katagiri T, Sugimori N, Ishiyama K, Sasaki Y, Seiki Y, et al. Favorable outcome of patients who have 13q deletion: a suggestion for revision of the WHO 'MDS-U' designation. Haematologica. 2012;97(12):1845–9.
34. Holbro A, Jotterand M, Passweg JR, Buser A, Tichelli A, Rovo A. Comment to "Favorable outcome of patients who have 13q deletion: a suggestion for revision of the WHO 'MDS-U' designation" Haematologica. 2012;97(12):1845–9. Haematologica. 2013;98(4):e46–7.

35. Chattopadhyay S, Lionel S, Selvarajan S, Devasia AJ, Korula A, Kulkarni U, et al. Relapse and transformation to myelodysplastic syndrome and acute myeloid leukemia following immunosuppressive therapy for aplastic anemia is more common as compared to allogeneic stem cell transplantation with a negative impact on survival. Ann Hematol. 2024;103(3):749–58.
36. Groarke EM, Patel BA, Shalhoub R, Gutierrez-Rodrigues F, Desai P, Leuva H, et al. Predictors of clonal evolution and myeloid neoplasia following immunosuppressive therapy in severe aplastic anemia. Leukemia. 2022;36(9):2328–37.
37. Babushok DV. A brief, but comprehensive, guide to clonal evolution in aplastic anemia. Hematology Am Soc Hematol Educ Program. 2018;2018(1):457–66.
38. Yoshizato T, Dumitriu B, Hosokawa K, Makishima H, Yoshida K, Townsley D, et al. Somatic mutations and clonal hematopoiesis in aplastic anemia. N Engl J Med. 2015;373(1):35–47.
39. Babushok DV, Perdigones N, Perin JC, Olson TS, Ye W, Roth JJ, et al. Emergence of clonal hematopoiesis in the majority of patients with acquired aplastic anemia. Cancer Genet. 2015;208(4):115–28.
40. Dufour C, Veys P, Carraro E, Bhatnagar N, Pillon M, Wynn R, et al. Similar outcome of upfront-unrelated and matched sibling stem cell transplantation in idiopathic paediatric aplastic anaemia. A study on behalf of the UK Paediatric BMT Working Party, Paediatric Diseases Working Party and Severe Aplastic Anaemia Working Party of EBMT. Br J Haematol. 2015;171(4):585–94.
41. Maury S, Balere-Appert ML, Chir Z, Boiron JM, Galambrun C, Yakouben K, et al. Unrelated stem cell transplantation for severe acquired aplastic anemia: improved outcome in the era of high-resolution HLA matching between donor and recipient. Haematologica. 2007;92(5):589–96.
42. Peffault de Latour R, Purtill D, Ruggeri A, Sanz G, Michel G, Gandemer V, et al. Influence of nucleated cell dose on overall survival of unrelated cord blood transplantation for patients with severe acquired aplastic anemia: a study by eurocord and the aplastic anemia working party of the European group for blood and marrow transplantation. Biol Blood Marrow Transplant. 2011;17(1):78–85.
43. Walne AJ, Dokal I. Dyskeratosis congenita: a historical perspective. Mech Ageing Dev. 2008;129(1–2):48–59.
44. Walne AJ, Dokal I. Advances in the understanding of dyskeratosis congenita. Br J Haematol. 2009;145(2):164–72.
45. Auerbach AD. Fanconi anemia and its diagnosis. Mutat Res. 2009;668(1–2):4–10.
46. Gutierrez-Rodrigues F, Munger E, Ma X, Groarke EM, Tang Y, Patel BA, et al. Differential diagnosis of bone marrow failure syndromes guided by machine learning. Blood. 2023;141(17):2100–13.
47. Barrett J, Saunthararajah Y, Molldrem J. Myelodysplastic syndrome and aplastic anemia: distinct entities or diseases linked by a common pathophysiology? Semin Hematol. 2000;37(1):15–29.
48. Bennett JM, Orazi A. Diagnostic criteria to distinguish hypocellular acute myeloid leukemia from hypocellular myelodysplastic syndromes and aplastic anemia: recommendations for a standardized approach. Haematologica. 2009;94(2):264–8.
49. Bonadies N, Rovo A, Porret N, Bacher U. When should we think of myelodysplasia or bone marrow failure in a thrombocytopenic patient? A practical approach to diagnosis. J Clin Med. 2021;10(5):1026.
50. Pu JJ, Mukhina G, Wang H, Savage WJ, Brodsky RA. Natural history of paroxysmal nocturnal hemoglobinuria clones in patients presenting as aplastic anemia. Eur J Haematol. 2011;87(1):37–45.
51. Greenberg PL, Tuechler H, Schanz J, Sanz G, Garcia-Manero G, Sole F, et al. Revised international prognostic scoring system for myelodysplastic syndromes. Blood. 2012;120(12):2454–65.
52. Feng X, Scheinberg P, Wu CO, Samsel L, Nunez O, Prince C, et al. Cytokine signature profiles in acquired aplastic anemia and myelodysplastic syndromes. Haematologica. 2011;96(4):602–6.

53. Zhang TJ, Feng M, Zheng YZ, Li XX, Xu ZF, Qin TJ, et al. Analysis of in vitro characteristics of colony-forming cells in myelodysplastic syndrome and comparison with that in non-severe aplastic anemia. Zhonghua Xue Ye Xue Za Zhi. 2012;33(7):516–21.
54. Nissen C, Wodnar-Filipowicz A, Slanicka Krieger MS, Slanicka Gratwohl A, Tichelli A, Speck B. Persistent growth impairment of bone marrow stroma after antilymphocyte globulin treatment for severe aplastic anaemia and its association with relapse. Eur J Haematol. 1995;55(4):255–61.
55. Sachdeva MU, Varma N, Chandra D, Bose P, Malhotra P, Varma S. Multiparameter FLAER-based flow cytometry for screening of paroxysmal nocturnal hemoglobinuria enhances detection rates in patients with aplastic anemia. Ann Hematol. 2015;94(5):721–8.
56. Parra D, Mekki Y, Durieu I, Broussolle C, Seve P. Clinical and biological manifestations in primary parvovirus B19 infection in immunocompetent adult: a retrospective study of 26 cases. Rev Med Interne. 2014;35(5):289–96.
57. Kaptan K, Beyan C, Ural AU, Ustun C, Cetin T, Avcu F, et al. Successful treatment of severe aplastic anemia associated with human parvovirus B19 and Epstein-Barr virus in a healthy subject with allo-BMT. Am J Hematol. 2001;67(4):252–5.
58. Agrawal M, Paul RT, Pamu P, Avmr N. Parvovirus B19 induced transient aplastic crisis in an immunocompetent child. Turk Patoloji Derg. 2015;31(2):158–60.
59. Kurtzman G, Young N. Viruses and bone marrow failure. Baillieres Clin Haematol. 1989;2(1):51–67.
60. Kurtzman GJ, Ozawa K, Cohen B, Hanson G, Oseas R, Young NS. Chronic bone marrow failure due to persistent B19 parvovirus infection. N Engl J Med. 1987;317(5):287–94.
61. Ramzan M, Prakash Yadav S, Sachdeva A. Post-dengue fever severe aplastic anemia: a rare association. Hematol Oncol Stem Cell Ther. 2012;5(2):122–4.
62. Jordan MB, Allen CE, Weitzman S, Filipovich AH, McClain KL. How I treat hemophagocytic lymphohistiocytosis. Blood. 2011;118(15):4041–52.
63. Min KW, Jung HY, Han HS, Hwang TS, Kim SY, Kim WS, et al. Ileal mass-like lesion induced by Epstein-Barr virus-associated hemophagocytic lymphohistiocytosis in a patient with aplastic anemia. APMIS. 2015;123(1):81–6.
64. Youssef MAM, Ahmed ES, Kamal DT, Elsayh KI, Abdelfattah MA, Mahran HH, et al. Clinical signs and treatment of new-onset bone marrow failure associated SARS-CoV-2 infection in children: a single institution prospective cohort study. Mediterr J Hematol Infect Dis. 2024;16(1):e2024034.
65. Wu X, Mo Y, Wen K, Ming R, Yin X, Hu L, et al. Acquired aplastic anaemia after SARS-CoV-2 infection in China: a case report. Front Pediatr. 2023;11:1277540.
66. Chatzikalil E, Kattamis A, Diamantopoulos P, Solomou EE. New-onset aplastic anemia after SARS-CoV-2 vaccination. Int J Hematol. 2023;118(6):667–81.
67. Aguilar JJ, Dhillon V, Balasubramanian S. Manifestation of pancytopenia associated with COVID-19 as paroxysmal nocturnal hemoglobinuria (PNH) and aplastic anemia (AA). Hematol Rep. 2024;16(1):42–9.
68. Kmira Z, Sabrine K, Monia G, Imen A, Dorra C, Rania B, et al. A case of acquired aplastic anemia after severe hepatitis- probably induced by the Pfizer/BioNTech vaccine: a case report and review of literature. Vaccines (Basel). 2023;11(7):1228.
69. Young NS. Flaviviruses and bone marrow failure. JAMA. 1990;263(22):3065–8.
70. Locasciulli A, Bacigalupo A, Bruno B, Montante B, Marsh J, Tichelli A, et al. Hepatitis-associated aplastic anaemia: epidemiology and treatment results obtained in Europe. A report of the EBMT aplastic anaemia working party. Br J Haematol. 2010;149(6):890–5.
71. Brown KE, Tisdale J, Barrett AJ, Dunbar CE, Young NS. Hepatitis-associated aplastic anemia. N Engl J Med. 1997;336(15):1059–64.
72. Wang H, Tu M, Fu R, Wu Y, Liu H, Xing L, et al. The clinical and immune characteristics of patients with hepatitis-associated aplastic anemia in China. PLoS One. 2014;9(5):e98142.
73. Nawaz MT, Hameed AN, Angez M, Ansari AH, Adil SN. Hepatitis-associated aplastic anaemia: surveillance of frequency,clinico-haematological features, and demographic distribution at a tertiary care hospital in Pakistan. J Pak Med Assoc. 2023;73(1):217–21.

74. Yamamoto M, Keino D, Sumii S, Yokosuka T, Goto H, Inui A, et al. Severe hepatitis-associated aplastic anemia following COVID-19 mRNA vaccination. Intern Med. 2023;62(12):1813–6.
75. Li J, Liu Y, Wang J, Wang Y, Pang A, Yang D, et al. Exploring strategies to optimise outcomes in hepatitis-associated aplastic anaemia patients following haematopoietic stem cell transplantation. Sci Rep. 2024;14(1):5178.
76. Karch SB, Mari F, Bartolini V, Bertol E. Aminorex poisoning in cocaine abusers. Int J Cardiol. 2012;158(3):344–6.
77. Josol CV, Buenaluz-Sedurante M, Sandoval MA, Castillo G. Successful treatment of methimazole-induced severe aplastic anaemia in a diabetic patient with other co-morbidities. BMJ Case Rep. 2010;2010:bcr0520102993.
78. Wusthof M, Smirnova A, Bacher U, Kroger N, Zander AR, Schuch G, et al. Severe aplastic anaemia following leflunomide therapy. Rheumatology (Oxford). 2010;49(5):1016–7.
79. Wiesen A, Wiesen J, Limaye S, Kaushik N. Mesalazine-induced aplastic anemia. Am J Gastroenterol. 2009;104(4):1063.
80. Chng WJ, Tan LH. Late-onset marrow aplasia due to imatinib in newly diagnosed chronic phase chronic myeloid leukaemia. Leuk Res. 2005;29(6):719–20.
81. Song MK, Choi YJ, Seol YM, Shin HJ, Chung JS, Cho GJ, et al. Nilotinib-induced bone marrow aplasia. Eur J Haematol. 2009;83(2):161–2.
82. Yan L, Shang J, Shi X, Kang H, Liu W, Xu N, et al. Successful treatment of marrow failure after CARTs for myeloma by the infusion of cryopreserved stem cells. Am J Hematol. 2020;95(1):E20–E3.
83. Lolli G, Ursi M, Dicataldo M, Casadei B, Storci G, Argnani L, et al. Allogeneic stem cell transplantation is capable of healing a case of bone marrow aplasia following CAR-T cell therapy in a lymphoma patient. Leuk Lymphoma. 2022;63(12):3012–4.
84. Kenkel TJ, Sridhar N, Hammons LR, Hintzke M, Shah NN. Bone marrow aplasia after CAR-T-cell therapy for relapsed/refractory Burkitt's lymphoma. Med Sci (Basel). 2023;11(4):67.
85. Penack O, Peczynski C, Koenecke C, Polge E, Kuhnl A, Fegueux N, et al. Severe cytopenia after CD19 CAR T-cell therapy: a retrospective study from the EBMT Transplant Complications Working Party. J Immunother Cancer. 2023;11(4):e006406.
86. Guo Q, Zhao JN, Liu T, Gao J, Guo H, Cheng JM. Immune checkpoint inhibitor-induced aplastic anaemia: case series and large-scale pharmacovigilance analysis. Front Pharmacol. 2023;14:1057134.
87. Dasari S, Tse W, Wang J. Real-world evidence of incidence and outcomes of aplastic anaemia following administration of immune checkpoint inhibitors. Br J Haematol. 2023;202(6):1205–8.
88. Issaragrisil S, Chansung K, Kaufman DW, Sirijirachai J, Thamprasit T, Young NS. Aplastic anemia in rural Thailand: its association with grain farming and agricultural pesticide exposure. Aplastic Anemia Study Group. Am J Public Health. 1997;87(9):1551–4.
89. Maluf EM, Pasquini R, Eluf JN, Kelly J, Kaufman DW. Aplastic anemia in Brazil: incidence and risk factors. Am J Hematol. 2002;71(4):268–74.
90. Muir KR, Chilvers CE, Harriss C, Coulson L, Grainge M, Darbyshire P, et al. The role of occupational and environmental exposures in the aetiology of acquired severe aplastic anaemia: a case control investigation. Br J Haematol. 2003;123(5):906–14.
91. Fleming LE, Timmeny W. Aplastic anemia and pesticides. An etiologic association? J Occup Med. 1993;35(11):1106–16.
92. Guiguet M, Baumelou E, Mary JY. A case-control study of aplastic anaemia: occupational exposures. The French Cooperative Group for Epidemiological Study of Aplastic Anaemia. Int J Epidemiol. 1995;24(5):993–9.
93. Prihartono N, Kriebel D, Woskie S, Thetkhathuek A, Sripaung N, Padungtod C, et al. Risk of aplastic anemia and pesticide and other chemical exposures. Asia Pac J Public Health. 2011;23(3):369–77.
94. Newman K, Owlia MB, El-Hemaidi I, Akhtari M. Management of immune cytopenias in patients with systemic lupus erythematosus – old and new. Autoimmun Rev. 2013;12(7):784–91.

95. Chalayer E, Ffrench M, Cathebras P. Aplastic anemia as a feature of systemic lupus erythematosus: a case report and literature review. Rheumatol Int. 2015;35(6):1073–82.
96. Al-Ghazawi Z, Al-Farajat A, Toubasi AA, Tawileh HBA, Qteish A, Aladily TN, et al. Pancytopenia with aplastic anemia in systemic lupus erythematosus: case series and literature review. Rheumatol Int. 2024;44(5):943–53.
97. Paquette RL, Meshkinpour A, Rosen PJ, Autoimmune myelofibrosis. A steroid-responsive cause of bone marrow fibrosis associated with systemic lupus erythematosus. Medicine (Baltimore). 1994;73(3):145–52.
98. Ungprasert P, Chowdhary VR, Davis MD, Makol A. Autoimmune myelofibrosis with pancytopenia as a presenting manifestation of systemic lupus erythematosus responsive to mycophenolate mofetil. Lupus. 2016;25(4):427–30.
99. Antic M, Lautenschlager S, Itin PH. Eosinophilic fasciitis 30 years after – what do we really know? Report of 11 patients and review of the literature. Dermatology. 2006;213(2):93–101.
100. Grey-Davies E, Hows JM, Marsh JC. Aplastic anaemia in association with coeliac disease: a series of three cases. Br J Haematol. 2008;143(2):258–60.
101. Hinterberger-Fischer M, Kier P, Forstinger I, Lechner K, Kornek G, Breyer S, et al. Coincidence of severe aplastic anaemia with multiple sclerosis or thyroid disorders. Report of 5 cases. Acta Haemat. 1994;92(3):136–9.
102. Stalder MP, Rovo A, Halter J, Heim D, Silzle T, Passweg J, et al. Aplastic anemia and concomitant autoimmune diseases. Ann Hematol. 2009;88(7):659–65.
103. Cesaro S, Marsh J, Tridello G, Rovo A, Maury S, Montante B, et al. Retrospective survey on the prevalence and outcome of prior autoimmune diseases in patients with aplastic anemia reported to the registry of the European group for blood and marrow transplantation. Acta Haematol. 2010;124(1):19–22.
104. Sugimori C, Yamazaki H, Feng X, Mochizuki K, Kondo Y, Takami A, et al. Roles of DRB1 *1501 and DRB1 *1502 in the pathogenesis of aplastic anemia. Exp Hematol. 2007;35(1):13–20.
105. Yoshida N, Yagasaki H, Takahashi Y, Yamamoto T, Liang J, Wang Y, et al. Clinical impact of HLA-DR15, a minor population of paroxysmal nocturnal haemoglobinuria-type cells, and an aplastic anaemia-associated autoantibody in children with acquired aplastic anaemia. Br J Haematol. 2008;142(3):427–35.
106. Song EY, Kang HJ, Shin HY, Ahn HS, Kim I, Yoon SS, et al. Association of human leukocyte antigen class II alleles with response to immunosuppressive therapy in Korean aplastic anemia patients. Hum Immunol. 2010;71(1):88–92.
107. Wang M, Nie N, Feng S, Shi J, Ge M, Li X, et al. The polymorphisms of human leukocyte antigen loci may contribute to the susceptibility and severity of severe aplastic anemia in Chinese patients. Hum Immunol. 2014;75(8):867–72.
108. Fernandez-Torres J, Flores-Jimenez D, Arroyo-Perez A, Granados J, Lopez-Reyes A. The ancestry of the HLA-DRB1*15 allele predisposes the Mexican mestizo to the development of aplastic anemia. Hum Immunol. 2012;73(8):840–3.
109. Liang L, Li N, Wang Y, Luo S, Song Y, Fang B. Human leukocyte antigen-DRB1 gene polymorphism and aplastic anemia: a meta-analysis. Medicine (Baltimore). 2023;102(20):e33513.
110. Shao Y, Liu B, He L, Liu C, Fu R. Molecular mechanisms underlying the role of HLA-DQ in systemic immune activation in severe aplastic anemia. Blood Cells Mol Dis. 2023;98:102708.
111. Poullot E, Zambello R, Leblanc F, Bareau B, De March E, Roussel M, et al. Chronic natural killer lymphoproliferative disorders: characteristics of an international cohort of 70 patients. Ann Oncol. 2014;25(10):2030–5.
112. Lamy T, Loughran TP Jr. How I treat LGL leukemia. Blood. 2011;117(10):2764–74.
113. Yang W, Qi J, Li Z, Liu W, Yi S, Xu Y, et al. Analysis of clinical characteristics for large granular lymphocytic leukemia. Zhonghua Yi Xue Za Zhi. 2014;94(4):276–9.
114. Jerez A, Clemente MJ, Makishima H, Koskela H, Leblanc F, Peng Ng K, et al. STAT3 mutations unify the pathogenesis of chronic lymphoproliferative disorders of NK cells and T-cell large granular lymphocyte leukemia. Blood. 2012;120(15):3048–57.

115. Fattizzo B, Bellani V, Pasquale R, Giannotta JA, Barcellini W. Large granular lymphocyte expansion in myeloid diseases and bone marrow failure syndromes: whoever seeks finds. Front Oncol. 2021;11:748610.
116. Zhang HF, Huang ZD, Wu XR, Li Q, Yu ZF. Comparison of T lymphocyte subsets in aplastic anemia and hypoplastic myelodysplastic syndromes. Life Sci. 2017;189:71–5.
117. Hartsock RJ, Smith EB, Petty CS. Normal variations with aging of the amount of hematopoietic tissue in bone marrow from the anterior iliac crest. A study made from 177 cases of sudden death examined by necropsy. Am J Clin Pathol. 1965;43:326–31.
118. Bain BJ. Bone marrow trephine biopsy. J Clin Pathol. 2001;54(10):737–42.
119. Camitta BM, Rappeport JM, Parkman R, Nathan DG. Selection of patients for bone marrow transplantation in severe aplastic anemia. Blood. 1975;45(3):355–63.
120. Bacigalupo A, Hows J, Gluckman E, Nissen C, Marsh J, Van Lint MT, et al. Bone marrow transplantation (BMT) versus immunosuppression for the treatment of severe aplastic anaemia (SAA): a report of the EBMT SAA working party. Br J Haematol. 1988;70(2):177–82.
121. Tichelli A, Schrezenmeier H, Socie G, Marsh J, Bacigalupo A, Duhrsen U, et al. A randomized controlled study in patients with newly diagnosed severe aplastic anemia receiving antithymocyte globulin (ATG), cyclosporine, with or without G-CSF: a study of the SAA Working Party of the European Group for Blood and Marrow Transplantation. Blood. 2011;117(17):4434–41.
122. Scheinberg P, Nunez O, Young NS. Retreatment with rabbit anti-thymocyte globulin and ciclosporin for patients with relapsed or refractory severe aplastic anaemia. Br J Haematol. 2006;133(6):622–7.
123. Scheinberg P, Wu CO, Nunez O, Young NS. Predicting response to immunosuppressive therapy and survival in severe aplastic anaemia. Br J Haematol. 2009;144(2):206–16.
124. Yoshida N, Yagasaki H, Hama A, Takahashi Y, Kosaka Y, Kobayashi R, et al. Predicting response to immunosuppressive therapy in childhood aplastic anemia. Haematologica. 2011;96(5):771–4.
125. Desmond R, Townsley DM, Dumitriu B, Olnes MJ, Scheinberg P, Bevans M, et al. Eltrombopag restores trilineage hematopoiesis in refractory severe aplastic anemia that can be sustained on discontinuation of drug. Blood. 2014;123(12):1818–25.
126. Olnes MJ, Scheinberg P, Calvo KR, Desmond R, Tang Y, Dumitriu B, et al. Eltrombopag and improved hematopoiesis in refractory aplastic anemia. N Engl J Med. 2012;367(1):11–9.
127. Wang M, Dong C, Gao Y, Li J, Han M, Wang L. A deep learning model for the automatic recognition of aplastic anemia, myelodysplastic syndromes, and acute myeloid leukemia based on bone marrow smear. Front Oncol. 2022;12:844978.
128. Xiang P, Wu X, Zeng Z, Lin Z, Guo Y, Ma X, et al. Quantitative analysis of pelvic bone marrow fat using an MRI-based machine learning method for distinguishing aplastic anaemia from myelodysplastic syndromes. Clin Radiol. 2023;78(6):e463–e8.
129. Rovo A, Tichelli A, Dufour C, Saa-Wp E. Diagnosis of acquired aplastic anemia. Bone Marrow Transplant. 2013;48(2):162–7.

Open Access This chapter is licensed under the terms of the Creative Commons Attribution 4.0 International License (http://creativecommons.org/licenses/by/4.0/), which permits use, sharing, adaptation, distribution and reproduction in any medium or format, as long as you give appropriate credit to the original author(s) and the source, provide a link to the Creative Commons license and indicate if changes were made.

The images or other third party material in this chapter are included in the chapter's Creative Commons license, unless indicated otherwise in a credit line to the material. If material is not included in the chapter's Creative Commons license and your intended use is not permitted by statutory regulation or exceeds the permitted use, you will need to obtain permission directly from the copyright holder.

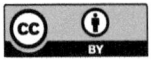

Chapter 5
Acquired Overlap Bone Marrow Failure Disorders

Jakob R. Passweg and Beatrice Drexler

Introduction

Diagnosis of aplastic anemia (AA) is a diagnosis of exclusion. This includes the notion that bone marrow failure with hypocellular marrow will be diagnosed as aplastic anemia if no other disease entity can be diagnosed [1–6]. Whereas some of the competing diagnoses, i.e., hereditary marrow failure, may be diagnosed based on tests that give a clear indication, such as a positive chromosomal breakage stress test, others are less conclusive, e.g., in the case of marrow failure with short telomeres but without a confirmed genetic diagnosis and without other clinical diagnostic features. Aplastic anemia may result in short telomeres based on replicative stress on the remaining hematopoietic stem cells [7, 8].

Hypoplastic myelodysplastic syndrome (MDS) is equally a diagnosis of exclusion; a set of criteria is used to separate hypoplastic MDS from aplastic anemia, but there is a large gray zone of overlapping entities [7–11]. These have been termed ICUS, idiopathic cytopenia of undetermined significance, i.e., a pre-MDS without sufficient alterations to warrant the diagnosis of MDS and Clonal hematopoiesis of indeterminate potential (CHIP), as it has been increasingly recognized that clonality

---

Discussing in particular: Hypoplastic MDS, including Idiopathic cytopenias of undetermined significance (ICUS) and Clonal hematopoiesis of indeterminate potential (CHIP), Single lineage cytopenias, e.g., pure red cell aplasia, or immune thrombocytopenia, Paroxysmal Nocturnal Hemoglobinuria, T-cell Large Granular Lymphocytes Leukemia (T-LGL) and undiagnosed Congenital marrow failure.

J. R. Passweg (✉) · B. Drexler
Division of Hematology, University Hospital Basel, Basel, Switzerland
e-mail: jakob.passweg@usb.ch

may be found in patients with aplastic anemia but also in healthy persons without signs of marrow failure [12–15].

All these reflections are to be included in the diagnostic workup of the cytopenic patient. Whereas diagnosis may be straightforward in the young patient with very severe aplastic anemia and a totally acellular marrow, the older patient with pancytopenia, a mildly hypocellular marrow, some dysplasia in erythropoiesis, no increase of blasts, no cytogenetic abnormality, and no other salient feature may pose a real challenge, and repetitive marrow examination may not carry the diagnosis forward, as disease progress may be slow.

Hypoplastic MDS

In particular, in older persons, the most important differential diagnosis is aplastic anemia versus hypoplastic myelodysplastic syndrome (MDS). MDS is 80–100 times more common than AA, and often the diagnosis is clear. According to the WHO classification, MDS are currently categorized according to the number of dysplastic lineages, the presence of ring sideroblasts, and the percentage of blasts in the bone marrow and the peripheral blood. The thresholds to define the percentage of dysplastic cells and of ringed sideroblasts as significant for diagnosis are somewhat arbitrary. A proportion of MDS patients will present with hypocellular marrow. When differentiating hypoplastic MDS from AA, features diagnostic of MDS are usually considered to be: marrow fibrosis, increased myeloid blasts, increased dysplastic megakaryopoiesis of myelopoiesis, and splenomegaly. Morphologic hot spots of erythropoiesis with some degree of dyserythropoiesis, as well as the presence of a PNH clone, can be seen in both diseases [6].

Aplastic anemia is known to have late clonal complications, of which MDS is the most frequently diagnosed disease [9]. Whether this represents a true transformation event or is an unmasking of preexisting MDS by immunosuppressive therapy and, probably more importantly, by the lapse of time is not known.

The WHO provisional entities of idiopathic cytopenias of undetermined significance (ICUS) and clonal hematopoiesis of indeterminate potential (CHIP) are not very helpful in the view of this author, as these include cases that are probably bona fide autoimmune cytopenias as well as clonal hematologic disease. The provisional category idiopathic cytopenia of undetermined significance (ICUS) has been introduced. To be classified in this, patients must have cytopenia in one or more lineages (hemoglobin <110 g/L, neutrophil count <1.5 × 10^9/L, platelet count <100 × 10^9/L) that is persistent for at least 6 months and cannot be explained by other disease and does not meet diagnostic criteria of MDS. Recent attempts at clarification by using the technology of next-generation sequencing have shown in patients with aplastic anemia that some mutations cluster around autoimmunity, whereas others around clonal myeloid disorders, and that the latter do have a poorer prognosis. Recurrent somatic mutations have been identified in several genes, including RNA splicing machinery (SF3B1, SRSF2, U2AF1, ZRSR2), DNA methylation (TET2, DNMT3A, IDH1/2), histone modification (ASXL1, EZH2), transcription regulation (RUNX1), DNA repair (TP53), signal transduction (CBL, NRAS, KRAS), and others. Myeloid precursor lesions have been added to the WHO 2022 classification, MDS has been renamed Myelodysplastic Neoplasia, and hypoplastic MDS is a defined entity. Hypoplastic MDS is a subset of MDS characterized by marrow hypocellularity, diagnosed in 10–15% of MDS patients. The pathogenesis shares features of aplastic anemia with activation of effector T cells against hematopoietic progenitor cells and high-risk MDS with acquisition of somatic mutations that provide a survival and growth advantage to these cells in the inflammatory bone marrow microenvironment. At the current time, there is, however, not enough evidence and no general agreement to reclassify all aplastic anemia cases with clonal hematopoiesis as hypoplastic MDS [13, 16]. The magnitude of the variant allele frequency may be useful in this situation, showing usually only small clones in AA but larger clones in MDS. In the past, patients with otherwise typical AA but clonal cytogenetic markers such as trisomy 8 or monosomy 7 have been diagnosed as AA and treated as AA, even though it was known that they were at increased risk of MDS and AML transformation.

In fact, over 40% of patients with acquired AA have expanded clones of paroxysmal nocturnal hemoglobinuria (PNH) cells as a result of somatic PIGA gene mutations arising in hematopoietic stem cells. In addition, cytogenetic abnormalities, sometimes transient, have been reported in AA without MDS. In a study with over 100 AA patients with no morphologic evidence of MDS, somatic mutations were detected in over 20% of cases. Most frequently mutated genes included ASXL1, DNMT3A, and BCOR, with a median mutant allele burden of 20%. Patients with somatic mutations had shorter telomere lengths and a higher risk of transformation to MDS compared with patients without mutations [16]. In a study already mentioned in the introduction, approximately one-third of patients had mutations in genes commonly affected in myeloid neoplasms. Most frequently mutated genes included PIGA, BCOR/BCORL1, DNMT3A, and ASXL1. However, a substantial diversity was observed in mutation frequencies compared with myeloid neoplasms, with mutations in PIGA and BCOR/BCORL1 being more common in AA [13]. The number of driver mutations per person and the mutant allele burden are increasing from CHIP and AA with clonal hematopoiesis to MDS, implicating that these small hematopoietic clones may have the potential to progress or represent small malignant clones at a preclinical stage. However, the mechanism by which a specific mutated gene is driving the transformation and the role of external factors need more research.

Finally, in the aging hematopoiesis, evidence of clonal hematopoiesis resulting from an expansion of cells harboring an initiating driver mutation may be found, and this suggests that these hematopoietic clones may represent a premalignant state. The spectrum of mutations is, however, similar.

Patients with MDS may respond to immunosuppressive therapy in a similar way as patients with AA, possibly more frequently if the marrow is hypoplastic, if HLA DR15 is present, and if the transfusion requirements are low [17–22]. This highlights the implication of the immune system in the pathophysiology of MDS and, hence, some similarities between AA and MDS.

Single Lineage Cytopenias, e.g., Pure Red Cell Aplasia (PRCA) or Immune Thrombocytopenia (ITP)

Aplastic anemia may present initially as a single lineage disorder with predominant hyporegenerative anemia or thrombocytopenia. Differentiating AA from PRCA and ITP is important as treatment strategies differ. ITP is defined as megakaryocytic thrombocytopenia with no other lineage abnormalities. Due to bleeding, there may be, however, anemia at initial presentation. Marrow aspirate and biopsy should be diagnostic. If this is of importance, however, be aware that in the elderly, subcortical marrow may be severely hypocellular and that only a biopsy of sufficient depth may clarify the situation.

PCRA is defined as a regenerative anemia with missing erythropoiesis in the marrow. Parvovirus infection has to be excluded. Causes of PRCA vary and may include parainfectious state as well as an equivalent of "single lineage" aplastic anemia with preservation of the other lineages. In addition, the congenital form, Diamond-Blackfan anemia, has to be excluded in young patients.

Agranulocytosis has a vast differential diagnosis covering toxic, autoimmune, and congenital causes. Discussion of all these entities is beyond the scope of this chapter.

T-cell Large Granular Lymphocytes

Large granular lymphocyte (LGL) leukemia is a rare lymphoproliferative neoplasia defined by clonal expansion of CD3 cytotoxic T-lymphocytes. It is a subgroup of mature peripheral T-cell neoplasms. Clinical features include neutropenia, anemia, and rheumatoid arthritis. Approximately one-third of patients are asymptomatic at diagnosis. Eighty-five percent of patients with LGL leukemia experience neutropenia, and 45% develop agranulocytosis. Recurrent bacterial infections are a hallmark of the disease. Transfusion-dependent hyporegenerative anemia is found more rarely. Thrombocytopenia may be found in some patients. Rheumatoid arthritis may occur and often precedes the diagnosis of T-LGL. Diagnosis of LGL leukemia is established by documentation of an increased number of clonal LGLs. Phenotypic analyses show terminal effector memory T cells; most patients with T-LGL leukemia show a CD3+ CD8+ CD57+ CD56− CD28−, TCR-alpha/beta phenotype. Clonality is confirmed by TCR gene rearrangement. LGL leukemia is thought to arise from chronic antigenic stimulation, with the long-term survival of LGL being promoted by constitutive activation of multiple survival signaling pathways. These lead to deregulation of apoptosis and resistance to normal pathways of cell death. Cytopenias are thought to be more often due to immune dysregulation and autoimmunity rather than to infiltration of the marrow with consecutive displacement of hematopoiesis in the marrow [23]. Overlap with other marrow failure disorders exists; in one study [24, 25], clonal effector T-cell expansion was demonstrated in patients with PNH based on V beta repertoires. Whether these clonal T-cell expansions reflect bona fide T-LGL or a reactive process is difficult to determine. Most common treatment options include Methotrexate and Cyclosporine. Detailed discussion of T-LGL leukemia is beyond the scope of this paragraph. Diagnosis of T-LGL requires attention to the differential diagnosis and, obviously, a search for the underlying lymphoid neoplasia.

Paroxysmal Nocturnal Hemoglobinuria (PNH)

Obviously, there is a large overlap between aplastic anemia and PNH, with AA patients often having a PNH clone detectable and patients with classical PNH evolving into a PNH aplastic anemia syndrome. For the discussion of PNH, we refer to Chap. 14. Patients with AA with PNH clones have been shown in some studies to have better responses to immunosuppressive treatment [26], possibly due to PNH clones representing rescue hematopoiesis in the face of autoimmune attack.

Congenital Marrow Failure Undiagnosed

Whereas congenital forms of marrow failure are discussed in detail in part II of this book, there are some considerations worth mentioning here. It is important to consider that many different types of inherited disorders may have a common end-organ failure, i.e., hematopoiesis. Mutations so diverse as to impact the machineries of DNA repair, telomere elongation, ribosome composition, and others may lead to marrow failure. The distinction of inherited forms of marrow failure from acquired forms is often difficult. Inherited forms of marrow failure have a great variability in expression of clinical manifestations and reliance on additional signs, e.g., of Fanconi anemia such as café au lait spots, microcephaly, skeletal abnormalities, and growth retardation, is not justified, as these may be completely absent. Furthermore, marrow failure may occur at an "advanced" age, and it is not unheard of to diagnose, e.g., Fanconi anemia in patients between 35 and 40 years of age. It is nevertheless reasonable to limit the diagnostic search for congenital forms to a certain age, e.g., 35 years, and perform such tests in older individuals only if a specific suspicion exists. It is not known how many patients with congenital forms of marrow failure have been treated by immunosuppressive therapy assuming acquired AA, but many hematologists interested in marrow failure disorders have encountered such cases. Therefore, maintaining a high degree of suspicion is important. In addition, there may be cases in which a congenital marrow disorder is suspected based on the combination of marrow failure with other features. Once the common congenital marrow failures have been ruled out, diagnosis is difficult. The NIH in the US is maintaining specialty clinics for rare and undiagnosed disorders and such clinics may contribute to widening the scope of inherited and acquired disorders of the hematopoietic system [27]. In the last years, data have accumulated, showing that inherited bone marrow failure (BMF) syndromes are genetically more diverse than thought; more than 100 genes have been associated with these syndromes, and the list continues to expand. Risk assessment and genetic counseling of patients with newly described BMF syndromes is difficult, as disease mechanisms, penetrance, genotype-phenotype associations, phenotypic heterogeneity, risk of hematologic malignancies, and clonal markers of disease progression are unknown. In addition, germline variants play a role to be clarified in the coming years.

Conclusion

As shown in Fig. 5.1, there is considerable overlap in the disorders discussed above. Some of the differential diagnoses have a major impact on treatment; congenital marrow failure should not be treated by immunosuppressive therapies, whereas it is of importance to know that hypocellular MDS and, for that matter, also MDS without increased blast counts may respond to immunosuppressive approaches similar to AA [17–19]. Ultimately ineffective hematopoiesis in MDS may in part be due to autoimmune T-cell clones driving hematopoiesis toward apoptosis. Marrow failure syndromes remain difficult to diagnose; often, more than one biopsy is required, and careful attention to details is required to narrow down the differential diagnosis. Finally, physicians need to be aware of the overlap in clinical presentation between many of these disease entities.

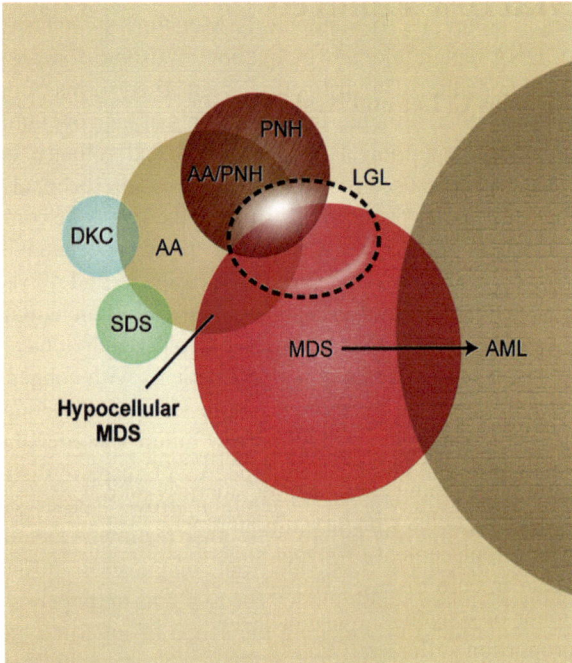

Fig. 5.1 The overlap of aplastic anemia with other clonal and congenital disorders

References

1. Young NS. The problem of clonality in aplastic anemia: Dr Dameshek's riddle, restated. Blood. 1992;79(6):1385–92.
2. Young NS, Barrett AJ. The treatment of severe acquired aplastic anemia. Blood. 1995;85(12):3367–77.
3. Young NS, Maciejewski J. The pathophysiology of acquired aplastic anemia. N Engl J Med. 1997;336(19):1365–72.
4. Young NS. Acquired aplastic anemia. JAMA. 1999;282(3):271–8.
5. Young NS, Calado RT, Scheinberg P. Current concepts in the pathophysiology and treatment of aplastic anemia. Blood. 2006;108(8):2509–19.
6. Rovó A, Tichelli A, Dufour C, SAA-WP EBMT. Diagnosis of acquired aplastic anemia. Bone Marrow Transplant. 2013;48(2):162–7.
7. Scheinberg P, Cooper JN, Sloand EM, Wu CO, Calado RT, Young NS. Association of telomere length of peripheral blood leukocytes with hematopoietic relapse, malignant transformation, and survival in severe aplastic anemia. JAMA. 2010;304(12):1358–64.
8. Kulasekararaj A, Cavenagh J, Dokal I, Foukaneli T, Gandhi S, Garg M, Griffin M, Hillmen P, Ireland R, Killick S, Mansour S, Mufti G, Potter V, Snowden J, Stanworth S, Zuha R, Marsh J, BSH Committee. Guidelines for the diagnosis and management of adult aplastic anaemia: a British Society for Haematology guideline. Br J Haematol. 2024;204(3):784–804.
9. Socie G, Mary JY, Schrezenmeier H, Marsh J, Bacigalupo A, Locasciulli A, Fuehrer M, Bekassy A, Tichelli A, Passweg J. Granulocyte-stimulating factor and severe aplastic anemia: a survey by the European Group for Blood and Marrow Transplantation (EBMT). Blood. 2007;109(7):2794–6.
10. Barrett J, Saunthararajah Y, Molldrem J. Myelodysplastic syndrome and aplastic anemia: distinct entities or diseases linked by a common pathophysiology? Semin Hematol. 2000;37(1):15–29. Review.
11. Malcovati L, Cazzola M. The shadowlands of MDS: idiopathic cytopenias of undetermined significance (ICUS) and clonal hematopoiesis of indeterminate potential (CHIP). Hematology Am Soc Hematol Educ Program. 2015;2015(1):299–307.
12. Maciejewski JP, Risitano A, Sloand EM, Nunez O, Young NS. Distinct clinical outcomes for cytogenetic abnormalities evolving from aplastic anemia. Blood. 2002;99(9):3129–35.
13. Yoshizato T, Dumitriu B, Hosokawa K, Makishima H, Yoshida K, Townsley D, Sato-Otsubo A, Sato Y, Liu D, Suzuki H, Wu CO, Shiraishi Y, Clemente MJ, Kataoka K, Shiozawa Y, Okuno Y, Chiba K, Tanaka H, Nagata Y, Katagiri T, Kon A, Sanada M, Scheinberg P, Miyano S, Maciejewski JP, Nakao S, Young NS, Ogawa S. Somatic mutations and clonal hematopoiesis in aplastic anemia. N Engl J Med. 2015;373(1):35–47.
14. Genovese G, Kähler AK, Handsaker RE, Lindberg J, Rose SA, Bakhoum SF, Chambert K, Mick E, Neale BM, Fromer M, Purcell SM, Svantesson O, Landén M, Höglund M, Lehmann S, Gabriel SB, Moran JL, Lander ES, Sullivan PF, Sklar P, Grönberg H, Hultman CM, McCarroll SA. Clonal hematopoiesis and blood-cancer risk inferred from blood DNA sequence. N Engl J Med. 2014;371(26):2477–87.
15. Jaiswal S, Fontanillas P, Flannick J, Manning A, Grauman PV, Mar BG, Lindsley RC, Mermel CH, Burtt N, Chavez A, Higgins JM, Moltchanov V, Kuo FC, Kluk MJ, Henderson B, Kinnunen L, Koistinen HA, Ladenvall C, Getz G, Correa A, Banahan BF, Gabriel S, Kathiresan S, Stringham HM, McCarthy MI, Boehnke M, Tuomilehto J, Haiman C, Groop L, Atzmon G, Wilson JG, Neuberg D, Altshuler D, Ebert BL. Age-related clonal hematopoiesis associated with adverse outcomes. N Engl J Med. 2014;371(26):2488–98.
16. Kulasekararaj AG, Jiang J, Smith AE, et al. Somatic mutations identify a subgroup of aplastic anemia patients who progress to myelodysplastic syndrome. Blood. 2014;124(17):2698–704.
17. Sloand EM, Wu CO, Greenberg P, Young N, Barrett J. Factors affecting response and survival in patients with myelodysplasia treated with immunosuppressive therapy. J Clin Oncol. 2008;26(15):2505–11.

18. Passweg JR, Giagounidis AA, Simcock M, Aul C, Dobbelstein C, Stadler M, Ossenkoppele G, Hofmann WK, Schilling K, Tichelli A, Ganser A. Immunosuppressive therapy for patients with myelodysplastic syndrome: a prospective randomized multicenter phase III trial comparing antithymocyte globulin plus cyclosporine with best supportive care–SAKK 33/99. J Clin Oncol. 2011;29(3):303–9.
19. Sloand EM, Olnes MJ, Shenoy A, Weinstein B, Boss C, Loeliger K, Wu CO, More K, Barrett AJ, Scheinberg P, Young NS. Alemtuzumab treatment of intermediate-1 myelodysplasia patients is associated with sustained improvement in blood counts and cytogenetic remissions. J Clin Oncol. 2010;28(35):5166–73.
20. Saunthararajah Y, Nakamura R, Nam JM, Robyn J, Loberiza F, Maciejewski JP, Simonis T, Molldrem J, Young NS, Barrett AJ. HLA-DR15 (DR2) is overrepresented in myelodysplastic syndrome and aplastic anemia and predicts a response to immunosuppression in myelodysplastic syndrome. Blood. 2002;100(5):1570–4.
21. Sloand EM, Kim S, Fuhrer M, Risitano AM, Nakamura R, Maciejewski JP, Barrett AJ, Young NS. Fas-mediated apoptosis is important in regulating cell replication and death in trisomy 8 hematopoietic cells but not in cells with other cytogenetic abnormalities. Blood. 2002;100(13):4427–32.
22. Karantanos T, DeZern AE. Biology and clinical management of hypoplastic MDS: MDS as a bone marrow failure syndrome. Best Pract Res Clin Haematol. 2021;34(2):101280. https://doi.org/10.1016/j.beha.2021.101280. Epub 2021 Jun 26. PMID:34404534.
23. Zhang D, Loughran TP Jr. Large granular lymphocytic leukemia: molecular pathogenesis, clinical manifestations, and treatment. Hematology Am Soc Hematol Educ Program. 2012;2012:652–9.
24. Saunthararajah Y, Molldrem JL, Rivera M, Williams A, Stetler-Stevenson M, Sorbara L, Young NS, Barrett JA. Coincident myelodysplastic syndrome and T-cell large granular lymphocytic disease: clinical and pathophysiological features. Br J Haematol. 2001;112(1):195–200.
25. Risitano AM, Maciejewski JP, Muranski P, Wlodarski M, O'Keefe C, Sloand EM, Young NS. Large granular lymphocyte (LGL)-like clonal expansions in paroxysmal nocturnal hemoglobinuria (PNH) patients. Leukemia. 2005;19(2):217–22.
26. Sugimori C, Chuhjo T, Feng X, Yamazaki H, Takami A, Teramura M, Mizoguchi H, Omine M, Nakao S. Minor population of CD55-CD59- blood cells predicts response to immunosuppressive therapy and prognosis in patients with aplastic anemia. Blood. 2006;107(4):1308–14.
27. Feurstein S. Emerging bone marrow failure syndromes-new pieces to an unsolved puzzle. Front Oncol. 2023;13:1128533. https://doi.org/10.3389/fonc.2023.1128533. eCollection 2023. PMID: 37091189.

Open Access This chapter is licensed under the terms of the Creative Commons Attribution 4.0 International License (http://creativecommons.org/licenses/by/4.0/), which permits use, sharing, adaptation, distribution and reproduction in any medium or format, as long as you give appropriate credit to the original author(s) and the source, provide a link to the Creative Commons license and indicate if changes were made.

The images or other third party material in this chapter are included in the chapter's Creative Commons license, unless indicated otherwise in a credit line to the material. If material is not included in the chapter's Creative Commons license and your intended use is not permitted by statutory regulation or exceeds the permitted use, you will need to obtain permission directly from the copyright holder.

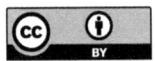

Part III
Non-transplant Treatment and Supportive Care

Chapter 6
Non-transplant Treatments for Acquired Bone Marrow Failure Disorders

Pedro H. Prata, Camilla Frieri, Antonio M. Risitano, and Régis Peffault de Latour

Introduction

Immune (idiopathic) aplastic anemia (IAA) is the prototypical presentation of acquired bone marrow failure disorders. It is characterized by pancytopenia and a fatty bone marrow [1]. Clinical findings are nonspecific and secondary to pancytopenia (e.g., fatigue, bleeding, and infection). IAA is a rare disease, with an incidence of two cases per million inhabitants and a prevalence of 0.0004% in Western countries [2, 3], with an incidence threefold higher in Southeast Asia [1]. It affects both genders equally and has a bimodal age distribution, with the first peak among young adults and the second among patients over 50.

The first evidence of immune pathophysiology for aplastic anemia came from a clinical observation: Mathé and Schwarzenberg noted an autologous reconstitution following allogeneic cell transplantation with antithymoglobulin (ATG) and deduced that immunosuppression was responsible for the response [4]. Subsequently, robust experimental data supported the immune-mediated pathophysiology of IAA [5–10]. By our current understanding, oligoclonal auto-reactive T cells are activated and expanded, possibly within a broader immune system derangement (i.e., reduced Tregs [11, 12] and increased Th17 cells [12, 13]). These pathogenic lymphocytes

P. H. Prata (✉)
Hematology and Cellular Therapy Department, CHU de Limoges, France
e-mail: pedro.prata@chu-limoges.fr

C. Frieri · A. M. Risitano
Hematology and Hematopoietic Transplant Unit, Azienda Ospedaliera di Rilievo Nazionale San Giuseppe Moscati, Avellino, Italy

R. Peffault de Latour
Hematology and Transplant Unit, Saint-Louis Hospital, AP-HP and Université Paris Cité, Paris, France

damage hematopoietic stem cells both directly and through cytokine production [14], leading to a decrease in the hematopoietic stem cell pool, hampering the production of blood cells. To date, the triggers of the autoimmune reaction leading to bone marrow failure remain unknown.

The expected long-term overall survival of IAA patients receiving an allogeneic hematopoietic stem cell transplant (HSCT) or immunosuppressive treatment (IST) is a testament to the significant progress made in recent decades, standing at around 80% [15, 16]. Survival has improved over the last decades primarily due to better supportive care (i.e., improved management and prevention of infectious complications, including relapsed/refractory patients) [8], better HLA-matching for unrelated donor selection, better strategies for using alternative donors, and higher efficacy of non-transplant strategies with the inclusion of eltrombopag into the therapeutic arsenal. In this chapter, we focus on non-transplant treatment for IAA.

Non-transplant Treatment Modalities

Specific treatment is indicated for patients meeting the Camitta severity criteria (Table 6.1) [17] or who are transfusion-dependent.

Watch and wait is an adequate strategy for non-severe patients who do not require transfusions. On the other hand, they must be regularly assessed with complete blood counts and screened for clonal evolution into myeloid neoplasms or paroxysmal nocturnal hemoglobinuria (PNH).

First-line treatment options for IAA include HSCT and IST. Both strategies deliver an appropriate immunosuppressive effect, allowing residual autologous hematopoietic stem cells (IST) or donor hematopoietic stem cells (HSCT) to expand.

The choice between these two options relies chiefly on patients' age and availability of an HLA-identical sibling donor: HSCT is the preferred front-line treatment for young (<40 years old) patients with a matched-HLA sibling donor, whereas IST is the standard choice for all other situations. The second and subsequent lines will depend on the availability of an allogeneic donor and the patient's eligibility for HSCT. For HSCT in the context of IAA, please see other chapters in the book discussing HSCT. Figure 6.1 presents a schematic algorithm for IAA treatment modalities. It is crucial to note that the field of non-transplant treatment for IAA is still evolving, and continued research is needed to improve outcomes and quality of life for patients with immune aplastic anemia.

Table 6.1 Camitta severity criteria

Severe	At least two among the three following criteria: Neutrophils <0.5×10^9/L Platelets <20×10^9/L Reticulocyte count <20×10^9/L (<60×10^9/L if automate) [15]
Non-severe	Patients not fulfilling the above criteria

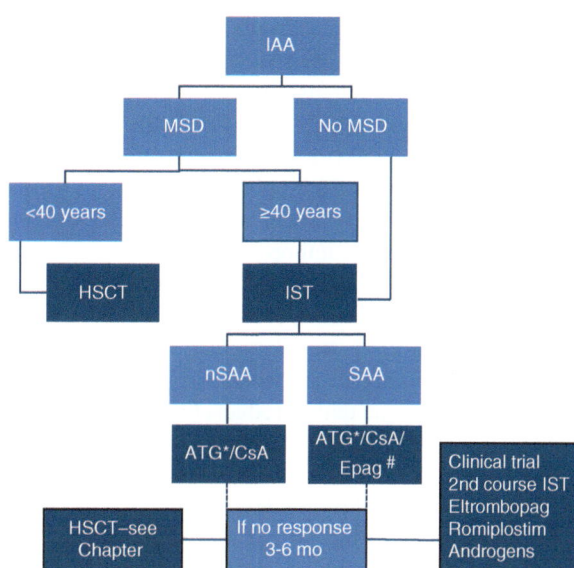

Fig. 6.1 Algorithm for newly diagnosed IAA immune aplastic anemia, MSD matched sibling donor, IST immunosuppressive therapy, nSAA non-severe aplastic anemia, SAA severe aplastic anemia, ATG antithymoglobulin, CsA cyclosporin, Epag eltrombopag. *Horse ATG is the preferred option. Rabbit ATG can be used instead if hATG is unavailable. #Eltrobopag is added for patients ≥15 years old

First-Line Immunosuppressive Treatment

Following the observations of Mathé and Schwarzenberg, immunosuppression with ATG is the cornerstone treatment for IAA. ATG consists of polyclonal, heterologous antihuman thymocyte antibodies obtained from pigs, horses, or rabbits [18–20]. The combination of ATG with the calcineurin-inhibitor cyclosporine A (CsA), which inhibits lymphocyte activation and clonal expansion, is the most widespread non-transplant treatment for IAA. A randomized controlled clinical trial demonstrated that the most effective lymphocyte-depleting agent is horse-ATG [21] (hATG, ATGAM®) when administered with ciclosporin, resulting in an overall hematologic response rate of 60–70% [9–11]. The median response time is 3 months; the 5-year OS can achieve 90% [22].

The authors propose hATG at 40 mg/kg/day for four consecutive days as an IV infusion lasting 12–18 hours. For obese patients, defined as a body weight higher than 1.3 times the ideal body weight (IBW), the dose will be between $1.3 \times$ IBW and actual body weight. If the calculated weight exceeds 100 kg, the infusion volume should be increased to at least 1 L. Premedication with paracetamol and anti-H1 medications might improve tolerance.

Clinicians must be aware that hATG might cause serum sickness, and concomitant prophylactic treatment with corticosteroids is warranted. Methylprednisolone is given at 1 mg/kg/day IV (fractioned in 2–3 infusions) starting the day before hATG. Oral prednisone 1 mg/kg/day can replace IV methylprednisolone from day 5. If no signs of serum sickness are present, steroids should be tapered from a third at day 10, two-thirds of the initial dose at day 20, and withdrawn at day 30. Cyclosporine is started on day 5 for better tolerance; nonetheless, starting on day 1 is also an acceptable strategy. It can be given orally (3 mg/kg PO twice a day) or IV (3 mg/kg in continuous perfusion or divided into two perfusions of 2 h 12 h apart). If coadministration with voriconazole or posaconazole is required, the cyclosporine dose should be reduced by 50%. The residual predose concentration 200–300 ug/L.

For patients with severe aplastic anemia (SAA), the SAA Working Party led a randomized controlled clinical trial (the RACE trial) that demonstrated the addition of eltrombopag, a thrombopoietin receptor agonist, to the hATG/CsA scheme yielded more rapid and effective responses with significantly higher complete responses than hATG/CsA alone for patients, without any difference in toxicity [15]. Eltrombopag is started on day 10 following IST, beginning at 75 mg and increasing to 150 mg after 2 weeks if there is good tolerance (risk of transaminitis). It is an oral drug, and dairy products highly affect its bioavailability. Patients should take tablets at least 2 hours before or after any meal. If the response is absent after 3 months, the dose can be further augmented to 225 mg.

Primary anti-mold prophylaxis (e.g., posaconazole or voriconazole) for neutropenic patients or during steroid therapy. This prophylaxis should be extended for neutropenic patients and kept until the neutrophil count is $>0.5 \times 10^9$/L. HSV/VZV (e.g., valacyclovir, acyclovir) and *Pneumocystis jirovecii* (e.g., co-trimoxazole, atovaquone) prophylaxis should be started with ATG and kept until 3 months following IST, or until total $CD4^+$ lymphocytes exceed 250/µL.

The triple therapy with hATG is now the standard of care for SAA patients older than 15 years of age who are not eligible for first-line HSCT or lack a matched sibling donor. For younger patients, the beneficial role of eltrombopag has not been confirmed [23].

Nonetheless, about one-third of IAA patients will not respond to IST. Furthermore, among responding patients, one-third will eventually relapse, and another third may require long-term cyclosporine maintenance. Therefore, effective rescue treatment for patients not eligible for HSCT remains an unmet clinical need.

Noteworthy, IST does not play a role in nonimmune acquired aplastic anemia (direct physical/chemical damage, idiosyncratic drug reactions, or inherited syndromes).

Patients Not Eligible for Standard Immunosuppressive Therapy

Comorbid or frail patients might not be fit for ATG-based or HSCT treatments because of unreasonable toxicity risk. In this scenario (or if ATG is unavailable), the association of ciclosporin with eltrombopag is an accepted option [24]. Eltrombopag can also be used in monotherapy if contraindication to cyclosporin [25]. Of note, age per se is not a contraindication to ATG-based treatment.

Second-Line Treatment Options

Eltrombopag

Eltrombopag monotherapy is also an option for patients who failed IST and are not eligible for HSCT if they did not receive it in the first-line regimen. A phase II trial, which included refractory, heavily pretreated patients, found an overall response rate of 40%. In some patients with trilineage response, eltrombopag could be discontinued without loss of response [26, 27]. Before starting a second line, it is imperative to assess marrow for clonal evolution in special monosomy 7 since there is a risk of clonal expansion [28].

Eltrombopag is a synthetic, orally available, non-peptide thrombopoietin (TPO) mimetic that binds to the TPO receptor c-mpl at the level of its transmembrane and juxtamembrane domains without competing with endogenous TPO, which binds to a distinct site [29]. TPO is a glycoprotein produced by the liver (and to a lesser extent by stromal marrow cells) that works as a hematopoietic growth factor, mainly stimulating megakaryopoiesis [30]. Fully functional c-mpl is also expressed on primitive hematopoietic stem and progenitor cells [31]. For instance, loss-of-function mutations of *c-MPL* are associated with congenital amegakaryocytic thrombocytopenia, a bone marrow failure syndrome (see others chapters in the discussing HSCT) [32].

TPO is a crucial cytokine for the proper functioning of the bone marrow. Still, it does not play a significant role in the pathophysiology of IAA since serum levels of TPO are highly increased in IAA [33]. In this setting, excess IFN-γ induces the formation of TPO: IFN-γ heteromers, perturbing TPO signaling. Eltrombopag bypasses this inhibition [34].

Androgens

From a historical perspective, androgens have been used for the treatment of IAA since the initial studies investigating the effect of IST [35], even if the actual role in promoting hematopoietic recovery is unclear [36]. In vitro data showed that androgens stimulate telomerase activity [37]. Since telomere attrition has been implicated in HSC exhaustion in inherited and possibly acquired forms of bone marrow failure [38–40], androgens may rescue hematopoiesis in some refractory patients.

To date, androgens should be reserved for refractory or relapsed patients who are not eligible or have failed other treatments [41], and the evidence supporting their use is unconvincing [41–43]. Patients receiving androgen treatment for longer than 12 months must be screened yearly for hepatic tumors even after the treatment is stopped. Close prostatic surveillance is required among men before, during, and after treatment.

Alternative Immunosuppressive Strategies

Over the last three decades, several alternative regimens of IST have been investigated to improve the results achieved by standard hATG and CsA [12, 13]. Three strategies to intensify IST have been exploited: (i) adding a third immunosuppressive agent on top of the platform hATG + CsA; (ii) replacing the key lymphocyte-depleting agent with alternative, more lymphotoxic, immunosuppressive agents; (iii) novel strategies without conventional lymphocyte depletion. Even if most of them (if not all) led to disappointing results, we describe the most relevant attempts. While they remain scientifically remarkable for the information they gave us, none of these strategies resulted in a change in the standard care of IAA. Nevertheless, because of the apparent biological activity of some of these regimens, an alternative IST strategy could be discussed for patients failing standard IST who are unsuitable for HSCT.

Adding a Third Immunosuppressive Agent

The addition of a third immunosuppressive agent, such as the anti-metabolite mycophenolate mofetil (MMF) or the inhibitor of mammalian target (mTOR), rapamycin/sirolimus, did not result in positive results.

Mycophenolate Mofetil
MMF is an inhibitor of purine synthesis, affecting T cell expansion; it was tested in a prospective single-arm, open-label study in combination with standard hATG + CsA. In a cohort of 104 untreated AA patients, this three-drug regimen resulted in a 6-month response rate of 62%; the relapse rate was 37% (despite maintenance IST with MMF and CsA), and clonal evolution was 9%. Compared with historical controls, adding MMF to standard IST did not confer any advantage in hematologic response, relapse, or clonal evolution [44].

Rapamycin/Sirolimus
Sirolimus is an mTOR inhibitor developed for several autoimmune conditions, including GvHD. It exerts its immunosuppressive effect through two different mechanisms of action. Indeed, sirolimus binds to immunophilins (FKBP12), blocking initial IL-2-dependent T cell activation, like calcineurin inhibitors. Furthermore, once bound to its target, sirolimus inhibits mTOR, modulating many intracellular pathways needed for cell-cycle progression toward the G1/S stage. Because of this mechanism of action, a strong rationale suggests that sirolimus might work synergistically with CsA [45]. In IAA, a prospective randomized controlled clinical trial compared the addition of sirolimus to the standard hATG/CsA and failed to show any benefit [46].

Replacing hATG with Another Lymphocyte-Depleting Agent

Studies exploring the intensification of IST by replacing hATG with more potent lymphocyte-depleting agents assumed it could lead to a better eradication of pathogenic T-cells, resulting in a better hematologic response. Altogether, the data did not show any benefit. Below, we describe the three agents that have been investigated.

Rabbit ATG

Rabbit ATG (rATG, Thymoglobuline®, Sanofi) was frequently used in IAA for many decades and is still used today in countries without access to hATG. RATG yields a more potent lymphocyte-depleting effect than hATG, as demonstrated in the transplant setting [47, 48]. It showed acceptable results as salvage therapy for patients relapsed/after hATG [49, 50].

With these premises, a prospective randomized clinical trial compared rATG/CsA to hATG/CsA. Quite surprisingly, rATG led to a significantly lower response rate than hATG (37% vs 68% at 6 months, $p < 0.001$), with a detrimental effect on overall survival at 3 years (70% vs 94%, $p = 0.008$) [21]. These observations were confirmed in a subsequent open-label EBMT study [51].

Horse ATG is more effective than rATG; however, if hATG is unavailable, rATG is an accepted alternative for standard upfront immunosuppressive therapy, including triple therapy [52].

Cyclophosphamide

Because of its strong anti-lymphocyte effect, cyclophosphamide has been considered a candidate lymphocyte-depleting agent for treating IAA. Cyclophosphamide at high doses (50 mg/kg for four consecutive days, intravenously) showed an overall response rate of 70% [53]. However, a subsequent randomized trial comparing cyclophosphamide combined with CsA to the hATG/CsA showed excess morbidity and mortality secondary to infectious complications (mostly fungal infections) in the cyclophosphamide arm, leading to the early termination of the trial [54]. Cyclophosphamide did not reduce the risk of relapse or clonal evolution [55]. Another trial exploring a moderate dose of cyclophosphamide further confirmed the unacceptable long-lasting neutropenia and high risk of severe fungal infections [56].

Alemtuzumab

Alemtuzumab is a recombinant, humanized anti-CD52 monoclonal antibody that provokes peripheral lymphoid depletion [57]. Different clinical trials explored alemtuzumab in refractory, relapsed, and untreated IAA. The overall response rate was 37% in refractory patients ($n = 54$) and 56% among relapsed patients ($n = 25$). Nevertheless, this activity as a second-line treatment did not translate into efficacy as a front-line treatment [35]. Indeed, in the prospective randomized trial for untreated IAA, the alemtuzumab arm was closed prematurely because of a lack of efficacy [35]. A smaller EBMT prospective trial exploring alemtuzumab in combination with CsA shows an overall response rate of 84% and a 3-year OS of 74% [36]. Subsequent studies confirmed the safety profile of alemtuzumab for IAA patients [58, 59].

The Lessons Learned from Alternative Lymphocyte-Depleting Agents

The use of lymphocyte killers other than hATG demonstrated their biological activity in IAA because of their lympholytic effect on T cells. In contrast with what was expected, even if they resulted in a more profound lymphocyte depletion, it did not translate into any clinical benefit. On the contrary, it might lead to unacceptable infectious-related morbidity. Nevertheless, the disappointing and unexpected results of these more potent immunosuppressive agents [21, 35, 55] conclude that they (or any other experimental drug) must be offered only within well-designed, prospective studies.

Other Hematopoietic Growth Factors

G-CSF
Adding G-CSF to IST has been a common practice for many years, with the risk of delaying appropriate treatment [60]. Following inconclusive observations from at least six small clinical trials [37, 61–65], the SAA WP conducted a prospective, controlled, randomized clinical trial comparing ATG/CsA with or without G-CSF, studying 192 patients not eligible for HSCT [66].

There was no difference in OS between groups; however, patients treated with G-CSF had fewer infectious episodes (24% vs. 36%, $p = 0.006$) and hospitalization days (82% vs. 87%, $p = 0.0003$). With a median follow-up of 11.7 years, G-CSF did not affect long-term survival nor the incidence of secondary neoplasms [67].

Romiplostim
Romiplostim is a recombinant analog of the TPO receptor (c-MPL) developed initially for chronic immune thrombocytopenic purpura [68]. Since hematopoietic stem cells express c-MPL (see discussion on eltrombopag), romiplostim was studied for IAA patients refractory to IST, titrating doses from 10 μg/kg up to 20 μg/kg [69]. A small ($n = 10$) prospective, single-arm, open-label trial found that 70% of patients with IAA who have failed eltrombopag increased at least one lineage following treatment with romiplostim [70]. With a median follow-up of two and a half years, the cumulative incidence of trilineage response increased to 55% by 1 year. It remained stable thereafter, demonstrating the presence of late responders [33]. Romiplostim is an option for patients who are refractory or ineligible for IST.

Conclusions

Over the decades, advancements in supportive care and treatment modalities have improved the long-term overall survival of IAA patients. More recently, eltrombopag has further ameliorated the prognosis of IAA patients.

In the journey to achieve the significant hematologic response rates and survival outcomes we have today, novel immunosuppressive strategies have been explored but with varying success rates and concerns regarding efficacy and safety. Attempts to intensify IST by adding a third immunosuppressive agent or replacing hATG with more potent lymphocyte-depleting agents have shown promising biological activity but have not translated into significant clinical benefits. Indeed, these alternative strategies may increase infectious-related morbidity. Consequently, they underscore the necessity for well-designed prospective studies to guide their use judiciously.

Combinations of ciclosporin with eltrombopag offer an acceptable option for elderly or fragile patients deemed unfit for standard treatments. Additionally, for those who fail IST and are ineligible for HSCT, eltrombopag monotherapy or other second-line options may be considered, albeit with caution and close monitoring for adverse events.

In essence, while significant strides have been made in understanding and treating IAA, challenges persist, particularly in identifying effective rescue treatments for nonresponders and addressing relapse. The evolving landscape of immunosuppressive strategies underscores the need for continued research to improve outcomes and quality of life for patients with IAA.

References

1. Young NS. Aplastic anemia. N Engl J Med. 2018;379:1643–56.
2. Maluf EMCP, Pasquini R, Eluf JN, Kelly J, Kaufman DW. Aplastic anemia in Brazil: incidence and risk factors. Am J Hematol. 2002;274:268–74.
3. Young N, Alter B. Epidemiology of acquired aplastic anemia. In: Aplastic anemia acquired and inherited. Philadelphia: W.B. Saunders; 1994. p. 24–31.
4. Mathe G, Schwarzenberg L. Treatment of bone marrow aplasia by mismatched bone marrow transplantation after conditioning with antilymphocyte globulin--long-term results. Transplant Proc. 1976;8:595–602.
5. Hoffman R, Zanjani ED, Lutton JD, Zalusky R, Wasserman LR. Suppression of erythroid-colony formation by lymphocytes from patients with aplastic anemia. N Engl J Med. 1977;296:10–3.
6. Zeng W, Maciejewski JP, Chen G, Young NS. Limited heterogeneity of T cell receptor BV usage in aplastic anemia. J Clin Invest. 2001;108:765–73.
7. Nakao S, et al. Isolation of a T-cell clone showing HLA-DRB1*0405-restricted cytotoxicity for hematopoietic cells in a patient with aplastic anemia. Blood. 1997;89:3691–9.
8. Risitano AM, et al. In-vivo dominant immune responses in aplastic anaemia: molecular tracking of putatively pathogenetic T-cell clones by TCR β-CDR3 sequencing. Lancet. 2004;364:355–64.
9. Melenhorst JJ, et al. T cells selectively infiltrate bone marrow areas with residual haemopoiesis of patients with acquired aplastic anaemia. Br J Haematol. 1997;99:517–9.
10. Maciejewski JP, Selleri C, Sato T, Anderson S, Young NS. Increased expression of Fas antigen on bone marrow CD34+ cells of patients with aplastic anaemia. Br J Haematol. 1995;91:245–52.
11. Solomou EE, et al. Deficient CD4+ CD25+ FOXP3+ T regulatory cells in acquired aplastic anemia. Blood. 2007;110:1603–6.
12. Kordasti S, et al. Functional characterization of CD4+ T cells in aplastic anemia. Blood. 2012;119:2033–43.
13. de Latour RP, et al. Th17 immune responses contribute to the pathophysiology of aplastic anemia. Blood. 2010;116:4175–84.
14. Laver J, et al. In vitro interferon-gamma production by cultured T-cells in severe aplastic anaemia: correlation with granulomonopoietic inhibition in patients who respond to anti-thymocyte globulin. Br J Haematol. 1988;69:545–50.

15. Peffault de Latour R, et al. Eltrombopag added to immunosuppression in severe aplastic anemia. N Engl J Med. 2022;386:11–23.
16. Gurnari C, et al. Clinical and molecular determinants of clonal evolution in aplastic anemia and paroxysmal nocturnal hemoglobinuria. J Clin Oncol. 2023;41:132–42.
17. Camitta B, Rappeport J, Parkman R, Nathan D. Selection of patients for bone marrow transplantation in severe aplastic anemia. Blood. 1975;45:355–63.
18. Scheinberg P, Young NS. How I treat acquired aplastic anemia. Blood. 2014;120:1185–96.
19. Bacigalupo A. How I treat acquired aplastic anemia. Blood. 2017;129:1428–36.
20. Peffault de Latour R. Transplantation for bone marrow failure: current issues. Hematology. 2016;2016:90–8. https://doi.org/10.1182/asheducation-2016.1.90.
21. Scheinberg P, et al. Horse versus rabbit antithymocyte globulin in acquired aplastic anemia. N Engl J Med. 2011;3365:430–8.
22. Peffault de Latour R, et al. Nationwide survey on the use of horse antithymocyte globulins (ATGAM) in patients with acquired aplastic anemia: a report on behalf of the French Reference Center for Aplastic Anemia. Am J Hematol. 2018;93:635–42.
23. Groarke EM, et al. Eltrombopag added to immunosuppression for children with treatment-naïve severe aplastic anaemia. Br J Haematol. 2021;192:605–14.
24. Scheinberg P, et al. Activity and safety of eltrombopag in combination with cyclosporin A as first-line treatment of adults with severe aplastic anaemia (SOAR): a phase 2, single-arm study. Lancet Haematol. 2024;11:e206–15.
25. Lengline E, et al. Nationwide survey on the use of eltrombopag in patients with severe aplastic anemia: a report on behalf of the french reference center for aplastic anemia. Haematologica. 2018;103:212–20.
26. Olnes MJ, et al. Eltrombopag and improved hematopoiesis in refractory aplastic anemia. N Engl J Med. 2012;367:11–9.
27. Townsley DM, et al. Eltrombopag restores trilineage hematopoiesis in refractory severe aplastic anemia that can be sustained on discontinuation of drug. Blood. 2013;123:1818–25.
28. Winkler T, et al. Eltrombopag for refractory severe aplastic anemia: dosing, duration, long term outcomes and clonal evolution. Blood. 2019;133:blood.2019000478.
29. Bussel JB, et al. Eltrombopag for the treatment of chronic idiopathic thrombocytopenic purpura. N Engl J Med. 2007;357:2237–47.
30. Garnock-Jones KP, Keam SJ. Eltrombopag. Drugs. 2009;69:567–76.
31. Zeigler FC, et al. In vitro megakaryocytopoietic and thrombopoietic activity of c-mpl ligand (TPO) on purified murine hematopoietic stem cells. Blood. 1994;84:4045–52.
32. Ihara K, et al. Identification of mutations in the c-mpl gene in congenital amegakaryocytic thrombocytopenia. Proc Natl Acad Sci USA. 1999;96:3132–6.
33. Mitani K, et al. Long-term efficacy and safety of romiplostim in refractory aplastic anemia: follow-up of a phase 2/3 study. Blood Adv. 2024;8:1415–9.
34. Alvarado LJ, et al. Eltrombopag maintains human hematopoietic stem and progenitor cells under inflammatory conditions mediated by IFN-γ. Blood. 2019;133:2043–55.
35. Scheinberg P, et al. Activity of alemtuzumab monotherapy in treatment-naive, relapsed, and refractory severe acquired aplastic anemia. Blood. 2012;119:345–54.
36. Risitano AM, et al. Alemtuzumab is safe and effective as immunosuppressive treatment for aplastic anaemia and single-lineage marrow failure: a pilot study and a survey from the EBMT WPSAA. Br J Haematol. 2010;148:791–6.
37. Teramura M, et al. Treatment of severe aplastic anemia with antithymocyte globulin and cyclosporin A with or without G-CSF in adults: a multicenter randomized study in Japan. Blood. 2007;110:1756–61.
38. Scheinberg P, et al. Association of telomere length of peripheral blood leukocytes with hematopoietic relapse, malignant transformation, and survival in severe aplastic anemia. JAMA. 2010;304:1358–64.
39. Calado RT, et al. Short telomeres result in chromosomal instability in hematopoietic cells and precede malignant evolution in human aplastic anemia. Leukemia. 2012;26:700–7.

40. Dumitriu B, et al. Telomere attrition and candidate gene mutations preceding monosomy 7 in aplastic anemia. Blood. 2015;125:706–9.
41. Pagliuca S, et al. Current use of androgens in bone marrow failure disorders: a report from the Severe Aplastic Anemia Working Party of the European Society of Blood and Marrow Transplantation. Haematologica. 2023;109:765. https://doi.org/10.3324/haematol.2023.282935.
42. Kaltwasser JP, Dix U, Schalk KP, Vogt H. Effect of androgens on the response to antithymocyte globulin in patients with aplastic anaemia. Eur J Haematol. 1988;40:111–8.
43. Champlin RE, et al. Do androgens enhance the response to antithymocyte globulin in patients with aplastic anemia? A prospective randomized trial. Blood. 1985;66:184–8.
44. Scheinberg P, Nunez O, Wu C, Young NS. Treatment of severe aplastic anaemia with combined immunosuppression: anti-thymocyte globulin, ciclosporin and mycophenolate mofetil. Br J Haematol. 2006;133:606–11.
45. Sehgal SN. Rapamune (RAPA, rapamycin, sirolimus): mechanism of action immunosuppressive effect results from blockade of signal transduction and inhibition of cell cycle progression. Clin Biochem. 1998;31:335–40.
46. Scheinberg P, et al. Treatment of severe aplastic anemia with a combination of horse antithymocyte globulin and cyclosporine, with or without sirolimus: a prospective randomized study. Haematologica. 2009;94:348–54.
47. Brennan DC, et al. A randomized, double-blinded comparison of Thymoglobulin versus Atgam for induction immunosuppressive therapy in adult renal transplant recipients. Transplantation. 1999;67:1011–8.
48. Gaber AO, et al. Results of the double-blind, randomized, multicenter, phase III clinical trial of Thymoglobulin versus Atgam in the treatment of acute graft rejection episodes after renal transplantation. Transplantation. 1998;66:29–37.
49. Di Bona E, et al. Rabbit antithymocyte globulin (r-ATG) plus cyclosporine and granulocyte colony stimulating factor is an effective treatment for aplastic anaemia patients unresponsive to a first course of intensive immunosuppressive therapy. Gruppo Italiano Trapianto di Midollo Osseo (GITMO). Br J Haematol. 1999;107:330–4.
50. Scheinberg P, Nunez O, Young NS. Retreatment with rabbit anti-thymocyte globulin and ciclosporin for patients with relapsed or refractory severe aplastic anaemia. Br J Haematol. 2006;133:622–7.
51. Marsh JC, et al. Prospective study of rabbit antithymocyte globulin and cyclosporine for aplastic anemia from the EBMT Severe Aplastic Anaemia Working Party. Blood. 2012;119:5391–6.
52. Imada K, et al. Eltrombopag in combination with rabbit anti-thymocyte globulin/cyclosporine A in immunosuppressive therapy-naïve patients with aplastic anemia in Japan. Intern Med. 2021;60:1159–68.
53. Brodsky RA, Sensenbrenner LL, Jones RJ. Complete remission in severe aplastic anemia after high-dose cyclophosphamide without bone marrow transplantation. Blood. 1996;87:491–4.
54. Tisdale JF, et al. High-dose cyclophosphamide in severe aplastic anaemia: a randomised trial. Lancet. 2000;356:1554–9.
55. Tisdale JF, Maciejewski JP, Nuñez O, Rosenfeld SJ, Young NS. Late complications following treatment for severe aplastic anemia (SAA) with high-dose cyclophosphamide (Cy): follow-up of a randomized trial. Blood. 2002;100:4668–70.
56. Scheinberg P, et al. Moderate-dose cyclophosphamide for severe aplastic anemia has significant toxicity and does not prevent relapse and clonal evolution. Blood. 2014;124:2820–3.
57. Hu Y, et al. Investigation of the mechanism of action of alemtuzumab in a human CD52 transgenic mouse model. Immunology. 2009;128:260–70.
58. Kim H, et al. A pilot dose-escalating study of alemtuzumab plus cyclosporine for patients with bone marrow failure syndrome. Leuk Res. 2009;33:222–31.
59. Gómez-Almaguer D, et al. Subcutaneous alemtuzumab plus cyclosporine for the treatment of aplastic anemia. Ann Hematol. 2010;89:299–303.

60. Marsh JC, et al. Haemopoietic growth factors in aplastic anaemia: a cautionary note. European Bone Marrow Transplant Working Party for Severe Aplastic Anaemia. Lancet. 1994;344:172–3.
61. Zheng Y, Liu Y, Chu Y. Immunosuppressive therapy for acquired severe aplastic anemia (SAA): a prospective comparison of four different regimens. Exp Hematol. 2006;34:826–31.
62. Shao Z, Chu Y, Zhang Y, Chen G, Zheng Y. Treatment of severe aplastic anemia with an immunosuppressive agent plus recombinant human granulocyte-macrophage colony-stimulating factor and erythropoietin. Am J Hematol. 1998;59:185–91.
63. Kojima S, et al. Immunosuppressive therapy using antithymocyte globulin, cyclosporine, and danazol with or without human granulocyte colony-stimulating factor in children with acquired aplastic anemia. Blood. 2000;96:2049–54.
64. Gordon-Smith EC, et al. Randomised placebo controlled study of RH-GM-CSF following ALG in the treatment of aplastic anaemia. Bone Marrow Transplant. 1991;7(Suppl 2):78–80.
65. Gluckman E, et al. Results and follow-up of a phase III randomized study of recombinant human-granulocyte stimulating factor as support for immunosuppressive therapy in patients with severe aplastic anaemia. Br J Haematol. 2002;119:1075–82.
66. Tichelli A, et al. A randomized controlled study in patients with newly diagnosed severe aplastic anemia receiving antithymocyte globulin (ATG), cyclosporine, with or without G-CSF: a study of the SAA Working Party of the European Group for Blood and Marrow Transplantation. Blood. 2011;117:4434–41.
67. Tichelli A, et al. Long-term outcome of a randomized controlled study in patients with newly diagnosed severe aplastic anemia treated with antithymocyte globulin and cyclosporine, with or without granulocyte colony-stimulating factor: a Severe Aplastic Anemia Working Party Trial from the European Group of Blood and Marrow Transplantation. Haematologica. 2020;105:1223–31.
68. Cersosimo RJ. Romiplostim in chronic immune thrombocytopenic purpura. Clin Ther. 2009;31:1887–907.
69. Lee JW, et al. Romiplostim in patients with refractory aplastic anaemia previously treated with immunosuppressive therapy: a dose-finding and long-term treatment phase 2 trial. Lancet Haematol. 2019;6:e562–72.
70. Ise M, et al. Romiplostim is effective for eltrombopag-refractory aplastic anemia: results of a retrospective study. Int J Hematol. 2020;112:787–94.

Open Access This chapter is licensed under the terms of the Creative Commons Attribution 4.0 International License (http://creativecommons.org/licenses/by/4.0/), which permits use, sharing, adaptation, distribution and reproduction in any medium or format, as long as you give appropriate credit to the original author(s) and the source, provide a link to the Creative Commons license and indicate if changes were made.

The images or other third party material in this chapter are included in the chapter's Creative Commons license, unless indicated otherwise in a credit line to the material. If material is not included in the chapter's Creative Commons license and your intended use is not permitted by statutory regulation or exceeds the permitted use, you will need to obtain permission directly from the copyright holder.

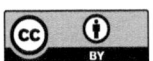

Chapter 7
Supportive Care in Severe and Very Severe Aplastic Anemia

Britta Höchsmann, Mahmoud Aljurf, Hubert Schrezenmeier, and Shaykhah AlOtaibi

Introduction

Survival rates in aplastic anemia have significantly improved over the past 30 years due to advances in immunosuppressive therapy and allogeneic bone marrow transplantation [1]. Importantly, this improvement is not restricted to responders to specific treatments but also extends to nonresponders, highlighting the role of optimized supportive care [2]. The individual risk of infection and other complications is primarily determined by neutrophil and monocyte counts [2–8]. Despite a reduction in infection-related mortality and invasive fungal infections over the past two decades, infections remain the leading cause of death in severe and very severe aplastic anemia. In major clinical trials, bacterial and fungal infections continue to be the most prevalent complications [3–5]. This chapter provides an overview of major aspects of supportive treatment in aplastic anemia, including infection prophylaxis and management, transfusion strategies, and iron overload treatment.

B. Höchsmann (✉)
Institute of Clinical Transfusion Medicine and Immunogenetics Ulm, German Red Cross Blood Transfusion Service Baden-Württemberg – Hessen and University Hospital Ulm, Ulm, Germany
e-mail: b.hoechsmann@blutspende.de

M. Aljurf · S. AlOtaibi
Department of Hematology, Stem Cell Transplant & Cellular Therapy, Cancer Centre of Excellence, King Faisal Specialist Hospital & Research Centre, Riyadh, Saudi Arabia

H. Schrezenmeier
Institute of Transfusion Medicine, University of Ulm and German Red Cross, Ulm, Germany

Prevention of Infections by General Precautions

Patients with neutrophil counts ≤0.5 G/L are at risk for severe infections, and management of these patients should therefore be restricted to experienced centers.

Most of the following recommendations are based on studies of neutropenic patients in the context of malignant disorders and chemotherapy or stem cell transplantation and have been adopted for patients with aplastic anemia. There are no randomized controlled trials on the effect of prophylactic interventions specifically in the group of aplastic anemia (AA) patients [1]. Therefore, it seems reasonable to deduce the recommendations from the large number of randomized controlled clinical trials and the respective meta-analyses that are available for other neutropenic conditions [2–7].

Since the 1960s, typical strategies to prevent neutropenic infections have been a protective environment, a special low-bacterial diet, and antibiotic prophylaxis, as well as protective clothing and isolation, but the evidence for most of them is weak.

Several recent studies showed that a low-bacterial diet did not significantly reduce the incidence of neutropenic infections, febrile neutropenia, days of antibiotic use, survival, and stool colonization by gram-negative bacilli as well as yeasts in hospitalized patients [8–10] and febrile admission in an outpatient setting [11]. Thus, the available data do not support the use of a special low-bacteria diet in neutropenic patients [12]. Additionally, a low-bacterial diet can adversely impact the patient's quality of life, increase the risk of infection, and possibly affect the gut microbiota. Further studies are needed to confirm that last finding [13]. Despite the lack of evidence, surveys showed that 43–78% of the hospitals use a special neutropenic diet. We recommend following the FDA-approved food safety guidelines, which involve certain recommendations related to food storage, food preparation, and safe cooking and serving of food without placing major restrictions on the type of food [14]. In case of severe mucositis, parenteral nutrition may be necessary to avoid negative nitrogen balance.

Prolonged neutropenia is a major risk factor for acquiring invasive mold infections. Other environmental factors associated with a higher risk of exposure should be avoided, like gardening and working or living in or near construction sites, as there are well-documented outbreaks of aspergillus infections in patients exposed to sites of construction [15, 16]. The data about the impact of using the HEPA filter in neutropenic patients are not consistent [17, 18]; the use of the HEPA filter in neutropenic non-transplant hospitalized patients was associated with less incidence of invasive aspergillosis [19].

During hospitalization, protective isolation, including air quality control, prophylactic antibiotics, and barrier isolation, brought about a significant reduction in all-cause mortality (RR 0.60 (95% CI 0.50–0.70)) in patients with cancer. However, inclusion of prophylactic antibiotics was necessary to show the effect on mortality. Control of air quality *and* barrier isolation alone (without prophylactic antibiotics) had no significant effect on mortality and overall occurrence of infection [7].

Even if no independent effect of barrier precautions and single-patient rooms can be proven, they might help to reduce the spread of (multi-) resistant bacteria [20]. Thus, barrier isolation and facilities with HEPA filtration, as well as single rooms with en-suite facilities, are not imperative but should be used if available.

Staff should follow local guidelines regarding clothing and hygienic routines. There should be procedures in place for the management of central and peripheral venous catheters. Staff handling venous lines should be taught about the correct practice.

Hand washing and rubbing with alcohol-based disinfection solutions must be used before and after handling the patient by the staff and by visitors. Optimal hand hygiene has been shown to be highly effective in reducing neutropenic infections [21, 22].

As the majority of neutropenic infections are caused by the entry of the microbial flora of the patient into the blood, individual hygiene rules should be explained to the patient. Mucositis and oral lesions are known causes for bacterial entry, resulting in morbidity and mortality of the patients [23]. Thus, especially oral hygiene is an important point: soft toothbrushes should be used to avoid bleeding and lesions of the mucosa. Additional usage of an antiseptic medical mouth rinse may be reasonable.

Early mobilization of the patient should avoid bedsores and guarantee good pulmonary function. Physical exercises are recommended if the patient is well enough. Especially in patients with anemia, training should be adapted to the heart rate. Additionally, passive mobilization and breathing exercises by a physical therapist may be helpful for hospitalized patients who are not able to do such activities.

Physical examination (especially infection and bleeding signs) and monitoring of vital parameters (blood pressure, heart frequency, temperature), as well as physical parameters like weight, respiration, stools, and diuresis, have to be evaluated daily in hospitalized patients.

Prevention and Treatment of Infections by Prophylactic Antimicrobial

Severe aplastic anemia patients with prolonged period of severe neutropenia are at risk of developing invasive fungal infection [24, 25], mold specifically is considered to be a leading cause of death in AA patients [2, 6, 7, 26–28]. A systematic review and meta-analysis analyzed 64 randomized controlled clinical trials comparing systemic antifungals with placebo in cancer patients receiving chemotherapy with more than 70% hematologic malignancies, including patients post-HSCT. Antifungal prophylaxis decreased all-cause mortality, fungal-related mortality, and documented invasive fungal infection in allogeneic hematopoietic stem cell recipients [29].

Based on the available data on the pattern of infection in aplastic anemia and the antifungal prophylaxis recommendations for patients with other hematological disorders, in addition to the expected prolonged neutropenia, which is known to be one of the strongest factors for invasive fungal infection in patients with hematologic disorders, prophylactic anti-mold antifungals are strongly recommended in patients with severe or very severe aplastic anemia [29]. There are no general recommendations for prophylaxis against *Pneumocystis jirovecii* pneumonia in aplastic anemia [25]. Treatment with CSA and antithymocyte globulin (ATG) has been observed to be associated with an increased risk of PCP; therefore, during immunosuppressive therapy and postbone marrow transplant, it is recommended to give PCP prophylaxis [30].

Neutropenic AA anemia patients are at risk of both Gram-negative and Grampositive sepsis; therefore, it is recommended to give antibacterial prophylaxis, which is based on several recommendations related to neutropenia management in cancer patients [31, 32]. In a meta-analysis of 95 randomized controlled clinical trials in afebrile neutropenic cancer patients, prophylactic antibiotics reduced mortality. Both quinolone antibiotics (such as ciprofloxacin) and a combination of nonabsorbable antibiotics (such as neomycin and colistin) can be effective. In this meta-analysis, mortality was substantially reduced when the analysis was limited to fluoroquinolones. However, prophylactic use of fluoroquinolones increased the risk for the development of antibacterial resistance. The patients most likely to benefit are those with vSAA; therefore, antibacterial prophylaxis could be considered in this group. The risk for severe infections decreases rapidly with increasing neutrophil counts, and in patients with ANC >0.5 × 10e9/l, antibacterial prophylaxis is not recommended [4].

It should be noted that there are no sufficient data about the potential negative effects of long-term usage of antibiotics and antimycotics on hematopoiesis [33].

There are only limited data on the risk for viral infection in patients with aplastic anemia and recommendations are variable. IST with cyclosporin and ATG is associated with a 4.8–6% risk of viral infection, mostly herpes [28, 34]; therefore, many centers use acyclovir in patients who have undergone intensive immunosuppressive therapy with ATG and cyclosporine. Patients who undergo allogeneic HSCT should follow standard procedures for the prevention and treatment of viral infections in HSCT [35].

IST is associated with an increase in the risk of CMV reactivation but with almost a negligible risk of CMV disease, as CMV level drops within a short period of time without antiviral treatment. Peak CMV level depends on the type of IST, with alemtuzumab being the IST associated with the highest peak level. As the risk of CMV disease is very low, CMV monitoring and preemptive therapy are not warranted outside the HSCT setting except in alemtuzumab-treated patients [31, 36, 37]. Most seropositive EBV patients will have reactivation post-immunosuppressive therapy; peak level and duration correlate with the type of immunosuppressive therapy, with rabbit ATG/CsA being the most common IST associated with the highest peak and longer duration. Despite the increased EBV reactivation risk, EBV disease is rare [36, 37]. Influenza is also a potentially severe infection in immunocompromised patients, and therapy with neuraminidase inhibitors (oseltamivir, zanamivir) should be considered in patients with proven influenza. In vSAA patients and patients early after ATG therapy, postexposure prophylaxis with neuraminidase inhibitors can also be considered.

Hematopoietic Growth Factors as Prophylaxis of Infections or in Combination with Immunosuppression to Improve Quality of Response

There is no indication for the treatment of aplastic anemia with growth factors alone [38–40]. The addition of G-CSF to triple immunosuppression with ATG, cyclosporine, and corticosteroids accelerates the recovery of neutrophils and reduces the rate of early infections and the length of hospital stay [41, 42]. Addition of G-CSF does not improve trilineage response, event-free survival, relapse rate, and overall survival [41, 42]. One study from Japan comparing immunosuppression with or without G-CSF reported a lower relapse rate in the G-CSF group [43]. This was not confirmed in a large European multicenter trial [41]. One must also consider the potential risk that G-CSF increases the incidence of secondary clonal disorders [44, 45]. There are currently no data to support the routine use of G-CSF in aplastic anemia, either alone or as an adjunct to immunosuppression.

TPO (thrombopoietin-receptor agonist) has been used in AA patients refractory to IST and found to be beneficial [46–48]. When eltrombopag was added to CSA + ATG in a randomized control trial, the CR rate was higher compared to CSA + ATG only, and the time to response was shorter. Adding eltrombopag did not impact the overall survival or relapse rate and was not associated with the risk of clonal evolution. Therefore, it is recommended to always consider adding eltrombopag to the frontline IST therapy [49].

Neutropenic Fever

Fever with neutropenia is an indication for immediate hospitalization. Diagnostic procedures should include careful physical examination, blood cultures, and cultures from other relevant sites; a chest X-ray is optional but often useful. However, treatment of infection must be started at once without waiting for culture results. Therefore, local hospital guidelines for the treatment of febrile neutropenia should be followed. In addition, patient history and recent medication should also be taken into consideration.

In cases of persisting fever or previous or suspected fungal infection, systemic antifungal therapy should be used early in the therapy of fever in neutropenic aplastic anemia patients. In these cases, CT scanning of the chest should be performed.

Adding G-CSF to the frontline IST results in fewer infectious episodes and shorter duration of hospitalization. It is not a standard of care, as it did not alter the hematological response, the need for bone marrow transplant, or the overall survival, but since the use of G-CSF was considered to be safe with no increase in secondary malignancy, it can always be considered during the AA treatment course. The use of short-term G-CSF may result in a temporary increase of neutrophils and may therefore be beneficial, as, even though there are no guidelines, it is clear from several studies that prophylactic growth factors do not improve overall results but growth factors are often given when treating infectious complications of AA.

In life-threatening infections during neutropenia, the use of irradiated granulocyte transfusions should be discussed with the awareness of limited data to support this procedure and possible side effects. They may have an adjunctive role to bridge the gap between specific treatment and neutrophil recovery [50]. RING, the randomized clinical trial, had failed to show a significant difference between the granulocyte transfusion group and control group, although the study was limited by the low accrual rate. Post hoc analysis showed a significant difference between the high- and low-dose granulocyte groups, as the high-dose group had higher survival and infection resolution [51]. A recently published single-center experience included AA anemia patients being treated with IST who experienced serious infection during their neutropenia phase and demonstrated a strong correlation between response to the granulocyte transfusion and survival with hematopoietic recovery. There has been concern that human leukocyte antigens (HLA) alloimmunization will inhibit the therapeutic activity of granulocyte concentrates. However, patients with or without HLA alloantibodies did not differ in mean post-transfusion neutrophil count [52].

Vaccination

Vaccination strategies for aplastic anemia patients are not well defined except for patients undergoing transplantation, where recommendations are well established [38, 53]. There have been concerns about immune activation of different patient cohorts with immune-mediated disorders, such as AA patients, patients with autoimmune hematologic disorders, and patients with rheumatic disorders. The support for these concerns is very limited and is only based on case reports [54–56]. While larger controlled studies in rheumatology patients have not shown an increased risk [57, 58]. On the other hand, the response to vaccination in patients with vSAA is likely to be poor. In less severely affected patients, vaccinations against pneumococci and influenza can be indicated since the risk/benefit ratio of vaccination is likely to be positive. Children with AA should receive their age-appropriate vaccines, with the exception of live vaccines (varicella, MMR, live influenza vaccine) while receiving immunosuppression.

Transfusion Therapy

Many patients require regular red blood cell (RBC) transfusions in order to maintain their quality of life and physical activity. However, frequent transfusions are associated with an increased risk of alloimmunization against RBC antigens and iron overload. Similarly, platelet transfusions can lead to immunization against human leukocyte antigens (HLA) or human platelet antigens (HPA). Aplastic anemia (AA) is associated with a higher risk of alloimmunization compared to malignant disorders, further compounding the immunization risk due to the frequent need for transfusions [55]. Additionally, the severity of AA is an independent risk factor for alloimmunization. Both of these findings may be attributed to the heightened immunogenicity observed in AA [56].

Several studies in the 1980s and 1990s have demonstrated a negative impact of the number of pretransplant transfusions on outcome after transplantation [59–61]. However, the quality of blood products has changed substantially since these studies were performed. With the current universal leuko-reduction of blood products, HLA alloimmunization remained frequent but reduced compared to the previous cohorts [62–64]. Retrospective analysis showed that allosensitization did not poorly impact the outcomes [65] but further studies are needed to confirm the impact on, e.g., outcome after stem cell transplantation. Allosensitization is mostly due to residual leukocytes in transfused blood products, although a study in mice indicates that minor histocompatibility antigens on donor erythrocytes may contribute to allosensitization. An erythrocyte-dependent immunization against minor histocompatibility antigens is not eliminated by leukocyte depletion [64].

A restrictive transfusion policy should be applied, in particular in patients who are candidates for allogenic bone marrow transplantation [59–61, 66]. However, a planned transplantation is no reason to withhold an otherwise indicated transfusion. The decision for transfusion and the safe hemoglobin level should be based on clinical symptoms, the comorbidities, and the physical state of the patient. In this context, the transfusion trigger in most aplastic anemia patients ranges between 80 and 85 g/L. [67] But patients with cardiac, pulmonary, or vascular comorbidities may require a higher transfusion trigger [68, 69]. To avoid hypoxic cell damage, hemoglobin levels $\leq 6,0$ g/dl are obligate transfusion triggers.

Bleeding due to thrombocytopenia is the second most common cause of death in aplastic anemia [70]. Aplastic anemia patients should receive prophylactic platelet transfusions in case of platelets $<10 \times 10^9/l$ without fever, bleeding signs (including petechial bleeding), or history of major bleeding events [71]. Based on data from a single-center study [72], in addition to some of the transfusion guidelines, a platelet level of $5 \times 10^9/l$ can be considered as a threshold for prophylactic transfusion in stable patients without bleeding signs (including petechial bleeding) [50]. This very low transfusion trigger requires regular measurement of platelet count and daily physical examination to closely monitor for any bleeding signs. To allow an immediate therapeutic transfusion in case of major bleeding, the availability of platelet concentrates must be assured. Aplastic anemia patients with fever, elderly or bleeding signs, or a history of relevant bleeding (WHO grade 3 or 4 bleeding; for example, cerebral bleeding) should receive prophylactic platelet transfusions if the platelet count is below <20 × 10^9/l. Fever was shown to be a risk factor for an increased bleeding risk; therefore, a platelet trigger of 20 was adopted in most centers. It can be observed in many patients that bleeding starts if the platelet count drops below a certain threshold. This patient-individual threshold, based on observation of the clinical course of the patients, must be taken into consideration. In particular, if a patient experienced a major bleeding complication (WHO grade 3 or 4) at a platelet count above 5 × 10^9/L.

For invasive procedures, platelet transfusions must be given to achieve the recommended levels [71]. Cross-reacting antibodies in ATG can bind to platelets and increase platelet consumption. In some patients, a rapid drop in platelet count during ATG infusion can be observed. Therefore, patients should be transfused optimally to achieve a platelet count of >20 × 10^9/l prior to ATG treatment [30, 73].

Immediate therapeutic transfusion is necessary in case of WHO grade 3 or grade 4 bleeding.

There is no data that the use of non-HLA-matched apheresis platelet concentrates is superior to pooled platelet concentrates in non-allosensitized patients [74].

In the case of inadequate platelet count increment after platelet transfusion, screening for HLA antibodies should be performed. If no HLA antibodies can be detected, a screening for HPA antibodies should also be performed. If HLA antibodies are detected, HLA-matched single-donor apheresis platelet concentrates should be used for further transfusions. Ideally, the platelet concentrates are identical in HLA-A and HLA-B antigens to the patient. If appropriate platelet donors are not available, the concentrates must be at least negative for the epitopes recognized by the HLA antibodies [57, 75]. All blood products must be leukodepleted [40]. Transfusions from family members should be strictly avoided [76].

There are two reasons for the use of irradiated blood products in aplastic anemia: Irradiation can avoid transfusion-associated graft-versus-host disease (TA-GvHD). Data from an animal model suggest that irradiation reduces the risk of allosensitization [40, 77].

In order to avoid a taGvHD, irradiation with 25–30 Gy is recommended for the following situations: [50, 76–78].

- During ATG treatment and thereafter until lymphocyte count recovers to at least 1×10^9/L.
- During and after other intensive immunosuppressive treatment, e.g., fludarabine or alemtuzumab.
- Patients receiving allogeneic stem cell transplantation [53]. Transfusion regimen has to be switched to irradiated blood products at the latest at the start of the conditioning.
- Some centers use irradiated blood products in all patients with aplastic anemia—irrespective of treatment. The aim of this strategy is the avoidance of alloimmunization. A European survey demonstrated substantial heterogeneity in the use of irradiated blood products for AA.

- HLA-matched apheresis platelet concentrates.
- Granulocyte concentrates.

Currently, many centers switch to pathogen-reduced platelet concentrates. The pathogen-reduction treatment seems to be even more effective than irradiation at abrogating leukocyte immune functions [79].

In general, there is no need for CMV-negative blood products if universal leukodepletion is applied [80–83]. However, some centers give only CMV-negative blood products for patients undergoing HSCT where both the patient and donor are CMV negative [84].

Iron Chelation Therapy

Aplastic anemia patients who are RBC transfusion-dependent over a long period of time are at risk of developing iron overload. Iron overload can significantly impact the morbidity and mortality of aplastic anemia [85–88]. In non-transplant settings, ferritin of more than 1000 ng/ml was found to be associated with poor outcomes; therefore, it is recommended by most guidelines to initiate iron chelation when ferritin is more than 1000 ng/ml [24, 40, 51, 89]. This applies in particular to candidates for allogeneic stem cell transplantation since iron overload is associated with higher transplant-related mortality and worse survival after transplantation [90–93]. However, the recommendation with a threshold of 1000 ng/ml in a transplant setting has been adopted from other disorders, e.g., myelodysplastic syndromes-related guidelines [94, 95]. Recently, a study showed a strong correlation between the response to the iron overload when initiated in the pretransplant period with deferasirox and the transplant outcome based on the response to deferasirox, suggesting that ferritin of >1000 ng/mL be considered as a cutoff to initiate iron chelation [96]. Iron chelation was associated with bone marrow recovery when used to treat iron overload in transfusion-dependent patients who failed to respond to immunosuppressive therapy; the same findings were previously described in MDS patients, suggesting that the bone marrow suppression associated with the iron overload is likely related to the production of reactive oxygen species (ROS), which consequently can lead to cellular damage [97–99]. An individual assessment should be performed in each aplastic anemia patient, taking into account the individual risk of complications of iron overload, the potential adverse events of iron chelators and the expected period with ongoing RBC transfusion dependence. Iron chelation can be performed with deferoxamine or deferasirox [100]. A relatively high incidence of agranulocytosis has been reported with deferiprone [100]. Therefore, this is not recommended for aplastic anemia patients. Only a few studies are available on the use of deferoxamine in aplastic anemia [88, 101, 102]. A sub-study of the EPIC trial

[103] analyzed 116 aplastic anemia patients with iron overloads who were treated with deferasirox. In this subgroup, the serum ferritin concentration fell significantly during one year of treatment and no drug-induced cytopenia was observed. A decrease occurred in chelation-naive and previously chelated patients.

Emerging research suggests that eltrombopag, commonly used to increase platelet counts, also exhibits iron-chelation properties. Studies have shown that eltrombopag can bind and reduce iron levels within cells, potentially aiding in conditions involving iron overload. Studies have also highlighted its ability to mobilize cellular iron and decrease reactive oxygen species.(R) These findings suggest eltrombopag may offer therapeutic benefits beyond its primary use [104–106].

Psychological Support

Aplastic anemia is a rare disease, and at the time of initial diagnosis, a thorough explanation of its nature, treatment options, prognosis, and social implications is essential for both patients and their families. The treating physician should allocate sufficient time for a comprehensive discussion, addressing all possible scenarios that may arise during treatment, with particular emphasis on the chronic nature of the disease and the potential for a slow response to therapy.

Since cytopenia may persist in a significant proportion of patients, it is crucial to highlight not only disease remission but also quality of life as a secondary therapeutic goal. In patients with persistent neutropenia, providing guidance on maintaining a functional social life can help prevent unnecessary isolation. Encouraging a lifestyle that is as normal as possible is vital for psychological well-being.

Given that an aplastic anemia diagnosis is a life-altering event, some patients may require professional psychological support. Additionally, connecting with other individuals affected by the disease can be beneficial for some patients, and information about relevant patient support groups should be provided.

Conflicts of Interest None.

References

1. Gafter-Gvili A, et al. Management of aplastic anemia: the role of systematic reviews and meta-analyses. Acta Haematol. 2011;125(1–2):47–54.
2. Gafter-Gvili A, et al. Antibiotic prophylaxis for bacterial infections in afebrile neutropenic patients following chemotherapy. Cochrane Database Syst Rev. 2005;4:CD004386.
3. Gafter-Gvili A, et al. Meta-analysis: antibiotic prophylaxis reduces mortality in neutropenic patients. Ann Intern Med. 2005;142(12 Pt 1):979–95.
4. Gafter-Gvili A, et al. Effect of quinolone prophylaxis in afebrile neutropenic patients on microbial resistance: systematic review and meta-analysis. J Antimicrob Chemother. 2007;59(1):5–22.

5. Gafter-Gvili A, et al. Antibiotic prophylaxis in neutropenic patients. Isr Med Assoc J. 2007;9(6):460–2.
6. Leibovici L, et al. Antibiotic prophylaxis in neutropenic patients: new evidence, practical decisions. Cancer. 2006;107(8):1743–51.
7. Schlesinger A, et al. Infection-control interventions for cancer patients after chemotherapy: a systematic review and meta-analysis. Lancet Infect Dis. 2009;9(2):97–107.
8. van Tiel F, et al. Normal hospital and low-bacterial diet in patients with cytopenia after intensive chemotherapy for hematological malignancy: a study of safety. Ann Oncol. 2007;18(6):1080–4.
9. Gardner A, et al. Randomized comparison of cooked and noncooked diets in patients undergoing remission induction therapy for acute myeloid leukemia. J Clin Oncol. 2008;26(35):5684–8.
10. Moody K, et al. Feasibility and safety of a pilot randomized trial of infection rate: neutropenic diet versus standard food safety guidelines. J Pediatr Hematol Oncol. 2006;28(3):126–33.
11. DeMille D, et al. The effect of the neutropenic diet in the outpatient setting: a pilot study. Oncol Nurs Forum. 2006;33(2):337–43.
12. Jubelirer SJ. The benefit of the neutropenic diet: fact or fiction? Oncologist. 2011;16(5):704–7.
13. Gulliver T, et al. The neutropenic diet and its impacts on clinical, nutritional, and lifestyle outcomes for people with cancer: a scoping review. J Nutr Sci. 2024;13:e60.
14. Moody KM, et al. A randomized trial of the effectiveness of the neutropenic diet versus food safety guidelines on infection rate in pediatric oncology patients. Pediatr Blood Cancer. 2018;65(1)
15. Oren I, et al. Invasive pulmonary aspergillosis in neutropenic patients during hospital construction: before and after chemoprophylaxis and institution of HEPA filters. Am J Hematol. 2001;66(4):257–62.
16. Caira M, et al. Pre-chemotherapy risk factors for invasive fungal diseases: prospective analysis of 1,192 patients with newly diagnosed acute myeloid leukemia (SEIFEM 2010-a multicenter study). Haematologica. 2015;100(2):284–92.
17. Eckmanns T, Rüden H, Gastmeier P. The influence of high-efficiency particulate air filtration on mortality and fungal infection among highly immunosuppressed patients: a systematic review. J Infect Dis. 2006;193(10):1408–18.
18. Menegueti MG, et al. Assessment of microbiological air quality in hemato-oncology units and its relationship with the occurrence of invasive fungal infections: an integrative review. Rev Soc Bras Med Trop. 2013;46(4):391–6.
19. Friese C, et al. Neutropenia-related aspergillosis in non-transplant haematological patients hospitalised under ambient air versus purified air conditions. Mycoses. 2023;66(6):505–14.
20. Mattner F, et al. Preventing the spread of multidrug-resistant gram-negative pathogens: recommendations of an expert panel of the German Society for Hygiene and Microbiology. Dtsch Arztebl Int. 2012;109(3):39–45.
21. Gould D. Nurses' hand decontamination practice: results of a local study. J Hosp Infect. 1994;28(1):15–30.
22. Hayes-Lattin B, Leis JF, Maziarz RT. Isolation in the allogeneic transplant environment: how protective is it? Bone Marrow Transplant. 2005;36(5):373–81.
23. Khan SA, Wingard JR. Infection and mucosal injury in cancer treatment. J Natl Cancer Inst Monogr. 2001;29:31–6.
24. Passweg JR, Marsh JC. Aplastic anemia: first-line treatment by immunosuppression and sibling marrow transplantation. Hematology Am Soc Hematol Educ Program. 2010;2010:36–42.
25. Torres HA, et al. Infections in patients with aplastic anemia: experience at a tertiary care cancer center. Cancer. 2003;98(1):86–93.
26. Valdez JM, et al. Decreased infection-related mortality and improved survival in severe aplastic anemia in the past two decades. Clin Infect Dis. 2011;52(6):726–35.
27. Valdez JM, et al. Infections in patients with aplastic anemia. Semin Hematol. 2009;46(3):269–76.

28. Weinberger M, et al. Patterns of infection in patients with aplastic anemia and the emergence of Aspergillus as a major cause of death. Medicine (Baltimore). 1992;71(1):24–43.
29. Robenshtok E, et al. Antifungal prophylaxis in cancer patients after chemotherapy or hematopoietic stem-cell transplantation: systematic review and meta-analysis. J Clin Oncol. 2007;25(34):5471–89.
30. Scheinberg P, Young NS. How I treat acquired aplastic anemia. Blood. 2012;120(6):1185–96.
31. NCCN. Prevention and treatment of cancer-related infections. 2024.
32. NICE. Neutropenic sepsis: prevention and management in people with cancer. 2012.
33. Neftel KA, Hauser SP, Müller MR. Inhibition of granulopoiesis in vivo and in vitro by beta-lactam antibiotics. J Infect Dis. 1985;152(1):90–8.
34. Lionel SA, et al. Profile and predictors of infection following anti-thymocyte globulin or anti-lymphocyte globulin with cyclosporine in aplastic anemia. Indian J Hematol Blood Transfus. 2023;39(3):419–28.
35. Tomblyn M, et al. Guidelines for preventing infectious complications among hematopoietic cell transplant recipients: a global perspective. *Preface*. Bone Marrow Transplant. 2009;44(8):453–5.
36. Scheinberg P, et al. Distinct EBV and CMV reactivation patterns following antibody-based immunosuppressive regimens in patients with severe aplastic anemia. Blood. 2007;109(8):3219–24.
37. Scheinberg P, et al. Activity of alemtuzumab monotherapy in treatment-naive, relapsed, and refractory severe acquired aplastic anemia. Blood. 2012;119(2):345–54.
38. Marsh JC, et al. Haemopoietic growth factors in aplastic anaemia: a cautionary note. European Bone Marrow Transplant Working Party for Severe Aplastic Anaemia. Lancet. 1994;344(8916):172–3.
39. Gurion R, et al. Hematopoietic growth factors in aplastic anemia patients treated with immunosuppressive therapy-systematic review and meta-analysis. Haematologica. 2009;94(5):712–9.
40. Marsh JC, et al. Guidelines for the diagnosis and management of aplastic anaemia. Br J Haematol. 2009;147(1):43–70.
41. Tichelli A, et al. A randomized controlled study in patients with newly diagnosed severe aplastic anemia receiving antithymocyte globulin (ATG), cyclosporine, with or without G-CSF: a study of the SAA Working Party of the European Group for Blood and Marrow Transplantation. Blood. 2011;117(17):4434–41.
42. Gluckman E, et al. Results and follow-up of a phase III randomized study of recombinant human-granulocyte stimulating factor as support for immunosuppressive therapy in patients with severe aplastic anaemia. Br J Haematol. 2002;119(4):1075–82.
43. Teramura M, et al. Treatment of severe aplastic anemia with antithymocyte globulin and cyclosporin A with or without G-CSF in adults: a multicenter randomized study in Japan. Blood. 2007;110(6):1756–61.
44. Socie G, et al. Granulocyte-stimulating factor and severe aplastic anemia: a survey by the European Group for Blood and Marrow Transplantation (EBMT). Blood. 2007;109(7):2794–6.
45. Ohara A, et al. Myelodysplastic syndrome and acute myelogenous leukemia as a late clonal complication in children with acquired aplastic anemia. Blood. 1997;90(3):1009–13.
46. Lengline E, et al. Nationwide survey on the use of eltrombopag in patients with severe aplastic anemia: a report on behalf of the French Reference Center for Aplastic Anemia. Haematologica. 2018;103(2):212–20.
47. Olnes MJ, et al. Eltrombopag and improved hematopoiesis in refractory aplastic anemia. N Engl J Med. 2012;367(1):11–9.
48. Desmond R, et al. Eltrombopag restores trilineage hematopoiesis in refractory severe aplastic anemia that can be sustained on discontinuation of drug. Blood. 2014;123(12):1818–25.
49. Peffault de Latour R, et al. Eltrombopag added to immunosuppression in severe aplastic anemia. N Engl J Med. 2022;386(1):11–23.

50. Cross-sectional guidelines for therapy with blood components and plasma derivatives. 2014: executive committee of the German medica; association on the recommendation of the scientific advisory board.
51. Price TH, et al. Efficacy of transfusion with granulocytes from G-CSF/dexamethasone-treated donors in neutropenic patients with infection. Blood. 2015;126(18):2153–61.
52. Quillen K, et al. Granulocyte transfusions in severe aplastic anemia: an eleven-year experience. Haematologica. 2009;94(12):1661–8.
53. Ljungman P, Small TN, V.R.W. Group. Vaccination of SCT recipients. Bone Marrow Transplant. 2011;46(4):621.
54. Jeong SH, Lee HS. Hepatitis A: clinical manifestations and management. Intervirology. 2010;53(1):15–9.
55. Viallard JF, et al. Severe pancytopenia triggered by recombinant hepatitis B vaccine. Br J Haematol. 2000;110(1):230–3.
56. Hendry CL, et al. Relapse of severe aplastic anaemia after influenza immunization. Br J Haematol. 2002;119(1):283–4.
57. Bengtsson C, et al. Common vaccinations among adults do not increase the risk of developing rheumatoid arthritis: results from the Swedish EIRA study. Ann Rheum Dis. 2010;69(10):1831–3.
58. Salemi S, D'Amelio R. Are anti-infectious vaccinations safe and effective in patients with autoimmunity? Int Rev Immunol. 2010;29(3):270–314.
59. Piccin A, et al. Outcome of bone marrow transplantation in acquired and inherited aplastic anaemia in the Republic of Ireland. Ir J Med Sci. 2005;174(3):13–9.
60. Champlin RE, et al. Graft failure following bone marrow transplantation for severe aplastic anemia: risk factors and treatment results. Blood. 1989;73(2):606–13.
61. Hernández-Boluda JC, et al. Bone marrow transplantation for severe aplastic anemia: the Barcelona hospital clinic experience. Haematologica. 1999;84(1):26–31.
62. Group, T.t.R.A.t.P.S. Leukocyte reduction and ultraviolet B irradiation of platelets to prevent alloimmunization and refractoriness to platelet transfusions. N Engl J Med. 1997;337(26):1861–9.
63. Dzik WH. Leukoreduction of blood components. Curr Opin Hematol. 2002;9(6):521–6.
64. Desmarets M, et al. Minor histocompatibility antigens on transfused leukoreduced units of red blood cells induce bone marrow transplant rejection in a mouse model. Blood. 2009;114(11):2315–22.
65. Julen K, et al. Transfusions in aplastic anemia patients cause HLA Alloimmunization: comparisons of current and past cohorts demonstrate progress. Transplant Cell Ther. 2021;27(11):939.e1–8.
66. Kaminski ER, et al. Pretransfused patients with severe aplastic anaemia exhibit high numbers of cytotoxic T lymphocyte precursors probably directed at non-HLA antigens. Br J Haematol. 1990;76(3):401–5.
67. Padhi S, et al. Blood transfusion: summary of NICE guidance. BMJ. 2015;351:h5832.
68. Carson JL, et al. Clinical trials evaluating red blood cell transfusion thresholds: an updated systematic review and with additional focus on patients with cardiovascular disease. Am Heart J. 2018;200:96–101.
69. Carson JL, et al. Transfusion thresholds for guiding red blood cell transfusion. Cochrane Database Syst Rev. 2021;12(12):CD002042.
70. Vaht K, et al. Incidence and outcome of acquired aplastic anemia: real-world data from patients diagnosed in Sweden from 2000–2011. Haematologica. 2017;102(10):1683–90.
71. Kulasekararaj A, et al. Guidelines for the diagnosis and management of adult aplastic anaemia: a British Society for Haematology guideline. Br J Haematol. 2024;204(3):784–804.
72. Sagmeister M, Oec L, Gmür J. A restrictive platelet transfusion policy allowing long-term support of outpatients with severe aplastic anemia. Blood. 1999;93(9):3124–6.
73. Scheinberg P, et al. Horse versus rabbit antithymocyte globulin in acquired aplastic anemia. N Engl J Med. 2011;365(5):430–8.

74. Schrezenmeier H, Seifried E. Buffy-coat-derived pooled platelet concentrates and apheresis platelet concentrates: which product type should be preferred? Vox Sang. 2010;99(1):1–15.
75. Laundy GJ, et al. Incidence and specificity of HLA antibodies in multitransfused patients with acquired aplastic anemia. Transfusion. 2004;44(6):814–25.
76. Shehata N. BSH guidelines for the use of irradiated blood components: guidance that is needed. Br J Haematol. 2020;191(5):658–60.
77. Bean MA, et al. Gamma-irradiation of pretransplant blood transfusions from unrelated donors prevents sensitization to minor histocompatibility antigens on dog leukocyte antigen-identical canine marrow grafts. Transplantation. 1994;57(3):423–6.
78. Marsh J, et al. Should irradiated blood products be given routinely to all patients with aplastic anaemia undergoing immunosuppressive therapy with antithymocyte globulin (ATG)? A survey from the European Group for Blood and Marrow Transplantation Severe Aplastic Anaemia Working Party. Br J Haematol. 2010;150(3):377–9.
79. Fast LD, DiLeone G, Marschner S. Inactivation of human white blood cells in platelet products after pathogen reduction technology treatment in comparison to gamma irradiation. Transfusion. 2011;51(7):1397–404.
80. Vamvakas EC. Is white blood cell reduction equivalent to antibody screening in preventing transmission of cytomegalovirus by transfusion? A review of the literature and meta-analysis. Transfus Med Rev. 2005;19(3):181–9.
81. Bowden RA, et al. Use of leukocyte-depleted platelets and cytomegalovirus-seronegative red blood cells for prevention of primary cytomegalovirus infection after marrow transplant. Blood. 1991;78(1):246–50.
82. Bowden RA, et al. A comparison of filtered leukocyte-reduced and cytomegalovirus (CMV) seronegative blood products for the prevention of transfusion-associated CMV infection after marrow transplant. Blood. 1995;86(9):3598–603.
83. Nichols WG, et al. Transfusion-transmitted cytomegalovirus infection after receipt of leukoreduced blood products. Blood. 2003;101(10):4195–200.
84. Pamphilon DH, et al. Prevention of transfusion-transmitted cytomegalovirus infection. Transfus Med. 1999;9(2):115–23.
85. Lee JW. Iron chelation therapy in the myelodysplastic syndromes and aplastic anemia: a review of experience in South Korea. Int J Hematol. 2008;88(1):16–23.
86. Kim KH, et al. Cost analysis of iron-related complications in a single institute. Korean J Intern Med. 2009;24(1):33–6.
87. Kushner JP, Porter JP, Olivieri NF. Secondary iron overload. Hematology Am Soc Hematol Educ Program. 2001;2001:47–61.
88. Takatoku M, et al. Retrospective nationwide survey of Japanese patients with transfusion-dependent MDS and aplastic anemia highlights the negative impact of iron overload on morbidity/mortality. Eur J Haematol. 2007;78(6):487–94.
89. Pawelec K, et al. Influence of iron overload on immunosuppressive therapy in children with severe aplastic anemia. Adv Exp Med Biol. 2015;866:83–9.
90. Armand P, et al. Prognostic impact of elevated pretransplantation serum ferritin in patients undergoing myeloablative stem cell transplantation. Blood. 2007;109(10):4586–8.
91. Pullarkat V, et al. Iron overload adversely affects outcome of allogeneic hematopoietic cell transplantation. Bone Marrow Transplant. 2008;42(12):799–805.
92. Koreth J, Antin JH. Iron overload in hematologic malignancies and outcome of allogeneic hematopoietic stem cell transplantation. Haematologica. 2010;95(3):364–6.
93. Deeg HJ, Spaulding E, Shulman HM. Iron overload, hematopoietic cell transplantation, and graft-versus-host disease. Leuk Lymphoma. 2009;50(10):1566–72.
94. Gattermann N. Guidelines on iron chelation therapy in patients with myelodysplastic syndromes and transfusional iron overload. Leuk Res. 2007;31(Suppl 3):S10–5.
95. Gattermann N. Overview of guidelines on iron chelation therapy in patients with myelodysplastic syndromes and transfusional iron overload. Int J Hematol. 2008;88(1):24–9.

96. Pan T, et al. Impact of iron overload and iron chelation with Deferasirox on outcomes of patients with severe aplastic anemia after allogeneic hematopoietic stem cell transplantation. Transplant Cell Ther. 2023;29(8):507.e1–8.
97. Jomen W. Analysis of hematological improvement with iron chelation therapy using Deferasirox in subject Ts with therapy-refractory severe aplastic anemia, vol. 122. Blood; 2013.
98. Hoeks M, et al. Impact of treatment with iron chelation therapy in patients with lower-risk myelodysplastic syndromes participating in the European MDS registry. Haematologica. 2020;105(3):640–51.
99. Pilo F, Angelucci E. A storm in the niche: iron, oxidative stress and haemopoiesis. Blood Rev. 2018;32(1):29–35.
100. Neufeld EJ. Oral chelators deferasirox and deferiprone for transfusional iron overload in thalassemia major: new data, new questions. Blood. 2006;107(9):3436–41.
101. Park SJ, Han CW. Complete hematopoietic recovery after continuous iron chelation therapy in a patient with severe aplastic anemia with secondary hemochromatosis. J Korean Med Sci. 2008;23(2):320–3.
102. Mwanda OW, Otieno CF, Abdalla FK. Transfusion haemosiderosis inspite of regular use of desferrioxamine: case report. East Afr Med J. 2004;81(6):326–8.
103. Lee JW, et al. Iron chelation therapy with deferasirox in patients with aplastic anemia: a subgroup analysis of 116 patients from the EPIC trial. Blood. 2010;116(14):2448–54.
104. Vlachodimitropoulou E, et al. Eltrombopag: a powerful chelator of cellular or extracellular iron(III) alone or combined with a second chelator. Blood. 2017;130(17):1923–33.
105. Fattizzo B, et al. Eltrombopag in immune thrombocytopenia, aplastic anemia, and myelodysplastic syndrome: from Megakaryopoiesis to immunomodulation. Drugs. 2019;79(12):1305–19.
106. Zhao Z, et al. Eltrombopag mobilizes iron in patients with aplastic anemia. Blood. 2018;131(21):2399–402.

Open Access This chapter is licensed under the terms of the Creative Commons Attribution 4.0 International License (http://creativecommons.org/licenses/by/4.0/), which permits use, sharing, adaptation, distribution and reproduction in any medium or format, as long as you give appropriate credit to the original author(s) and the source, provide a link to the Creative Commons license and indicate if changes were made.

The images or other third party material in this chapter are included in the chapter's Creative Commons license, unless indicated otherwise in a credit line to the material. If material is not included in the chapter's Creative Commons license and your intended use is not permitted by statutory regulation or exceeds the permitted use, you will need to obtain permission directly from the copyright holder.

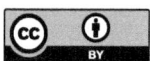

Part IV
Management of Aplastic Anemia in Children and Elderly

Chapter 8
Management of Acquired Aplastic Anemia in Children

Maurizio Miano, Gianluca Dell'Orso, and Carlo Dufour

Diagnosis and Clinical Characteristics

Acquired aplastic anemia (AA) is a rare disease with an estimated incidence of 2 cases in one million per year in Caucasian populations and a first peak in adolescents. Incidence is reported 2- to three-fold higher in Asia [1]. Formal data on epidemiology in childhood are not available, but the incidence is estimated to be lower than in adult age.

The association of bone marrow cellularity below 30% and the significant reduction in one or more peripheral blood cell lines define AA. Severe (SAA) or very severe aplastic anemia (VSAA) is defined according to the presence of at least two conditions among neutrophil counts <500/uL in SAA or < 200/uL in VSAA, platelets <20,000/uL, and reticulocytes <20,000/uL (or 60,000/uL if an automated counter is used) [2]. Thrombocytopenia and anemia with reticulocytopenia are the typical presenting symptoms [2] in the absence of detectable blast infiltration in the BM evaluation. Less frequently, neutropenia-related infections or single-lineage cytopenia can be present at diagnosis. A history of seronegative hepatitis can be documented and suggests a diagnosis of hepatitis-associated AA.

The main differential diagnoses of pediatric acquired AA are with hypocellular leukemia and with myelodysplasia (MDS) with low blast count, or with refractory cytopenia of childhood, and are based on bone marrow trephine biopsy findings (no blasts, no increase of CD34+ cells, no dysplastic features mainly in the magakaryocyte lineage) and with inherited bone marrow failure syndromes (IBMFS). Recent evidence also recommends differential diagnosis with inborn errors of immunity (IEI), often characterized by an immune-mediated pathogenesis. A pediatric-adapted diagnostic work-up for the diagnosis of AA is provided in Table 8.1.

M. Miano (✉) · G. Dell'Orso · C. Dufour
Hematology Unit, IRCCS Istituto Giannina Gaslini, Genoa, Italy
e-mail: mauriziomiano@gaslini.org; carlodufour@gaslini.org

Table 8.1 Diagnostic work-up of aplastic anemia in children

Recommended diagnostic tools
Full blood count with differential count and reticulocyte count
Peripheral blood smear
Liver function tests
Hepatitis virus tests (antibodies and DNA/RNA)
EBV, CMV, parvovirus, HHV6, HSV, HIV, adenovirus, and varicella-zoster virus tests
Bone marrow aspirate for morphology (dysplastic changes), cytogenetics (monosomy 7, trisomy 8, deletion of 5q, etc.), immunophenotype, pearl's staining (for intra-cytoplasmic iron)
Bone marrow trephine biopsy with immunostaining for CD34 and CD117 antigens and iron staining (gold standard test for AA diagnosis)
Flow cytometry for PNH clones
BM and PB flow cytometry analysis of B and T lymphocytes and related subsets, NK cells and monocytes. Monoclonal populations and/or blast search, evolution of abnormal maturation/differentiation patterns as a sign of dysplasia.
Immunoglobulin levels, antibody titers to vaccines, autoantibody screening (anti-nucleus and anti-DNA for SLE detection)
Vitamin B12 and folate serum levels
Fibrinogen and serum ferritin (detection of HLH)
Stool pancreatic elastase, serum pancreatic amylase, and lipase (for identification of Shwachman syndrome)
Serum bilirubin and LDH, HbF assay
Chest X-ray
Abdomen US scan and echocardiography (for liver, spleen, lymph node enlargement, and malformations)
Patient and family HLA typing
Differential diagnosis of IBMFS
Chromosomal fragility tests (MMC or DEB, gold standard for the diagnosis of Fanconi anemia). To be performed on fibroblasts if needed to identify somatic mosaicism
Flow FISH analysis for TL measurement
Sequencing of major genes or NGS panels, including genes associated with bone marrow failure syndrome as TBD, FA, DBA, SBDS, CAMT, SCN, GATA2 deficiency, SAMD9/SAMD9L, ETV6, MECOM, other congenital marrow failure syndrome, and inborn errors of immunity (IEI)
WES/WGS, if NGS/ turns out negative
Ancillary tests for the diagnosis of AA
Bone marrow culture and stain for mycobacteria infection (atypical mycobacteria more frequently than TB mycobacteria)
Marrow progenitor assay (not available in all centers)
MRI of the vertebral column
NGS panel to detect somatic mutations
Diagnostic work-up might be performed in a stepwise mode according to the severity of the clinical picture

History should explore exposure to medications, radiation, chemical agents, or drugs. Moreover, the history of infections due to hepatitis viruses, EBV, CMV, parvovirus B19, herpetic viruses, HIV, adenovirus, varicella-zoster, and mycobacteria should be taken into consideration since they may also cause marrow hypoplasia and pancytopenia.

An underlying congenital defect can be suspected in the presence of a positive family history for cytopenia, infections, hematologic or solid malignancies, particularly in atypical ages, or consanguinity, short stature, facial dysmorphisms, cleft palate, cardiac or renal/genitourinary tract malformations, skeleton, nail, teeth, skin, or eye abnormalities, and liver, lung, or CNS involvement [3]. Nonetheless, even in the absence of such elements because of the phenotypic variability of these disorders, it is mandatory to perform specific diagnostic tests to exclude a cryptic IBMFS.

Fanconi Anemia (FA) can be ruled out by a chromosomal fragility test (DEB or MMC test). Telomere length (TL) analysis in leukocytes below the first centile for age is strongly suggestive of Telomere Biology Disorder (TBD), which must be confirmed by genetic analysis. TL between the first and tenth centiles is suggestive of atypical forms of telomeropathies but can also be observed in diseases associated with increased cell turnover, such as AA and immune dysfunctions, or other IBMFSs like FA, Diamond-Blackfan Anemia (DBA), and Schwachman-Diamond syndrome (SDS). Genetic testing is needed in these circumstances to confirm the correct diagnosis. Additionally, telomere length is considered a powerful predictor of response to immunosuppressive therapy (IST) [4] and of evolution into MDS/AML [5]. As for the potential association of AA with IEIs, peripheral blood lymphocyte subset counts, including TCRαβ+ CD3 + CD4-CD8- T-cells (double-negative T cells, DNTs) and Tregs, and a wide immunological screening are also important diagnostic tools.

Over the years, the advent of Next Generation Sequencing (NGS) panels and of Whole Exome Sequencing (WES) increased the chance to detect cryptic IBMFS and to tailor appropriate conditioning regimens for Hematopoietic Stem cell Transplantation (HSCT). Nowadays, the use of NGS panels including genes involved in TBD, FA, DBA, SBDS, and Congenital Amegakaryocytic Thrombocytopenia (CAMT), and Severe Congenital Neutropenia (SCN) should be considered mandatory. Panels should also include some IEI genes known to be related to marrow failure, such as Deficiencies of Adenosine Deaminase type 2 (DADA 2) or GATA2, SAMD9/SAMD9L, and ETV6. Whole Exome Sequencing (WES) and Whole Genome Sequencing (WGS) are additional useful diagnostic tools in case of negative NGS panels.

Although at risk for false negative results in the presence of leukopenia, PNH clone analysis is also recommended, as it may result in positive up to 41% of newly diagnosed children with AA [6] even without hemolysis [11]. In non-transplanted patients, the PNH clone search can be repeated once the neutrophil count has risen.

Clonal hematopoiesis, defined by a large fraction of hematopoietic cells arising from a single stem cell or a multipotent hematopoietic progenitor, characterized by a specific genetic signature, is common in AA [7] and needs to be differentiated from "malignant clonal evolution" as an expression of progression to secondary malignancy. Transient or persistent chromosomal abnormalities may develop during the disease course. Monosomy of chromosome 7 or complex karyotypes are associated with persistence of low blood counts or further worsening of cytopenia, progression to MDS, and poor prognosis [8]. On the contrary, trisomy of chromosome 8 is associated with a good hematologic response to IST, whereas when occurring in primary MDS, this anomaly is typically associated with a poor prognosis, thus suggesting a different pathway between trisomy 8 of late AA and of primary MDS [9]. Among somatic mutations occurring over the course of the disease, BCOR/BCORL1 and PIG-A are associated with stability or spontaneous regression, whereas DNMT3A and ASXL1, although less frequent, are associated with poorer response to IST, inferior overall survival, and more frequent progression to MDS/AML [10]. Apart from mutations in these two and in the RUNX1 gene, the impact of somatic mutations on therapeutic decisions in idiopathic AA is currently rather limited [11], given also that a minority of patients can also progress without detection of any somatic mutation, suggesting the presence of small subclones below the limit of detection or in other untested/unknown genes [10, 12]. Overall, the incidence of malignant clonal evolution in the cohort of patients treated with IST is estimated at 5 years at 2–4%, rising up to 15–26% at 10 years [7, 10], and tends to increase in case of prolonged disease or in association with shorter TL or the loss of selected HLA class I alleles, such as HLA-B*14:02 and HLA-B*40:02, through mitotic recombination and 6p loss-of-heterozygosity, or through loss-of-function mutations [7]. "Malignant" clonal evolution is typically announced by worsening of blood counts in responders to immunosuppression or by the appearance of new marrow dysplastic changes and/or non-transient cytogenetic abnormalities. Therefore, a close monitoring of clonal hematopoiesis must be combined with clinical and morphological evaluation.

Patient and family HLA typing must be performed at diagnosis in order to have a matched family or an unrelated donor [13–16] available at any time.

Overall, the chances of a successful treatment depend on an early referral to centers with expertise in AA and marrow failure disorders to guarantee an accurate diagnostic work-up, a full treatment and follow-up program.

Supportive Treatment

Anemia should not be treated to maintain hemoglobin above the lower limit for age: transfusion of packed AB0 and Kell compatible red blood cells [17] is indicated only to manage symptoms related to anemia. Iron overload secondary to frequent transfusions should be avoided and regular monitoring through liver iron concentration (LIC) assessed by MRI (T2* or R2*) or through ferritin serum levels [18] is required. Iron chelation based on oral deferasirox [19] has to be started when ferritin levels are higher than 1000 ng/mL, with the additional aim to improve the probability of success of the transplant [20, 21].

Thrombocytopenia should be treated with platelet transfusion only when the count drops below 10 × 10^9/L or if bleeding occurs. The threshold is higher (20 × 10^9/L) during fever or ATG administration) [3].

All blood products should be leukodepleted and irradiated to reduce the risk of sensitization to HLA and non-HLA antigens, to avoid posttransfusion Graft-versus-Host Disease (GvHD) in the recipient, and to prevent CMV transmission in immunosuppressed patients (e.g., lymphocytes <1000/mmc or treated with immunosuppressant agents) [22–24].

Additionally, blood products from related donors are contraindicated because they may sensitize the recipient to minor HLA or leukocyte antigens of the potential HSCT donor.

Prophylaxis for Pneumocystis pneumonia should be started in lymphopenic patients. Although no data from clinical studies are available, antifungal and antibiotic prophylaxis may be considered when the neutrophil count is persistently <200/mmc [3].

G-CSF can be useful to increase neutrophil count and to reduce both infections and days of hospitalization in IST-treated patients [25]. G-CSF may also help to predict IST responders, i.e., those patients who, under G-CSF, experience a neutrophil count ≥0.5 × 10^9/L on day +30 of IST [26]. Neither increased risk of clonal evolution nor of second solid cancer or nonmalignant late event was associated with G-CSF use [25].

General Concepts for Specific Treatment

A limited observation period is recommended prior to establishing the diagnosis and the severity of the disease, during which supportive therapy, aimed at minimizing risks of bleeding and infection, should be provided. Steroids should not be used in this timeframe.

Specific treatment is based on restoration of hematopoiesis either by HSCT or IST. The treatment algorithm is shown in Fig. 8.1.

Non-severe forms (NSAA) can have different clinical courses: among non-transfusion-dependent cases, about 1/3 can experience spontaneous remission, while the remaining 2/3 may either remain stable for months to years or progress to SAA [3]. Due to the unpredictable course, it is debated if and when to start a specific treatment. Overall, a careful evaluation of the cost/benefit ratio is mandatory, weighing treatment-related toxicities and severe clinical comorbidities that can affect treatment efficacy. NSAA patients requiring transfusions tend more frequently to evolve to severe or very severe forms. Since diagnostic delay can worsen prognosis [3], usually the indication is to treat them as if they were subjects with severe aplastic anemia (SAA) (IST and HSCT) [3, 17, 27].

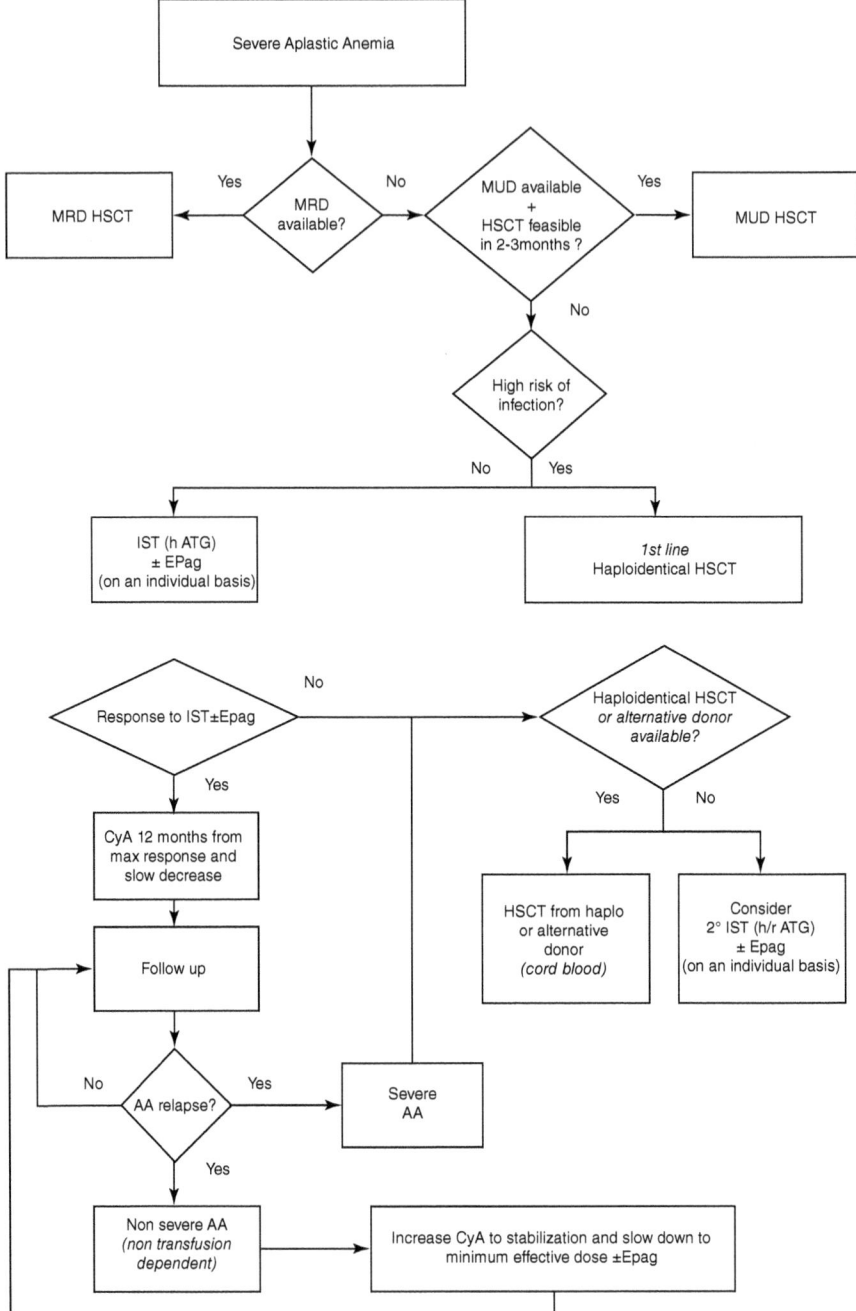

Fig. 8.1 Treatment algorithm for children affected by severe aplastic anemia. (From Guarina et al. [3])

Options for First-Line Treatment

Figure 8.1 shows a treatment algorithm for children with aplastic anemia suggested by the Marrow Failure Group of the Pediatric Haemato-Oncology Italian Association (AIEOP).

Given the improved outcomes of both matched related (MRD) and matched unrelated donor (MUD), particularly in young patients without comorbidities [3, 17], currently HSCT has overtaken IST as the main treatment strategy available for pediatric AA patients.

HSCT from MSD

In the presence of an available MRD, HSCT has a probability of success in above 90% of patients [13, 14]. Although based on retrospective studies, the significantly superior event-free survival (EFS) of MRD-HSCT [13, 14], the better hematopoietic reconstitution [28], and the lower risk of secondary malignancies [13, 14] over IST support the role of this transplantation strategy as first-line treatment. Of note, when ATG is used in the conditioning regimen, the grade II-IV acute and chronic GvHD incidence of upfront MRD-HSCT was below 15%, far lower than the 30–40% [13, 14] observed in adults. Bone marrow is the preferred stem cell source [29] because of the reduced risk of GvHD.

The conditioning regimen recommended by the European Blood and Marrow Transplantation (EBMT) Society is based on cyclophosphamide (Cy) (200 mg/kg) given in 4 days and ATG over 3 days [27, 30] or on fludarabine (30 mg/kg/day for 4 days) plus lower doses of Cy (300 mg/m^2/day for 4 days) combined with ATG or alemtuzumab [31]. Graft-versus-Host Disease (GvHD) prophylaxis with methotrexate and CsA was superior to CsA alone [27, 32]. In patients receiving alemtuzumab, MTX can be omitted [33]. Tacrolimus can replace CsA in case of intolerance, toxicity, or allergy [34].

HSCT from MUD

Thanks to the improvement of supportive therapies, conditioning regimens, HLA typing, and donor selection, the outcome of MUD HSCT in children and adolescents has improved remarkably over the last decade. Indeed, overall survival (OS) is similar to that obtained with MRD-HSCT, and, in retrospective studies, EFS, a qualitative indicator of survival, turned out to be superior [20, 21, 39] to IST. Based on these findings, in recent years, the indication for HSCT from MUD has gained importance in the treatment algorithm and is now recommended as a first-line option if an MSD is not available and if the transplant can be performed within 2 or, at the latest, 3 months since diagnosis. Indeed, in the absence of an MSD, MUD HSCT upfront proved, in retrospective studies, to be superior to the same treatment performed as a rescue option after failure of IST [15]. In addition, it has to be highlighted that MUD HSCT infers a lower risk of secondary malignancies compared to IST-refractory AA patients who require repeated treatment courses [13, 14, 16]. All these findings underline the importance of a very early HLA typing of patients and quick registry donor research if no HLA-matched donor is available in the family in order to perform an MUD HSCT within 3 months, preferably from a BM source [3, 35].

The most widely used conditioning regimen is fludarabine 120 mg/m2 (30 mg/m2/day × 4) in combination with cyclophosphamide 120 mg/kg (30 mg/kg/day × 4) plus ATG (FCA regimen). CsA and short-term MTX are indicated for GvHD prophylaxis [3, 30, 36]. A valid alternative regimen is the combination of fludarabine, cyclophosphamide, and alemtuzumab 0.2 mg/kg/day given for 4 or 5 days (FCC regimen) and CsA alone for GvHD prophylaxis, which is associated with low rates of acute and chronic grade GvHD [3, 15, 33, 36]. Low-dose (200 cGy) TBI should be added in patients older than 14 years of age, multi-transfused (>20 transfusions), or in case of partial HLA mismatch (1 or 2 Ag) to reduce the risk of rejection [3, 36, 37].

A recent study showed that a longer telomere length of the donor (and not in the recipient) is associated with better post-HSCT survival, thus highlighting the telomere length measurement as a potential new criterion for donor selection that may further improve the outcome of these transplants [38].

Options for Second-Line Treatments

Patients considered for second-line treatments are those who can not access a frontline MRD or MUD HSCT or who failed a first-line HSCT.

Of note, only a small proportion (4%) of patients who rejected first-line HSCT experience a spontaneous autologous recovery [39]. As a consequence, a second HSCT, although being a high-risk procedure due to infections and organ toxicity, has been proven to be a good rescue option in about 60% of cases [40]. OS and failure-free survival (FFS) were independent of age, donor type, conditioning regimen, and GvHD prophylaxis, thus suggesting the possibility of selecting either the same or a different donor. The use of non-myeloablative conditioning and a low dose of TBI (2–4 Gy) is recommended to reduce the toxicity related to a second transplant procedure and the risk of GF [41].

Haploidentical HSCT

HSCT from an HLA-haploidentical family donor has been previously considered only in the absence of an MRD/MUD, in nonresponders to IST, or after rejection of an MSD/MUD HSCT [42, 43]. Haploidentical HSCT nowadays is increasingly used in clinical practice both in children and adults [44] in the setting of nonmalignant diseases with satisfactory results [45]. However, the evidence in support of this strategy as a first-line treatment for severe AA, although quite encouraging, is still rather limited.

A single-center retrospective analysis of 89 patients who underwent HSCT from a haploidentical family donor or from a MUD after failure of first-line IST demonstrated a 3-year OS of 80.3% and GvHD/failure-free survival of 79% [46].

An EBMT retrospective analysis found a 92% OS in a pediatric subcohort of SAA patients who received haploidentical HSCT based on posttransplantation cyclophosphamide (PTCy, given 50 mg/kg on days +3 and + 4). In the whole cohort, the use of the Baltimore conditioning regimen (fludarabine total dose 150 mg/m2 over days from −6 to −2, cyclophosphamide 14.5 mg/kg/day from day −6 to −5, and TBI 200 cGy on day −1) was associated with a superior OS of 93% compared with 64% of the non-Baltimore regimens [47].

In a prospective phase 2 trial, the PTCy approach with the same reduced-intensity conditioning but increased TBI dose (400 vs 200 cGy) provided an OS around 90% at 3 years and lower rates of both acute and chronic GvHD [48].

The ongoing prospective trial (NCT02833805) comparing Haplo vs MUD HSCT in newly diagnosed patients may strengthen the evidence for the use of this transplant strategy as a first-line option.

Immunosuppressive Therapy

Excellent outcomes of HSCT in pediatric patients with AA in terms of OS and improved EFS favored this strategy over IST [13, 14]. Therefore, nowadays IST is mainly recommended as a first-line strategy only in patients who cannot undergo HSCT within 2 or 3 months of diagnosis or who are not fit for HSCT due to comorbidities and do not have a high risk of infections.

The association of horse ATG (hATG) and CsA is considered the standard first-line regimen [49]. Horse ATG at the dose of 40 mg/kg/day for 4 days proved to be superior to rabbit ATG (rATG) in a prospective National Institutes of Health (NIH) trial with a hematologic response of 68% and OS of 96% that favorably compared with 37% and 76%, respectively, obtained with rATG [50]. In a meta-analysis comparing the efficacy and safety of horse and rabbit ATG in 13 studies, hATG was associated with a better overall response rate (ORR) at six months, whereas early mortality at 3 months was higher in the rATG group, with deaths mainly due to infection and bleeding [51].

Response should be assessed on day +120 from the start of treatment [52] and it is recommended that oral CsA be started on day +1 at the dose of 5 mg/kg/day in order to reach serum levels around 200 ng/mL and be continued at the same dose for at least 12 months after the maximum response, with subsequent tapering (5–10% of the dose each month) until discontinuation, not earlier than 24 months after maximum response [3]. This is based on a retrospective study in children that showed that a slow tapering of CsA (0.3–0.7 mg/kg/month) was associated with a lower relapse incidence when compared to a rapid drop (>0.8 mg/kg) with no evidence of additional significant side effects [53].

Steroids (prednisone 2 mg/kg/day) should also be associated for at least 14 days, only with the aim to prevent serum sickness.

Most responses to IST are seen during the first 3–4 months after ATG, with few patients experiencing a slower response within 6 months or even afterward [54].

Failure of AA patients to respond to IST may also be explained by the presence of a still undiagnosed IBMFS.

Eltrombopag

Eltrombopag is an agonist of the thrombopoietin (TPO) receptor class, proposed in the treatment of AA because of its stimulatory effect on megakaryocytes and hematopoietic stem cell proliferation, and reported as an effective combination with standard IST in adults affected by AA [55]. However, eltrombopag associated with standard IST in patients below 18 years of age failed to demonstrate a significant advantage in overall response rate (ORR) in comparison with a historical cohort treated with standard IST [55].

A prospective randomized trial comparing classical IST with classical IST + eltrombopag showed an advantage for the eltrombopag arm only in complete response (CR) and ORR for SAA patients, but 3-year OS, EFS, ORR at 4 months, PR, and time to CR were not significantly different in the two arms [56].

Overall, the addition of eltrombopag to hATG and CsA in front-line treatment in children, despite the absence of significant adverse effects, does not generate the same advantages observed in the adult population. Reasons for different responses to eltrombopag associated with classical IST in adults and children are still largely misunderstood.

Options for Further-Line Treatments

In children not eligible for an early HSCT and with no satisfactory response to IST, limited third-line options are available. Not many comparative studies exist to clearly establish the superiority of one strategy over another. Therefore, the choice of the best treatment for these patients should rely on major driving factors like patients' age and comorbidities and drug availability [57].

A second course of horse or rabbit ATG ± eltrombopag can be performed in patients refractory/relapsed after IST and with no transplant strategy available. Chances of response at a second IST course with rATG/CsA are lower than 60% and down to 30% in those refractory (never responding) to first-line treatment [58].

Umbilical cord transplantation (UCT) was previously considered as an option for patients who lacked an MSD and an MUD. Nowadays, the results of haploidentical HSCT have moved its role to a third-line opportunity because the risk of graft failure in advanced and sensitized AA patients is higher when using a potentially rather poor cell source [59]. To overcome cell dose limitations, double -unit CBTs have also been used in AA, but although 2-year OS was good (80%), the incidence of acute GvHD was very high (71%) [60].

Among other potential immunosuppressive therapies, mycophenolate mofetil (MMF) was not demonstrated to be effective in a phase II trial conducted at the NIH [61]. According to one report [62], rapamycin/sirolimus may be helpful in cases of nephrotoxicity when CsA cannot be used.

Alemtuzumab was associated with a partial response rate of 56% in patients relapsing after IST, which is superior to what was seen in patients refractory (never responding) to the first course of IST (37%) [63]. However, alemtuzumab in monotherapy appears to have very limited space in AA in children.

Romiplostim was proposed as an alternative option to eltrombopag due to its binding on a more external TPO receptor domain. It was associated with hematologic response in pediatric age only in case series on a very small number of patients [64, 65].

References

1. Montane E, Ibanez L, Vidal X, Ballarin E, Puig R, Garcia N, et al. Epidemiology of aplastic anemia: a prospective multicenter study. Haematologica. 2008;93(4):518–23.
2. Rovó A, Tichelli A, Dufour C, on behalf of the SAA-WP EBMT. Diagnosis of acquired aplastic anemia. Bone Marrow Transplant. 2013;48(2):162–7.
3. Guarina A, Farruggia P, Mariani E, Saracco P, Barone A, Onofrillo D, et al. Diagnosis and management of acquired aplastic anemia in childhood. Guidelines from the Marrow Failure Study Group of the Pediatric Haemato-Oncology Italian Association (AIEOP). Blood Cells Mol Dis. 2024;108:102860.
4. Narita A, Muramatsu H, Sekiya Y, Okuno Y, Sakaguchi H, Nishio N, et al. Paroxysmal nocturnal hemoglobinuria and telomere length predicts response to immunosuppressive therapy in pediatric aplastic anemia. Haematologica. 2015;100(12):1546–52.
5. Calado RT, Cooper JN, Padilla-Nash HM, Sloand EM, Wu CO, Scheinberg P, et al. Short telomeres result in chromosomal instability in hematopoietic cells and precede malignant evolution in human aplastic anemia. Leukemia. 2012;26(4):700–7.
6. Timeus F, Crescenzio N, Longoni D, Doria A, Foglia L, Pagliano S, et al. Paroxysmal nocturnal hemoglobinuria clones in children with acquired aplastic anemia: a multicentre study. Ellis SR, editor. PLoS One. 2014;9(7):e101948.
7. Babushok DV. A brief, but comprehensive, guide to clonal evolution in aplastic anemia. Hematology Am Soc Hematol Educ Program. 2018;2018(1):457–66.
8. Hartung HD, Olson TS, Bessler M. Acquired aplastic anemia in children. Pediatr Clin N Am. 2013;60(6):1311–36.
9. Maciejewski JP, Risitano A, Sloand EM, Nunez O, Young NS. Distinct clinical outcomes for cytogenetic abnormalities evolving from aplastic anemia. Blood. 2002;99(9):3129–35.
10. Yoshizato T, Dumitriu B, Hosokawa K, Makishima H, Yoshida K, Townsley D, et al. Somatic mutations and clonal hematopoiesis in aplastic anemia. N Engl J Med. 2015;373(1):35–47.

11. Peffault De Latour R, Kulasekararaj A, Iacobelli S, Terwel SR, Cook R, Griffin M, et al. Eltrombopag added to immunosuppression in severe aplastic anemia. N Engl J Med. 2022;386(1):11–23.
12. Kulasekararaj AG, Jiang J, Smith AE, Mohamedali AM, Mian S, Gandhi S, et al. Somatic mutations identify a subgroup of aplastic anemia patients who progress to myelodysplastic syndrome. Blood. 2014;124(17):2698–704.
13. Dufour C, Pillon M, Passweg J, Socié G, Bacigalupo A, Franceschetto G, et al. Outcome of aplastic anemia in adolescence: a survey of the Severe Aplastic Anemia Working Party of the European Group for Blood and Marrow Transplantation. Haematologica. 2014;99(10):1574.
14. Dufour C, Pillon M, Sociè G, Rovò A, Carraro E, Bacigalupo A, et al. Outcome of aplastic anaemia in children. A study by the severe aplastic anaemia and paediatric disease working parties of the European group blood and bone marrow transplant. Br J Haematol. 2015;169(4):565–73.
15. Dufour C, Veys P, Carraro E, Bhatnagar N, Pillon M, Wynn R, et al. Similar outcome of upfront-unrelated and matched sibling stem cell transplantation in idiopathic paediatric aplastic anaemia. A study on behalf of the UK Paediatric BMT Working Party, Paediatric Diseases Working Party and Severe Aplastic Anaemia Working Party of EBMT. Br J Haematol. 2015;171(4):585–94.
16. Petit AF, Kulasekararaj AG, Eikema D, Maschan A, Adjaoud D, Kulagin A, et al. Upfront unrelated donor hematopoietic stem cell transplantation in patients with idiopathic aplastic anemia: a retrospective study of the Severe Aplastic Anemia Working Party of European Bone Marrow Transplantation. Am J Hematol [Internet] 2022 Jan [cited 2024 May 15];97(1). Available from: https://onlinelibrary.wiley.com/doi/10.1002/ajh.26354
17. Killick SB, Bown N, Cavenagh J, Dokal I, Foukaneli T, Hill A, et al. Guidelines for the diagnosis and management of adult aplastic anaemia. Br J Haematol. 2016;172(2):187–207.
18. Coates TD. Iron overload in transfusion-dependent patients. Hematology. 2019;2019(1):337–44.
19. Ko BS, Chang MC, Chiou TJ, Chang TK, Chen YC, Lin SF, et al. Long-term safety and efficacy of deferasirox in patients with myelodysplastic syndrome, aplastic anemia and other rare anemia in Taiwan. Hematology. 2019;24(1):247–54.
20. Marsh JCW, Ball SE, Cavenagh J, Darbyshire P, Dokal I, Gordon-Smith EC, et al. Guidelines for the diagnosis and management of aplastic anaemia. Br J Haematol. 2009;147(1):43–70.
21. Koreth J, Antin JH. Iron overload in hematologic malignancies and outcome of allogeneic hematopoietic stem cell transplantation. Haematologica. 2010;95(3):364–6.
22. Vamvakas EC. Is white blood cell reduction equivalent to antibody screening in preventing transmission of cytomegalovirus by transfusion? A review of the literature and meta-analysis. Transfus Med Rev. 2005;19(3):181–99.
23. Killick SB, Win N, Marsh JCW, Kaye T, Yandle A, Humphries C, et al. Pilot study of HLA alloimmunization after transfusion with pre-storage leucodepleted blood products in aplastic anaemia. Br J Haematol. 1997;97(3):677–84.
24. Treleaven J, Gennery A, Marsh J, Norfolk D, Page L, Parker A, et al. Guidelines on the use of irradiated blood components prepared by the British Committee for Standards in Haematology blood transfusion task force. Br J Haematol. 2011;152(1):35–51.
25. Tichelli A, De Latour RP, Passweg J, Knol-Bout C, Socié G, Marsh J, et al. Long-term outcome of a randomized controlled study in patients with newly diagnosed severe aplastic anemia treated with antithymocyte globulin and cyclosporine, with or without granulocyte colony-stimulating factor: a Severe Aplastic Anemia Working Party Trial from the European Group of Blood and Marrow Transplantation. Haematologica. 2020;105(5):1223–31.
26. Socie G, Mary JY, Schrezenmeier H, Marsh J, Bacigalupo A, Locasciulli A, et al. Granulocyte-stimulating factor and severe aplastic anemia: a survey by the European Group for Blood and Marrow Transplantation (EBMT). Blood. 2007;109(7):2794–6.
27. Korthof ET, Békássy AN, Hussein AA, on behalf of the SAA-WP of the EBMT. Management of acquired aplastic anemia in children. Bone Marrow Transplant. 2013;48(2):191–5.

28. Podesta M, Piaggio G, Frassoni F, Pitto A, Zikos P, Sessarego M, et al. The assessment of the hematopoietic reservoir after immunosuppressive therapy or bone marrow transplantation in severe aplastic anemia. Blood. 1998;91(6):1959–65.
29. Bacigalupo A, Socie G, Schrezenmeier H, Tichelli A, Locasciulli A, Fuehrer M, et al. Bone marrow versus peripheral blood as the stem cell source for sibling transplants in acquired aplastic anemia: survival advantage for bone marrow in all age groups. Haematologica. 2012;97(8):1142–8.
30. Bejanyan N, Kim S, Hebert KM, Kekre N, Abdel-Azim H, Ahmed I, et al. Choice of conditioning regimens for bone marrow transplantation in severe aplastic anemia. Blood Adv. 2019;3(20):3123–31.
31. Samarasinghe S, Clesham K, Iacobelli S, Sbianchi G, Knol C, Hamladji R, et al. Impact of T-cell depletion strategies on outcomes following hematopoietic stem cell transplantation for idiopathic aplastic anemia: a study on behalf of the European blood and marrow transplant severe aplastic anemia working party. Am J Hematol. 2019;94(1):80–6.
32. Locatelli F, Bruno B, Zecca M, Van-Lint MT, McCann S, Arcese W, et al. Cyclosporin A and short-term methotrexate versus cyclosporin A as graft versus host disease prophylaxis in patients with severe aplastic anemia given allogeneic bone marrow transplantation from an HLA-identical sibling: results of a GITMO/EBMT randomized trial. Blood. 2000;96(5):1690–7.
33. Marsh JC, Pearce RM, Koh MBC, Lim Z, Pagliuca A, Mufti GJ, et al. Retrospective study of alemtuzumab vs ATG-based conditioning without irradiation for unrelated and matched sibling donor transplants in acquired severe aplastic anemia: a study from the British Society for Blood and Marrow Transplantation. Bone Marrow Transplant. 2014;49(1):42–8.
34. Inamoto Y, Flowers MED, Wang T, Urbano-Ispizua A, Hemmer MT, Cutler CS, et al. Tacrolimus versus cyclosporine after hematopoietic cell transplantation for acquired aplastic anemia. Biol Blood Marrow Transplant. 2015;21(10):1776–82.
35. Samarasinghe S, Veys P, Vora A, Wynn R. Paediatric amendment to adult BSH guidelines for aplastic anaemia. Br J Haematol. 2018;180(2):201–5.
36. Iftikhar R, Chaudhry QUN, Anwer F, Neupane K, Rafae A, Mahmood SK, et al. Allogeneic hematopoietic stem cell transplantation in aplastic anemia: current indications and transplant strategies. Blood Rev. 2021;47:100772.
37. Bacigalupo A, Socie' G, Lanino E, Prete A, Locatelli F, Locasciulli A, et al. Fludarabine, cyclophosphamide, antithymocyte globulin, with or without low dose total body irradiation, for alternative donor transplants, in acquired severe aplastic anemia: a retrospective study from the EBMT-SAA working party. Haematologica. 2010;95(6):976–82.
38. Gadalla SM, Wang T, Haagenson M, Spellman SR, Lee SJ, Williams KM, et al. Association between donor leukocyte telomere length and survival after unrelated allogeneic hematopoietic cell transplantation for severe aplastic anemia. JAMA. 2015;313(6):594.
39. Piccin A, McCann S, Socié G, Oneto R, Bacigalupo A, Locasciulli A, et al. Survival of patients with documented autologous recovery after SCT for severe aplastic anemia: a study by the WPSAA of the EBMT. Bone Marrow Transplant. 2010;45(6):1008–13.
40. Cesaro S, De Latour RP, Tridello G, Pillon M, Carlson K, Fagioli F, et al. Second allogeneic stem cell transplant for aplastic anaemia: a retrospective study by the severe aplastic anaemia working party of the European society for blood and marrow transplantation. Br J Haematol. 2015;171(4):606–14.
41. Kudo K, Muramatsu H, Yoshida N, Kobayashi R, Yabe H, Tabuchi K, et al. Second allogeneic hematopoietic stem cell transplantation in children with severe aplastic anemia. Bone Marrow Transplant. 2015;50(10):1312–5.
42. Bacigalupo A. How I treat acquired aplastic anemia. Blood. 2017;129(11):1428–36.
43. Bacigalupo A, Sica S. Alternative donor transplants for severe aplastic anemia: current experience. Semin Hematol. 2016;53(2):115–9.

44. Passweg JR, Baldomero H, Chabannon C, Basak GW, De La Cámara R, Corbacioglu S, et al. Hematopoietic cell transplantation and cellular therapy survey of the EBMT: monitoring of activities and trends over 30 years. Bone Marrow Transplant. 2021;56(7):1651–64.
45. Xu ZL, Xu LP, Wu DP, Wang SQ, Zhang X, Xi R, et al. Comparable long-term outcomes between upfront haploidentical and identical sibling donor transplant in aplastic anemia: a national registry-based study. Haematologica. 2022;107(12):2918–27.
46. Lu Y, Sun RJ, Zhao YL, Xiong M, Cao XY, Zhang JP, et al. Unmanipulated haploidentical hematopoietic stem cell transplantation achieved outcomes comparable with matched unrelated donor transplantation in Young acquired severe aplastic anemia. Biol Blood Marrow Transplant. 2018;24:1881.
47. Prata PH, Eikema DJ, Afansyev B, Bosman P, Smiers F, Diez-Martin JL, et al. Haploidentical transplantation and posttransplant cyclophosphamide for treating aplastic anemia patients: a report from the EBMT Severe Aplastic Anemia Working Party. Bone Marrow Transplant. 2020;55(6):1050–8.
48. DeZern A, Zahurak ML, Symons HJ, Cooke KR, Huff CA, Jain T, et al. Alternative donor BMT with post-transplant cyclophosphamide as initial therapy for acquired severe aplastic anemia. Blood J. 2023:blood.2023020435.
49. Locasciulli A, Oneto R, Bacigalupo A, Socie G, Korthof E, Bekassy A, et al. Outcome of patients with acquired aplastic anemia given first line bone marrow transplantation or immunosuppressive treatment in the last decade: a report from the European Group for Blood and Marrow Transplantation. Haematologica. 2007;92(1):11–8.
50. Scheinberg P, Nunez O, Weinstein B, Scheinberg P, Biancotto A, Wu CO, et al. Horse versus rabbit antithymocyte globulin in acquired aplastic anemia. N Engl J Med. 2011;365(5):430–8.
51. Hayakawa J, Kanda J, Akahoshi Y, Harada N, Kameda K, Ugai T, et al. Meta-analysis of treatment with rabbit and horse antithymocyte globulin for aplastic anemia. Int J Hematol. 2017;105(5):578–86.
52. Scheinberg P, Wu CO, Nunez O, Young NS. Predicting response to immunosuppressive therapy and survival in severe aplastic anaemia. Br J Haematol. 2009;144(2):206–16.
53. Saracco P, Quarello P, Iori AP, Zecca M, Longoni D, Svahn J, et al. Cyclosporin A response and dependence in children with acquired aplastic anaemia: a multicentre retrospective study with long-term observation follow-up. Br J Haematol. 2008;140(2):197–205.
54. Jeong DC, Chung NG, Cho B, Zou Y, Ruan M, Takahashi Y, et al. Long-term outcome after immunosuppressive therapy with horse or rabbit antithymocyte globulin and cyclosporine for severe aplastic anemia in children. Haematologica. 2014;99(4):664–71.
55. Groarke EM, Patel BA, Gutierrez-Rodrigues F, Rios O, Lotter J, Baldoni D, et al. Eltrombopag added to immunosuppression for children with treatment-naïve severe aplastic anaemia. Br J Haematol. 2021;192(3):605–14.
56. Goronkova O, Novichkova G, Salimova T, Kalinina I, Baidildina D, Petrova U, et al. Efficacy of combined immunosuppression with or without eltrombopag in children with newly diagnosed aplastic anemia. Blood Adv. 2023;7(6):953–62.
57. Pierri F, Dufour C. Management of aplastic anemia after failure of frontline immunosuppression. Expert Rev Hematol. 2019;12(10):809–19.
58. Scheinberg P, Nunez O, Young NS. Retreatment with rabbit anti-thymocyte globulin and ciclosporin for patients with relapsed or refractory severe aplastic anaemia. Br J Haematol. 2006;133(6):622–7.
59. Peffault De Latour R, Purtill D, Ruggeri A, Sanz G, Michel G, Gandemer V, et al. Influence of nucleated cell dose on overall survival of unrelated cord blood transplantation for patients with severe acquired aplastic anemia: a study by Eurocord and the Aplastic Anemia Working Party of the European Group for Blood and Marrow Transplantation. Biol Blood Marrow Transplant. 2011;17(1):78–85.
60. Ruggeri A, Peffault De Latour R, Rocha V, Larghero J, Robin M, Rodrigues CA, et al. Double cord blood transplantation in patients with high risk bone marrow failure syndromes. Br J Haematol. 2008;143(3):404–8.

61. Scheinberg P, Nunez O, Wu C, Young NS. Treatment of severe aplastic anaemia with combined immunosuppression: anti-thymocyte globulin, ciclosporin and mycophenolate mofetil. Br J Haematol. 2006;133(6):606–11.
62. Niu H, Qi W, Wang Y, Xing L, Fu R, Shao Z, et al. Successful sirolimus therapy of an aplastic anemia patient with chronic kidney disease: a case report. Medicine. 2020;99(23):e20669.
63. Scheinberg P, Nunez O, Weinstein B, Scheinberg P, Wu CO, Young NS. Activity of alemtuzumab monotherapy in treatment-naive, relapsed, and refractory severe acquired aplastic anemia. Blood. 2012;119(2):345–54.
64. Yoshinari H, Kawahara Y, Niijima H, Oh Y, Hirata Y, Okada N, et al. Rapid blood cell recovery with immunosuppressive therapy combined with romiplostim in a patient with very severe hepatitis-associated aplastic anemia who underwent liver transplantation. Int J Hematol. 2021;114(4):524–7.
65. Al-Huniti A, Rathi N, Modi A, Bhagavathi S, Mitten R, Sharathkumar AA. Up-front treatment with Romiplostim in children with acquired bone marrow failure: a single institutional pediatric case series. J Pediatr Hematol Oncol. 2021;43(3):e431–5.

Open Access This chapter is licensed under the terms of the Creative Commons Attribution 4.0 International License (http://creativecommons.org/licenses/by/4.0/), which permits use, sharing, adaptation, distribution and reproduction in any medium or format, as long as you give appropriate credit to the original author(s) and the source, provide a link to the Creative Commons license and indicate if changes were made.

The images or other third party material in this chapter are included in the chapter's Creative Commons license, unless indicated otherwise in a credit line to the material. If material is not included in the chapter's Creative Commons license and your intended use is not permitted by statutory regulation or exceeds the permitted use, you will need to obtain permission directly from the copyright holder.

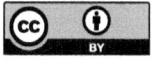

Chapter 9
Treatment of Elderly Patients with Aplastic Anemia

André Tichelli, Alicia Rovó, Constantijn J. M. Halkes, and Austin Kulasekararaj

Introduction

Aplastic anemia (AA) is a rare disease occurring in all age groups but with two peak incidences from 10 to 20 years and over 60 years. Particularly in the elderly, myelodysplastic syndrome (MDS) is a relatively common bone marrow disorder, and it can be difficult to distinguish between AA and hypocellular MDS [1, 2]. Hence, a careful review of the history of the patient and an examination of the blood film and bone marrow aspirates, along with trephine, cytogenetics, and next-generation sequencing (NGS), is needed, as discussed in the chapter "Diagnosis of Acquired Aplastic Anemia." Age, per se, is not a reason to forgo definitive treatment in patients with AA who are >60 years old, or even older than 80 years. But, in contrast to younger patients, the treatment decision-making process is not only based on disease-related factors but also on the functional status of the patient.

A. Tichelli (✉)
Division of Hematology, University Hospital Basel, Basel, Switzerland

A. Rovó
Department of Hematology and Central Hematology Laboratory, Inselspital, Bern University Hospital, University of Bern, Bern, Switzerland
e-mail: alicia.rovo@insel.ch

C. J. M. Halkes
Department of Hematology, Leiden University Medical Centre, Leiden, The Netherlands
e-mail: c.j.m.halkes@lumc.nl

A. Kulasekararaj
Department of Hematological Medicine, King's College Hospital NHS Foundation Trust, London, UK
e-mail: austin.kulasekararaj@nhs.net

© The Author(s) 2026
M. Aljurf et al. (eds.), *Textbook of Bone Marrow Failure*,
https://doi.org/10.1007/978-3-032-02386-5_9

General Treatment Considerations of Elderly Patients with Aplastic Anemia

Untreated, many patients with AA will die from bleeding or infection. The risk of life-threatening bleeding and serious infections increases substantially in older patients. Comparatively, in chronic immune thrombocytopenia (ITP) patients with persistent low platelet counts, the risk for major and fatal hemorrhage increases from 0.4% in younger ages up to 13% per year in patients over 60 years of age [3]. Moreover, the age-related decline of the immune system is contributing to the increased susceptibility to infectious diseases [4].

Once the eligibility for treatment is ascertained, the type of treatment for the AA has to be defined. Supportive measures, including treatment of infections and cell replacement with transfusions of red blood cells and platelets when indicated, are essential in all cases. For some patients with non-severe AA and minimal need for supportive measures, transfusions alone can be considered, as long as the disease status remains stable.

Immunosuppressive treatment (IST) is the standard option, although the response rate at 6 months to ATG-based treatment seems to be lower in older patients [5], and this treatment is associated with increased morbidity and mortality in older patients. The treatment decision in the elderly, and the type of IST to use, should be based therefore on several factors, including (i) severity of the disease, especially the severity of neutropenia, and its associated clinical complications, especially infections; (ii) the general health condition and the presence of comorbidities; (iii) the willingness of the patient and/or their family members to be treated with specific therapy other than supportive care; and (iv) the availability of specific medication for the treatment in different countries.

Immunosuppressive Therapy in the Elderly

In younger adults, the combination including anti-thymocyte globulin (ATG) and cyclosporine (CSA) with or without thrombopoietin receptor agonists (TPO-RAs) is considered the gold standard treatment [6]. For elderly patients eligible for IST, the choice of first-line IST should be based on the risk of severe infections and the need for rapid hematological recovery. Patients with severe disease or those requiring rapid response because of an imminent risk of a lethal complication should be treated, whenever possible, with the combination of ATG and CSA. This combination results in a faster and more complete response as compared to ATG alone [7] or an ATG-free immunosuppression. The drawback of a treatment including ATG is the need for hospitalization and the increased risk of infections and cardiac complications, while adding CSA is associated with delayed toxicity, such as nephrotoxicity, hypertension, and osteonecrosis [8].

Response to treatment and relapse rate of AA after IST are partly dependent on age, as treatment with ATG and CSA is associated with increased mortality with advancing age, due mainly to an increased risk of infection and bleeding [9]. In a prospective randomized study comparing ATG and CSA with or without granulocyte colony-stimulating factor (G-CSF), overall survival at 12 years of patients older than 60 years was 32%, as compared to 55% for patients aged 40–59 years and 81% for those aged 20–40 years (Fig. 9.1) [8]. In patients older than 60 years, the early death rate was 41%, compared to 15% for patients younger than 60 years [10]. The main cause of death in patients ≥60 years was infection (63%), followed by cardiovascular disease (12%), nonresponse (8%), and malignancies (8%). In patients younger than 60 years, the same causes of death were 45%, 5%, 30%, and 5%, respectively (unpublished data from the G-CSF study) [10].

A retrospective analysis from two prospective clinical trials of IST compared the outcome after first-line treatment with ATG and CSA with or without eltrombopag in severe AA patients ≥60 years to patients below 60 years. Older patients had a similar frequency of adverse events, except for higher cardiac events, not resulting in death. However, the relapse rate (71% versus 34%) and the cumulative incidence of clonal evolution (28% versus 17%) at 4 years were significantly higher in the

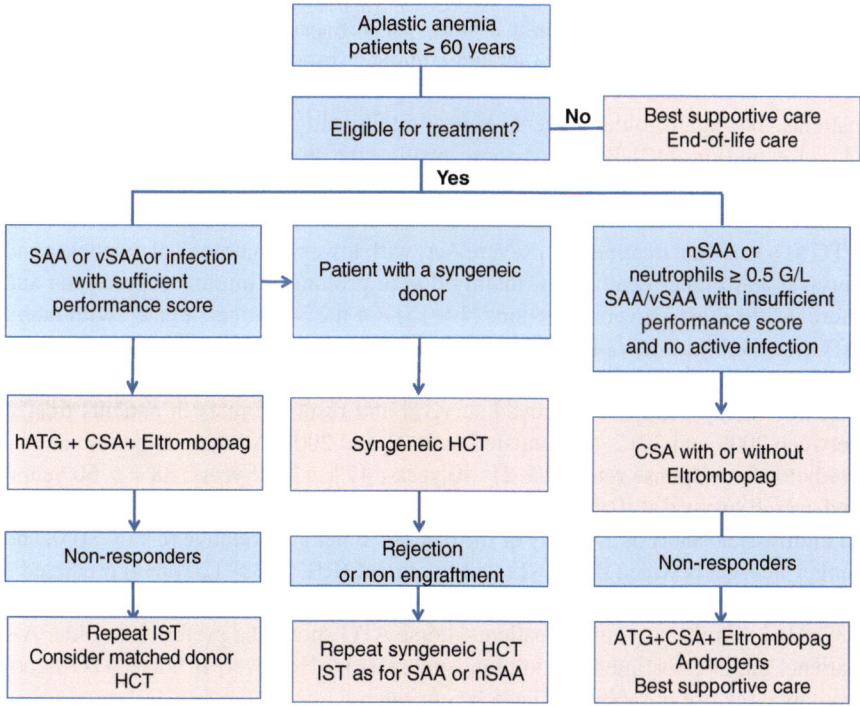

Fig. 9.1 Overall survival of 192 patients with SAA from the randomized G-CSF study, treated with hATG and cyclosporine with or without G-CSF. (Here, all patients are included and stratified according to age groups from [10] with permission)

older patients. This study is an argument not to withhold intensive immunosuppressive treatment in older fit patients, with caution on those with a significant cardiac history [11]. As even patients aged above 60 with significant comorbidities can be treated in specialized centers with ATG and CSA without irreversible side effects, the decision whether to offer this treatment to an elderly patient should be case-based and can differ between patients [12].

As for adult patients with severe AA, the addition of a TPO-RA to standard IST is an attractive option in the elderly, particularly because of its low toxicity profile. The European prospective randomized RACE (Randomized, Multicenter Trial Comparing Horse ATG plus Cyclosporine with or without Eltrombopag as First-Line) study demonstrated the advantage of the combination of ATG and CSA with eltrombopag over the standard IST in respect of response rate at 3 and 6 months, the faster hematopoietic recovery, earlier transfusion independency, and the lower pancytopenia-related complications. The median age of patients was 53 years (range 15–81), including 23% of patients who were 65 years of age or older (24/96 in the eltrombopag arm; 22/101 in the control arm). Despite comparable improvement of the outcome in the older patients of treatment with eltrombopag, the multivariate analysis demonstrated a worse overall response rate (ORR) at 6 months and overall survival and a higher relapse risk in the older patient group [5]. The long-term outcome of patients with severe AA treated with ATG, CSA, and eltrombopag was evaluated in a prospective phase 2 study on 178 patients, with 17% older than 60 years. The overall response rate and complete response of all patients were significantly higher in the eltrombopag-treated patients compared to the historical IST patients, but again, older patients had a significantly higher risk of relapse and clonal evolution. [13] Based on these results, the treatment schedule of patients >60 years eligible for an ATG and CSA combination should include eltrombopag.

In two prospective studies, rabbit ATG has been shown to be inferior to horse ATG as a first-line treatment for severe AA, with lower hematological responses and survival and higher death rates, mainly due to prolonged immunosuppression and more deaths due to severe infections [14, 15]. Of the 34 patients treated with rabbit ATG, 11 died (32%), 7/24 (29%) in the 21–60 age group, and 4/7 (57%) in patients >60 years. Meanwhile, a large retrospective analysis of rabbit ATG and CSA as first-line therapy showed improved survival and response rates in patients treated between 2009 and 2012, as compared to 2001 and 2008. Advanced age remained a predictor for response rate (52% 21–40 years; 47% 41–60 years; 38% > 60 years) and overall survival at 10 years (70% 21–40 years; 49% 41–60 years; 38% > 60 years). In multivariate analysis, severity of the disease, older age (relative risk of 5.05), and longer interval between diagnoses and treatment (RR 1.62 > 120 days) predicted a higher death rate. Patients older than 70 years (n = 30) had an early mortality rate of 33% [16]. Similar to younger patients, horse ATG should be preferred in older AA patients eligible for intensive immunosuppression. However, if horse ATG is not available, the use of rabbit ATG can be considered.

Could an attenuated ATG dose in older patients at risk for ATG toxicity decrease the risk of complications without reducing the response rate? The currently available data show conflicting results. In a single-center experience, 24 elderly patients, aged between 61 and 78 years (median age 70 years), were treated with ATG and CSA, 17 with an attenuated dose of ATG (≤ 50% of the normal dosage), and seven with a standard dose. There was no difference in response rate and overall survival between the two groups, but patients receiving an attenuated ATG dose had fewer serious events during treatment (77% versus 43%; not statistically significant) [17]. Also, discordant results have been reported in a study on 14 elderly patients, aged between 62 and 74 years, and treated with one-third of the standard dose of ATG, but without CSA. Only one of the 14 patients responded to the attenuated dose of ATG [18]. In a more recent retrospective analysis, 20 of 53 elderly patients (>60 years) received the attenuated ATG (50% dose) with CSA and in 80% of them, with eltrombopag. There was no statistical difference in overall survival and response rate between patients with attenuated ATG compared to those receiving a total dose of ATG. However, patients receiving attenuated ATG presented fewer infectious complications compared to patients treated with a standard ATG dose [19]. Despite not being conclusive, these data suggest that an attenuated ATG dose in combination with CSA and/or eltrombopag could be a reasonable option for elderly patients at risk for ATG toxicity. This should preferably be done as part of a clinical study.

For patients who are not at immediate risk of severe infections and who can therefore be managed as outpatients and receive supportive care, first-line treatment with CSA without ATG is recommended. This concerns mainly patients with non-severe AA, particularly those presenting with anemia and thrombocytopenia, without severe neutropenia. In a randomized study, CSA alone was associated with an inferior response rate and disease-free survival than the combination of ATG and CSA, although overall survival was not affected, because CSA-refractory patients responded to second-line treatment with ATG and CSA [20]. Therefore, patients who respond to first-line CSA alone are not exposed to the treatment toxicity of ATG and avoid hospitalization for administration of ATG. CSA nonresponders, if in acceptable condition, can still be re-treated with a more intensive immunosuppression, without additional risk due to the delay.

In a phase 2, single-arm study, the combination of eltrombopag with CSA was evaluated in 43 patients with severe AA as first-line treatment. The ATG-free therapy was chosen because the patients did not have access to ATG or were unable to tolerate ATG. Twenty-three (42%) patients were 60 years of age or older. Compared to patients younger than 60 years (response rate of 52%), patients aged 60 years or older had lower overall response rates (39%), mainly due to early withdrawals and deaths in patients who did not have a response [21]. Eltrombopag was also used in a single-center retrospective analysis of 45 AA patients, mainly because of their advanced age (median age 76 years) or comorbidity. In 43 of the patients, eltrombopag was combined with CSA. This treatment was effective, leading to a unilineage and trilineage response in 66% and 33%, respectively [22]. In a retrospective single-center study of 52 patients older than 60 years, adding Avatrombopag + CSA (26 patients)significantly improved the overall and complete response compared to CSA alone (26 patients) [23]. TPO-RAs with CSA might be beneficial for older patients with AA, ineligible for ATG, or when ATG is not available.

A real-life management study in the elderly AA from France showed a great heterogeneity in the choice of treatment, which was not based on objective selection criteria. For first-line treatment, the combination of ATG and CSA represented the majority, followed by CSA alone, and androgen or eltrombopag [24].

Hematopoietic Cell Transplantation in the Elderly

There is no place for allogeneic HCT as first-line treatment in patients >60 years of age. This does not apply to patients with a syngeneic donor, in whom transplantation should be the first-line therapy, even in advanced age, although there are no specific data on patients aged 60 years or more. The largest retrospective study on syngeneic HCT in AA reported on 88 patients with a median age of 21 years and an upper range of 68 years; however, it lacked specific details on patients >60 years of age [25]. This approach, however, seems reasonable, since patients with AA receiving syngeneic HCT can be conditioned with reduced intensity and will not present Graft-versus-Host disease (GVHD) complications. A potential issue for syngeneic transplantation in older patients is the age of the donor and, therefore, a higher probability of not being medically suitable for stem cell donation. Experience with adult-related donors is available up to a donor age of 75 years. The physician assessing the donor's suitability should be aware of the higher risk due to the prevalence of many age-related health disorders [26]. Complications of hematopoietic stem cell collection have been more often observed in HCT with older age donors [27].

The results of allogeneic HCT remain unsatisfactory and over decades have not improved in patients with AA older than 40 years of age and refractory to IST [28]. For unexplained reasons, age has a stronger negative impact after transplantation in SAA than in leukemia [29]. Many studies on so-called older AA patients reported on patients over 40 years, with only isolated cases over 60 years [30–32]. More recently, there are some data available on patients 60 years of age or older. In a retrospective analysis from the EBMT, the 5-year overall survival of 95 patients >60 years transplanted between 2010 and 2015 was 45%, significantly worse than that of patients aged 50–59 years (58%) and those aged 40–49 years (67%). Predictors for improved 5-year survival were age below 60 years, experienced centers, and the use of ATG or alemtuzumab [28]. Another study reported on HCT in 79 patients (16% of the whole cohort), aged between 65 and 77 years, and refractory to IST. The 3-year overall survival after matched related or unrelated HCT was 50%. A higher mortality risk was observed in patients with a performance score less than 90% (33% versus 68% with a higher score) and after unrelated donor transplantation [33]. There is no study comparing HCT with IST in the elderly, but the overall survival at 3 and 6 years of the patients >60 years from the prospective randomized study treated with ATG and CSA with or without G-CSF was 65% and 56%, respectively [10], and therefore quite comparable to the outcome after HCT. Another recent small retrospective study compared the outcome of patients aged 51 years or older to a younger cohort. Fifteen patients of the older group were aged 60–71 years. The 5-year overall survival, as well as the one-year GVHD-free and relapse-free survival, was excellent (86% and 84%) and not statistically different from the younger cohort. The low incidence of GVHD and the good outcome were possibly due to the conditioning regimen including fludarabine, low-dose cyclophosphamide, and alemtuzumab, as well as carefully selected patients with good performance state [34]. From these data, it can be deduced that allogeneic HCT deserves consideration for selected fit patients with a good performance score after a treatment failure with ATG, CSA, and eltrombopag.

First-Line Treatment Strategy of Elderly Aplastic Anemia Patients

Age, per se, is not a limiting factor for IST in elderly patients with AA who are >60 years old, even older than 80 years (Fig. 9.2). For patients in a reasonable physical condition, standard immunosuppression with the combination of ATG and CSA, with eltrombopag, remains the standard first-line treatment. This combination is of particular importance when a fast and more complete hematopoietic recovery is needed, as for patients with severe infection or with a very high risk of developing severe infections (neutrophils <0.2 G/L) and/or needing any hospitalization. The prerequisite for such intensive immunosuppression is a reasonable health condition. For patients ineligible for ATG treatment, an ATG-free IST based on CSA might be a less aggressive alternative but with a higher probability of delayed response or even refractoriness. Although the data is not yet conclusive, the use of attenuated ATG, as part of the standard immunosuppressive treatment with CSA and eltrombopag, could be a reasonable option in patients in whom there are concerns about ATG-related complications. Any delay in hematopoietic response may expose these

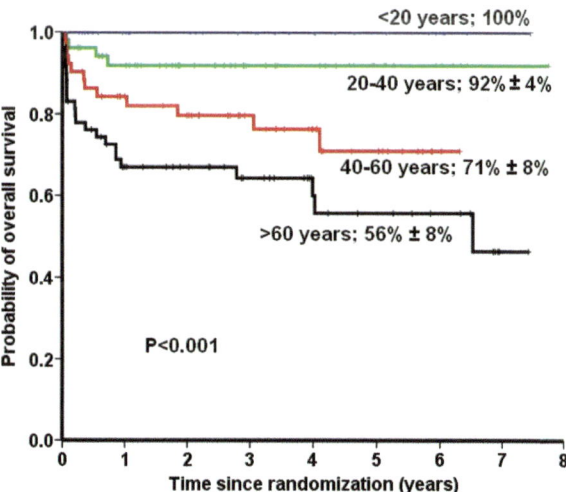

Fig. 9.2 Algorithm of treatment of aplastic anemia patients aged >60 years. (Modified from [37]). IS: immunosuppression; AA: aplastic anemia; SAA: severe aplastic anemia; vSAA: very severe aplastic anemia; ATG: anti-thymocyte globulin; CSA: cyclosporine; BMT: bone marrow transplantation

high-risk AA patients to serious infections, with an increased risk of death. In elderly patients with high-risk AA, the potential benefits from a fast and complete response to treatment have to be balanced with the risk of toxicity due to higher intensity immunosuppression.

For patients who are not at immediate risk for severe infections and who can be managed as outpatients with supportive care until response, first-line treatment with CSA with or without a TPO-RA can be considered [21–23]. It concerns mainly patients with non-severe AA and some patients with SAA but with a neutrophil count above 0.5 G/L and without severe infection (Fig. 9.2). Severe thrombocytopenia and anemia alone are not usually an indication for hospitalization. The use of low-dose subcutaneous alemtuzumab [35] or androgens, particularly in men, can be considered in case of unacceptable side effects or unavailability of CSA or eltrombopag. However, androgens are associated with hepatotoxicity, congestive cardiac failure, prostatic enlargement, elevated blood lipids, mood changes, and other side effects and require careful monitoring of the patient. Patients not responding to CSA and/or eltrombopag after 6 months but still eligible for intensive IST may be considered for second-line treatment with the combination of ATG and CSA, with eltrombopag.

With the exception of syngeneic transplantation, there is no place for HCT as a first-line treatment in patients ≥60 years of age. For patients who failed to respond to the standard combination with ATG, CSA, and eltrombopag, and who are still fit with a good performance score, allogeneic HCT can be considered on an individual basis (Fig. 9.2).

Patients unfit for or intolerant to IST, and those declining treatment, should be offered the best supportive care [6].

The functional ability, comorbidity, nutritional status, and social support, rather than the chronological age of the patient, decide whether to treat and what type of treatment should be considered. In geriatric medicine, the decision to treat always concerns two levels: function and disease. The functional ability of the patient determines the eligibility to be treated, and the disease determines the therapeutic possibilities [36].

References

1. Steensma DP, Bejar R, Jaiswal S, et al. Clonal hematopoiesis of indeterminate potential and its distinction from myelodysplastic syndromes. Blood. 2015;126(1):9–16.
2. Scheinberg P, Bruemmendorf TH, Peffault de Latour R, et al. Analysis of real-world data to identify predictors for earlier diagnosis of aplastic anemai. EHA Library. 2024;2024:PB2674.
3. Cohen YC, Djulbegovic B, Shamai-Lubovitz O, Mozes B. The bleeding risk and natural history of idiopathic thrombocytopenic purpura in patients with persistent low platelet counts. Arch Intern Med. 2000;160(11):1630–8.
4. Derhovanessian E, Solana R, Larbi A, Pawelec G. Immunity, ageing and cancer. Immun Ageing. 2008;5:11.
5. Peffault de Latour R, Kulasekararaj A, Iacobelli S, et al. Eltrombopag added to immunosuppression in severe aplastic anemia. N Engl J Med. 2022;386(1):11–23.
6. Kulasekararaj A, Cavenagh J, Dokal I, et al. Guidelines for the diagnosis and management of adult aplastic anaemia: a British Society for Haematology guideline. Br J Haematol. 2024;204(3):784–804.

7. Frickhofen N, Heimpel H, Kaltwasser JP, Schrezenmeier H, German Aplastic Anemia Study G. Antithymocyte globulin with or without cyclosporin a: 11-year follow-up of a randomized trial comparing treatments of aplastic anemia. Blood. 2003;101(4):1236–42.
8. Tichelli A, de Latour RP, Passweg J, et al. Long-term outcome of a randomized controlled study in patients with newly diagnosed severe aplastic anemia treated with antithymocyte globulin and cyclosporine, with or without granulocyte colony-stimulating factor: a Severe Aplastic Anemia Working Party Trial from the European Group of Blood and Marrow Transplantation. Haematologica. 2020;105(5):1223–31.
9. Tichelli A, Socie G, Henry-Amar M, et al. Effectiveness of immunosuppressive therapy in older patients with aplastic anemia. European Group for Blood and Marrow Transplantation Severe Aplastic Anaemia Working Party. Ann Intern Med. 1999;130(3):193–201.
10. Tichelli A, Schrezenmeier H, Socie G, et al. A randomized controlled study in patients with newly diagnosed severe aplastic anemia receiving antithymocyte globulin (ATG), cyclosporine, with or without G-CSF: a study of the SAA Working Party of the European Group for Blood and Marrow Transplantation. Blood. 2011;117(17):4434–41.
11. Prabahran A, Durrani J, Coelho-Da Silva J, et al. Safety and efficacy of immunosuppressive therapy for elderly patients with severe aplastic anaemia. Br J Haematol. 2024;205:1170.
12. Tjon JM, de Groot MR, Sypkens Smit SMA, et al. Short-term efficacy and safety of antithymocyte globulin treatment in elderly patients with acquired aplastic anaemia. Br J Haematol. 2018;180(3):459–62.
13. Patel BA, Groarke EM, Lotter J, et al. Long-term outcomes in patients with severe aplastic anemia treated with immunosuppression and eltrombopag: a phase 2 study. Blood. 2022;139(1):34–43.
14. Marsh JC, Bacigalupo A, Schrezenmeier H, et al. Prospective study of rabbit antithymocyte globulin and cyclosporine for aplastic anemia from the EBMT Severe Aplastic Anaemia Working Party. Blood. 2012;119(23):5391–6.
15. Scheinberg P, Nunez O, Weinstein B, et al. Horse versus rabbit antithymocyte globulin in acquired aplastic anemia. N Engl J Med. 2011;365(5):430–8.
16. Bacigalupo A, Oneto R, Schrezenmeier H, et al. First line treatment of aplastic anemia with thymoglobuline in Europe and Asia: outcome of 955 patients treated 2001-2012. Am J Hematol. 2019;94(1):165.
17. Kao SY, Xu W, Brandwein JM, et al. Outcomes of older patients (> or = 60 years) with acquired aplastic anaemia treated with immunosuppressive therapy. Br J Haematol. 2008;143(5):738–43.
18. Killick SB, Cavenagh JD, Davies JK, Marsh JC. Low dose antithymocyte globulin for the treatment of older patients with aplastic anaemia. Leuk Res. 2006;30(12):1517–20.
19. Foucar CE, Foley DH, Aldous J, et al. Real-world outcomes with immunosuppressive therapy for aplastic anemia in patients treated at the University of Michigan. Eur J Haematol. 2024;112(3):424–32.
20. Marsh J, Schrezenmeier H, Marin P, et al. Prospective randomized multicenter study comparing cyclosporin alone versus the combination of antithymocyte globulin and cyclosporin for treatment of patients with nonsevere aplastic anemia: a report from the European Blood and Marrow Transplant (EBMT) Severe Aplastic Anaemia Working Party. Blood. 1999;93(7):2191–5.
21. Scheinberg P, Finelli C, Montano-Figueroa EH, et al. Activity and safety of eltrombopag in combination with cyclosporin A as first-line treatment of adults with severe aplastic anaemia (SOAR): a phase 2, single-arm study. Lancet Haematol. 2024;11(3):e206–e15.
22. Iino M, Jinguji A, Sato T, Nakadate A. Real-world experience of treatment with thrombopoietin receptor agonists in anti-thymocyte globulin-naive patients with aplastic anemia: an observational retrospective analysis in a single institution. Hematology. 2022;27(1):360–6.
23. Zhang Z, Hu Q, Wang LS, Yang C, Chen M, Han B. Cyclosporine plus avatromopag versus cyclosporine alone for first-line treatment of elderly patients with transfusion-dependent non-severe aplastic anemia: a single center, retrospective study. EHA Library. 2024;2024:P1919.

24. Contejean A, Resche-Rigon M, Tamburini J, et al. Aplastic anemia in the elderly: a nationwide survey on behalf of the French reference Center for Aplastic Anemia. Haematologica. 2019;104(2):256–62.
25. Gerull S, Stern M, Apperley J, et al. Syngeneic transplantation in aplastic anemia: pretransplant conditioning and peripheral blood are associated with improved engraftment: an observational study on behalf of the Severe Aplastic Anemia and Pediatric Diseases Working Parties of the European Group for Blood and Marrow Transplantation. Haematologica. 2013;98(11):1804–9.
26. Worel N, Buser A, Greinix HT, et al. Suitability criteria for adult related donors: a consensus statement from the worldwide network for blood and marrow transplantation standing committee on donor issues. Biol Blood Marrow Transplant. 2015;21(12):2052–60.
27. Lysák D, Kořístek Z, Gašová Z, Skoumalová I, Jindra P. Efficacy and safety of peripheral blood stem cell collection in elderly donors; does age interfere? J Clin Apher. 2011;26(1):9–16.
28. Giammarco S, Peffault de Latour R, Sica S, et al. Transplant outcome for patients with acquired aplastic anemia over the age of 40: has the outcome improved? Blood. 2018;131(17):1989–92.
29. Bacigalupo A. Antithymocyte globulin and cyclosporin: standard of care also for older patients with aplastic anemia. Haematologica. 2019;104(2):215–6.
30. Gupta V, Eapen M, Brazauskas R, et al. Impact of age on outcomes after bone marrow transplantation for acquired aplastic anemia using HLA-matched sibling donors. Haematologica. 2010;95(12):2119–25.
31. Sangiolo D, Storb R, Deeg HJ, et al. Outcome of allogeneic hematopoietic cell transplantation from HLA-identical siblings for severe aplastic anemia in patients over 40 years of age. Biol Blood Marrow Transplant. 2010;16(10):1411–8.
32. Marsh JC, Gupta V, Lim Z, et al. Alemtuzumab with fludarabine and cyclophosphamide reduces chronic graft-versus-host disease after allogeneic stem cell transplantation for acquired aplastic anemia. Blood. 2011;118(8):2351–7.
33. Rice C, Eikema DJ, Marsh JCW, et al. Allogeneic hematopoietic cell transplantation in patients aged 50 years or older with severe aplastic anemia. Biol Blood Marrow Transplant. 2018;25:488.
34. Sheth VS, Potter V, Gandhi SA, et al. Similar outcomes of alemtuzumab-based hematopoietic cell transplantation for SAA patients older or younger than 50 years. Blood Adv. 2019;3(20):3070–9.
35. Thota S, Patel BJ, Sadaps M, et al. Therapeutic outcomes using subcutaneous low dose alemtuzumab for acquired bone marrow failure conditions. Br J Haematol. 2018;183(1):133–6.
36. Stähelin HB. Besonderheiten der Geriatrie. In: Zöllner N, Gresser U, Hehlmann R, editors. Innere Medizin. Berlin, Heidelberg: Springer Berlin Heidelberg; 1991. p. 657–68.
37. Tichelli A, Marsh JC. Treatment of aplastic anaemia in elderly patients aged >60 years. Bone Marrow Transplant. 2013;48(2):180–2.

Open Access This chapter is licensed under the terms of the Creative Commons Attribution 4.0 International License (http://creativecommons.org/licenses/by/4.0/), which permits use, sharing, adaptation, distribution and reproduction in any medium or format, as long as you give appropriate credit to the original author(s) and the source, provide a link to the Creative Commons license and indicate if changes were made.

The images or other third party material in this chapter are included in the chapter's Creative Commons license, unless indicated otherwise in a credit line to the material. If material is not included in the chapter's Creative Commons license and your intended use is not permitted by statutory regulation or exceeds the permitted use, you will need to obtain permission directly from the copyright holder.

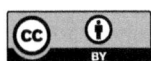

Part V
Hematopoietic Stem Cell Transplantation for Aplastic Anemia

Chapter 10
Matched Sibling Donor Transplantation in Aplastic Anemia

Ali. D. Alahmari, Riad El Fakih, Constantijn J. M. Halkes, Simone Cesaro, and Mahmoud Aljurf

History of SAA HSCT

In 1957, E. Donnall Thomas and his group reported the first evidence of human hematopoietic stem cell engraftment and the safety of intravenous bone marrow infusion after total body irradiation (TBI) [1]. This success story followed decades of different transplant attempts in animals and humans [2, 3]. The first successful transplant for a severe aplastic anemia (SAA) patient using a syngeneic donor was reported in 1961 [4]. Between the mid-1950s and early 1960s, 200 transplants were reported worldwide; 73 of them were for SAA patients [5]. During that same period, human leukocyte antigen (HLA) typing was developed, and the success of HSCT was clearly related to the degree of HLA matching between recipient and donor [6]. In 1972, Thomas et al. reported the first successful transplant for SAA patients from matched sibling donors (MSD) following cyclophosphamide (Cy) conditioning [7]. The Seattle group published the first randomized trial for SAA in 1976. The trial showed a higher survival benefit after MSD transplantation compared to the standard of care (supportive transfusions and androgens) [8]. Currently, MSD transplantation is the standard of care as frontline therapy for young patients (<40–50 years) versus immunosuppressive therapy for older patients or young patients with unavailable MSD. A recommendation is supported by major guidelines. Published data

A. D. Alahmari (✉) · R. El Fakih · M. Aljurf
Department of Hematology, Stem Cell Transplant & Cellular Therapy, Cancer Centre of Excellence, King Faisal Specialist Hospital & Research Centre, Riyadh, Saudi Arabia
e-mail: aalahmari7@kfshrc.edu.sa

C. J. M. Halkes
Department of Hematology, Leiden University Medical Centre, Leiden, The Netherlands

S. Cesaro
Pediatric Hematology and Oncology, Department of the Mother and the Child, Azienda Ospedaliera Universitaria Integrata, Verona, Italy

show that the failure-free survival after MSD transplant declines with increasing age due to higher mortality after transplant in older patients [9–12].

HSCT Indication in SAA

Aplastic anemia (AA) is thought to be an immune-related hematopoietic stem cell destruction. The disease is defined as pancytopenia with hypocellular bone marrow [<25% (or 25–50% if <30% of residual cells are hematopoietic)] in the absence of marrow infiltrates or fibrosis [13–18]. The severity is defined by the degree of cytopenia, and severity is important to guide therapy [12–14]. Patients with severe or very severe forms need urgent intervention [12–14, 19]. The choice of frontline therapy is guided by the patient's age, the comorbidities, and the availability of an MSD. Transplant is a curative option that aims to re-establish hematopoiesis, ideally with good engraftment and absence of graft-versus-host disease (GvHD). Presently, with the standardization of conditioning regimens, better supportive care, and diagnostic abilities, the cure rate of allogeneic HSCT for younger patients can reach 90% [20, 21]. The superiority of allogeneic HSCT compared to immunosuppressive therapy (IST) derives from the decrease in relapse risk and the onset of late clonal disorders, such as myelodysplastic syndrome (MDS) and paroxysmal nocturnal hemoglobinuria (PNH). However, the risk of acute GvHD (aGvHD) and chronic GvHD (cGvHD), poor graft function, and graft failure (GF) remains a challenge after HSCT [22]. Considering the potential toxicities associated with the conditioning and the higher risk of GvHD in older patients, allogeneic HSCT is typically recommended for individuals within the age of 40–50 years with an available MSD. Matched sibling transplant can be selectively offered to biologically fit older patients who have indicators of poor response to immunosuppressive therapy [23–25]. HSCT is recommended as a second-line treatment for older patients who have not responded effectively to prior IST [20, 21, 26].

A large European Group for Blood and Marrow Transplantation (EBMT) study (1500 patients spanning from 1991 to 2002) showed that the best survival rate is achieved with young patients (<20 years), an interval from diagnosis to HSCT (<180 days), use of bone marrow (BM) as a stem cell source, and use of antithymocyte globulin (ATG) in the conditioning regimen. Patients under the age of 16 years had a remarkable survival rate of 91% as compared to a 74% survival rate for patients older than 16 years [21]. A pediatric study from Japan showed a notably lower 10-year overall survival (OS) rate of 55% for an upfront IST (n = 63), compared to 97% OS in 37 patients who underwent HSCT, with 26 (70%) of them receiving upfront HSCT from MSD [27].

Pre-HSCT Factors

A number of pretransplant factors can potentially influence the outcomes of HSCT in SAA:

Age

Long-term follow-up of young patients transplanted from MSD invariably revealed a 10-year survival rate of more than 80% [28–32]. In recent decades, with the improvement of supportive care and better tailoring of the conditioning regimens, this survival is around 90% in young patients [20, 21]. Registry-level data from large registries (EBMT and Center for International Blood and Marrow Transplant Research [CIBMTR]) consistently show worse outcomes for older patients [21, 33, 34]. However, with modern tailored regimens, a 5-year OS rate ranging between 86 and 88% has been reported irrespective of age [35, 36].

Severity

AA severity is defined according to the modified Camitta criteria into non-severe/moderate (MAA), severe (SAA), and very severe AA (vSAA). SAA is defined as marrow cellularity <25% (or 25–50% with <30% residual hematopoietic cells), plus at least two of the following peripheral blood findings: neutrophils $<0.5 \times 10^9$/L, platelets $<20 \times 10^9$/L, and reticulocytes $<60 \times 10^9$/L [37, 38]. Very severe AA fulfills the same criteria as SAA, except neutrophils are $<0.2 \times 10^9$/L [39, 40]. Without effective treatment, patients with SAA are at high risk of death from infection or hemorrhage [41]. Without immediate transplant, patients with vSAA do worse than those with SAA when they are treated with IST [20, 42–45].

HLA

During the early days of transplant, the success of HSCT was clearly correlated with the degree of HLA matching between the recipient and the donor. The discovery of the immunologic reactivity of the host (graft rejection) and/or of the graft (graft-versus-host disease) and its relationship to the HLA matching led to the standardization of HLA testing. Currently, many techniques are available and offer better accuracy compared to the serologic methods. Minimizing this bidirectional alloreactivity is very important in benign disorders and specifically in AA, as the GF and GvHD define the long-term success of the transplant procedure in this disease.

Pre-HSCT Blood Product Transfusion

Higher transfusion history prior to transplant correlates with poor outcomes in patients with AA [46]. In one study, patients transfused with >32 packed red blood cells (PRBC) before the transplant had a higher incidence of acute GvHD (grades II–IV) compared to the low-transfusion group ($p = 0.04$). Additionally, the high-transfusion group had higher 5-year transplant-related mortality (TRM) (24.8% vs 6.8%, $p < 0.001$) and lower OS (72.3% vs 91.9%, $p < 0.001$) [47]. Higher GF rates were reported with higher transfusions from multiple groups [48–50].

Pre-HSCT Infection

The presence of active infections or a history of prior infections negatively affects transplant outcomes and increases the risk of infectious complications post-HSCT [51]. This is particularly important in low- and middle-income countries, where the time from diagnosis to transplant is typically longer compared to high-income countries.

Conditioning Regimen

In SAA, the objective of HSCT is to achieve successful engraftment without GvHD. GF represents a challenge in these patients. Multiple mechanisms account for this complication, including the underlying autoimmune etiology, alloimmunization from prior transfusions, abnormalities of the recipient bone marrow microenvironment, the use of non-myeloablative regimens for conditioning, the bone marrow stem cell source, and an intact recipient immune system in SAA patients compared to a weakened recipient immune system in leukemia patients due to prior lines of chemotherapy. As such, a potent immunosuppressive preparative regimen is a prerequisite in SAA patients [20]. Below is a summary of the frequently used regimens.

Cyclophosphamide

During early transplant days, in the 1970s, GF was reported in up to 30% of patients with the use of Cy single-agent conditioning and methotrexate (MTX) for GvHD prophylaxis, particularly among heavily transfused patients [52]. Some of these patients regained hematopoiesis as a result of the immunosuppressive action of the conditioning (autologous recovery) [53]. Substantial regimen modifications significantly decreased the incidence of GF with modern conditioning regimens [22, 54]. Single-agent Cy may still be considered in very selected cases, like MSD transplant minimally transfused patients [54].

Total Body Irradiation (TBI) Plus Cy

The addition of TBI to Cy resulted in less GF at the cost of radiation-related toxicities. This combination did not confer any survival benefit and, as such, is only used in highly selected cases currently [48, 55–57].

Cy Plus ATG

The Seattle group added horse ATG (hATG) at a dose of 30 mg/kg/day for 3 days to Cy, along with MTX and cyclosporine (CsA) for GvHD prophylaxis. The combination led to 100% primary engraftment, a 3-year OS rate of 92%, aGvHD of 15%, and 6% secondary GF [58–60]. This protocol (CY200-hATG) with an unmanipulated bone marrow graft was introduced more than four decades ago and is still a standard for young AA patients undergoing MSD transplant. Although only one randomized trial compared this regimen to single-agent Cy and showed 5-year survival rates of 74% for the Cy-alone group and 80% for the Cy and ATG group, the difference was not statistically significant ($P = 0.44$) [54]. Many groups subsequently reported their experience with this regimen, showing good engraftment and low incidence of secondary malignancies, as well as preserved fertility.

Fludarabine (Flu) Plus Cy

This regimen was associated with better tolerance and fewer infections as compared to Cy/ATG [61–66]. Moreover, ATG is frequently unavailable, especially in resource-restricted countries. Thus, it is a suitable alternative in resource-restricted settings and for patients at higher risk of infection (e.g., older patients).

Flu Cy with ATG or Alemtuzumab

Adding ATG or alemtuzumab to the conditioning regimen may result in lower bidirectional immunoreactivity and, as such, better control of GF and GvHD. In a study of older patients undergoing transplant for AA (48% from MSD), factors associated with improved outcomes included the use of ATG or alemtuzumab [24]. In an

EBMT study, for patients older than 30, the addition of Flu to Cy/ATG was associated with a higher probability of OS compared to the control group of Cy-ATG ($p = 0.04$) [67]. In another study, where alemtuzumab was added to Flu/Cy, durable engraftment and low cGvHD were reported [68]. Many other reports showed better engraftment with the addition of ATG or alemtuzumab; however, many of these studies suffer from the heterogeneity of patients, conditioning, type of ATG used, and type of donors [69–73].

Syngeneic HSCT in SAA

Syngeneic HSCT represents a rare yet invaluable treatment option in aplastic anemia, characterized by remarkable long-term survival and minimal TRM. It stands as a unique opportunity when accessible. A study involving 40 patients who underwent syngeneic graft transplantation between 1964 and 1992 showed better engraftment with the use of Cy conditioning versus no conditioning (engraftment rate 64% versus 30%). This result supports the immune hypothesis of acquired aplastic anemia (AA); there was no difference in OS between patients who received or did not receive conditioning [74]. In a retrospective study from EBMT, a conditioning regimen was administered to three-quarters of patients, and 50% received post-HSCT immunosuppression. GF was more frequent in patients who did not receive conditioning and those who received a bone marrow graft, as compared to peripheral blood [75]. It may be reasonable in this scenario to use a peripheral blood graft, as the risk of GvHD is minimal, if any.

Stem Cell Source

Across all age groups, unmanipulated BM is the preferred stem cell source as it is associated with a lower incidence of GvHD and better survival [76, 77]. It is recommended to aim for a dose of at least 3×10^8 mononuclear cells/kg or 2×10^6 CD34+ cells/kg of the recipient, as lower doses are associated with a higher risk of GF. Peripheral blood can be used exceptionally where faster engraftment is needed (patients with ongoing severe infection) or an optimal dose cannot be secured from marrow. Of note, granulocyte-colony-stimulating factor-primed bone marrow (G-BM) is linked to faster engraftment compared to unmanipulated BM and a lower incidence of GvHD compared to peripheral blood [78, 79].

GvHD Prophylaxis

Adequate post-transplant immunosuppression is essential to control the bidirectional alloreactivity (both in the GF and GvHD direction) [4]. In the earlier trials, MTX alone was used for post-transplant immunosuppression. The addition of calcineurin inhibitors to MTX decreased the incidence of both GF and GvHD (and eventually TRM) and is still, as of now, the standard of care [80, 81]. For patients with renal impairment or other contraindications for calcineurin inhibitors, mycophenolate mofetil (MMF) can be considered as an alternative. Two cases of SAA with significant renal impairment reported in the literature demonstrated the feasibility of HSCT with the use of MMF for GvHD prophylaxis [82]. Graft engineering with selective T-cell depletion is experimental and cannot be recommended for the standard of care. Typically, post-transplant immunosuppression should be continued for at least one year, with a slow taper along with careful monitoring of blood count.

Post-HSCT Care

Engraftment and Chimerism

Chimerism stands as an essential tool for tracking engraftment kinetics periodically post-transplant. Transient mixed chimerism is frequently observed. In one study, 60% of patients exhibited mixed chimerism, with two-thirds of these individuals ultimately transitioning to complete donor-type hematopoietic cells, while the remaining third experienced graft rejection (although some of these recovered normal blood count, a phenomenon known as autologous recovery) [63, 83]. In another study, 45% had mixed chimerism, and those had a higher risk for GF [84]. There is no standard approach to address mixed chimerism. In general, when mixed chimerism is associated with declining cell counts, bone marrow assessment is warranted. Intensification of immunosuppressive therapy is recommended if the decline in chimerism primarily affects the lymphoid component. Alternatively, low doses of donor lymphocyte infusion may be considered, with careful monitoring for GvHD while maintaining immunosuppression prophylaxis. However, if the decline in chimerism affects the myeloid component, it indicates impending GF. In such cases, stem cell boosting with selected CD34 cells is contemplated, although there is limited published data on this approach.

Survival

The OS for SAA showed marked improvement over the past three decades. In the 1970s, survival rates typically ranged from 40% to 60%, whereas current survival rates range from 60% to 100% [60, 85]. In a large retrospective EBMT study, both the transplant year and the patient's age were predictive of outcomes. Notably, there has been a significant improvement in the 5-year survival rates when comparing patients transplanted before and after 1990 [21]. Another large CIBMTR study showed hemorrhage (33%), infection (32%), organ failure (22%), GF (14%), and GvHD (10%) as the major causes of death post-transplant for AA patients [86].

Infertility

Gonadal function typically returns to normal in patients conditioned with Cy alone. Among 65 women aged between 13 and 25 years who underwent Cy-only conditioning, all exhibited evidence of ovarian function recovery. However, in women aged 26–38 years, 37% experienced primary ovarian failure [87, 88]. Likewise, another study indicated that testicular function returned to normal in most men aged 14–41 years who received Cy-only conditioning [89].

Secondary Malignancy

Secondary malignancies following AA transplant are traditionally rare. An analysis of transplant outcomes in 700 patients with AA who underwent transplantation using total body irradiation (TBI)-based conditioning revealed an estimated incidence of secondary malignancies of 14% at 20 years [90]. However, this incidence decreased to 1.4% at 10 years when the regimen did not include radiation [91]. These findings were further validated by the aforementioned CIBMTR study conducted in 2012 [86].

Conclusion

- HSCT is the standard therapy for SAA in young patients with an available MSD.
- HSCT should be carried out urgently to minimize TRM.
- BM is the preferred stem cell source for HSCT in SAA.
- The Cy-ATG conditioning regimen remains the standard approach.
- Flu Cy-ATG is comparable to Cy-ATG but may be the preferred option for older patients or those with higher risk profiles.

- Flu-based regimens (flu with or without Cy) can be considered for patients older than 40 years.
- MTX with calcineurin inhibitors (CsA or tacrolimus) is the standard immunosuppression post-transplant regimen.

Prolonged IST post-HSCT is crucial to reduce the risk of graft failure.

References

1. Thomas ED, Lochte HL Jr, Lu WC, Ferrebee JW. Intravenous infusion of bone marrow in patients receiving radiation and chemotherapy. N Engl J Med. 1957;257(11):491–6.
2. Blume KG, Thomas ED. A history of allogeneic and autologous hematopoietic cell transplantation. Thomas' Hematopoietic Cell Transpl Stem Cell Transplant. 2015;1:1–11.
3. El Fakih R, Lazarus HM, Muffly L, Altareb M, Aljurf M, Hashmi SK. Historical perspective and a glance into the antibody-based conditioning regimens: a new era in the horizon? Blood Rev. 2022;52:100892.
4. Robins MM, Noyes WD. Aplastic anemia treated with bone-marrow transfusion from an identical twin. N Engl J Med. 1961;265:974–9.
5. Bortin MM. A compendium of reported human bone marrow transplants. Transplantation. 1970;9(6):571–87.
6. van Rood JJ. The detection of transplantation antigens in leukocytes. Semin Hematol. 1968;5(2):187–214.
7. Thomas ED, Storb R, Fefer A, et al. Aplastic anaemia treated by marrow transplantation. Lancet. 1972;1(7745):284–9.
8. Camitta BM, Thomas ED, Nathan DG, et al. Severe aplastic anemia: a prospective study of the effect of early marrow transplantation on acute mortality. Blood. 1976;48(1):63–70.
9. Bacigalupo A, Brand R, Oneto R, et al. Treatment of acquired severe aplastic anemia: bone marrow transplantation compared with immunosuppressive therapy-The European Group for Blood and Marrow Transplantation experience. Paper presented at: Seminars in hematology 2000.
10. Socié G, Rosenfeld S, Frickhofen N, Gluckman E, Tichelli A. Late clonal diseases of treated aplastic anemia. Paper presented at: Seminars in hematology 2000.
11. Yoshida N, Kobayashi R, Yabe H, et al. First-line treatment for severe aplastic anemia in children: bone marrow transplantation from a matched family donor versus immunosuppressive therapy. Haematologica. 2014;99(12):1784–91.
12. Young NS. Aplastic anemia. N Engl J Med. 2018;379(17):1643–56.
13. Killick SB, Bown N, Cavenagh J, et al. Guidelines for the diagnosis and management of adult aplastic anaemia. Br J Haematol. 2016;172(2):187–207.
14. Bacigalupo A, Hows J, Gluckman E, et al. Bone marrow transplantation (BMT) versus immunosuppression for the treatment of severe aplastic anaemia (SAA): a report of the EBMT* SAA Working Party. Br J Haematol. 1988;70(2):177–82.
15. Montané E, Ibáñez L, Vidal X, et al. Epidemiology of aplastic anemia: a prospective multicenter study. Haematologica. 2008;93(4):518–23.
16. Mary J, Baumelou E, Guiguet M. Epidemiology of aplastic anemia in France: a prospective multicentric study. The French Cooperative Group for Epidemiological Study of Aplastic. Anemia. 1990;75:1646.
17. Heimpel H. Incidence of aplastic anemia: the relevance of diagnostic criteria. Blood. 1987;70(6):1718–21.
18. Issaragrisil S, Kaufman DW, Anderson T, et al. The epidemiology of aplastic anemia in Thailand. Blood. 2006;107(4):1299–307.
19. Höchsmann B, Moicean A, Risitano A, Ljungman P, Schrezenmeier H. Supportive care in severe and very severe aplastic anemia. Bone Marrow Transplant. 2013;48(2):168–73.

20. Armand P, Antin JH. Allogeneic stem cell transplantation for aplastic anemia. Biol Blood Marrow Transplant. 2007;13(5):505–16.
21. Bacigalupo A, Brand R, Oneto R, et al. Treatment of acquired severe aplastic anemia: bone marrow transplantation compared with immunosuppressive therapy--The European Group for Blood and Marrow Transplantation experience. Semin Hematol. 2000;37(1):69–80.
22. DeZern AE, Guinan EC. Aplastic anemia in adolescents and young adults. Acta Haematol. 2014;132(3–4):331–9.
23. Aljurf M, Al-Zahrani H, Van Lint MT, Passweg JR. Standard treatment of acquired SAA in adult patients 18-40 years old with an HLA-identical sibling donor. Bone Marrow Transplant. 2013;48(2):178–9.
24. Giammarco S, Peffault de Latour R, Sica S, et al. Transplant outcome for patients with acquired aplastic anemia over the age of 40: has the outcome improved? Blood. 2018;131(17):1989–92.
25. Iftikhar R, Chaudhry QUN, Anwer F, et al. Allogeneic hematopoietic stem cell transplantation in aplastic anemia: current indications and transplant strategies. Blood Rev. 2021;47:100772.
26. Locasciulli A, Oneto R, Bacigalupo A, et al. Outcome of patients with acquired aplastic anemia given first line bone marrow transplantation or immunosuppressive treatment in the last decade: a report from the European Group for Blood and Marrow Transplantation (EBMT). Haematologica. 2007;92(1):11–8.
27. Kojima S, Horibe K, Inaba J, et al. Long-term outcome of acquired aplastic anaemia in children: comparison between immunosuppressive therapy and bone marrow transplantation. Br J Haematol 2000;111(1):321–328.
28. Kahl C, Leisenring W, Deeg HJ, et al. Cyclophosphamide and antithymocyte globulin as a conditioning regimen for allogeneic marrow transplantation in patients with aplastic anaemia: a long-term follow-up. Br J Haematol. 2005;130(5):747–51.
29. Anasetti C, Doney KC, Storb R, et al. Marrow transplantation for severe aplastic anemia. Long-term outcome in fifty "untransfused" patients. Ann Intern Med. 1986;104(4):461–6.
30. Kiem HP, McDonald GB, Myerson D, et al. Marrow transplantation for hepatitis-associated aplastic anemia: a follow-up of long-term survivors. Biol Blood Marrow Transplant. 1996;2(2):93–9.
31. Eapen M, Ramsay NK, Mertens AC, Robison LL, DeFor T, Davies SM. Late outcomes after bone marrow transplant for aplastic anaemia. Br J Haematol. 2000;111(3):754–60.
32. Deeg HJ, Leisenring W, Storb R, et al. Long-term outcome after marrow transplantation for severe aplastic anemia. Blood. 1998;91(10):3637–45.
33. Gupta V, Eapen M, Brazauskas R, et al. Impact of age on outcomes after bone marrow transplantation for acquired aplastic anemia using HLA-matched sibling donors. Haematologica. 2010;95(12):2119–25.
34. Bacigalupo A. How I treat acquired aplastic anemia. Blood. 2017;129(11):1428–36.
35. Sheth VS, Potter V, Gandhi SA, et al. Similar outcomes of alemtuzumab-based hematopoietic cell transplantation for SAA patients older or younger than 50 years. Blood Adv. 2019;3(20):3070–9.
36. Shin SH, Jeon YW, Yoon JH, et al. Comparable outcomes between younger (⩽40 years) and older (>40 years) adult patients with severe aplastic anemia after HLA-matched sibling stem cell transplantation using fludarabine-based conditioning. Bone Marrow Transplant. 2016;51(11):1456–63.
37. Camitta BM, Thomas ED, Nathan DG, et al. A prospective study of androgens and bone marrow transplantation for treatment of severe aplastic anemia. Blood. 1979;53(3):504–14.
38. Yoon HH, Huh SJ, Lee JH, et al. Should we still use Camitta's criteria for severe aplastic anemia? Korean J Hematol. 2012;47(2):126–30.
39. Camitta BM, Storb R, Thomas ED. Aplastic anemia (first of two parts): pathogenesis, diagnosis, treatment, and prognosis. N Engl J Med. 1982;306(11):645–52.
40. Camitta BM, Storb R, Thomas ED. Aplastic anemia (second of two parts): pathogenesis, diagnosis, treatment, and prognosis. N Engl J Med. 1982;306(12):712–8.
41. Babushok DV, DeZern AE, de Castro C, et al. Modified Delphi panel consensus recommendations for Management of Severe Aplastic Anemia. Blood Adv. 2024;8:3946.

42. Horowitz MM. Current status of allogeneic bone marrow transplantation in acquired aplastic anemia. Semin Hematol. 2000;37(1):30–42.
43. Tichelli A, Socie G, Henry-Amar M, et al. Effectiveness of immunosuppressive therapy in older patients with aplastic anemia. European Group for Blood and Marrow Transplantation Severe Aplastic Anaemia Working Party. Ann Intern Med. 1999;130(3):193–201.
44. Doney K, Leisenring W, Storb R, Appelbaum FR. Primary treatment of acquired aplastic anemia: outcomes with bone marrow transplantation and immunosuppressive therapy. Seattle Bone Marrow Transplant Team. Ann Intern Med. 1997;126(2):107–15.
45. Marsh JC, Hows JM, Bryett KA, Al-Hashimi S, Fairhead SM, Gordon-Smith EC. Survival after antilymphocyte globulin therapy for aplastic anemia depends on disease severity. Blood. 1987;70(4):1046–52.
46. Zhang X, Shi Y, Huang Y, et al. Serum ferritin is a different predictor from transfusion history for allogeneic transplantation outcome in patients with severe aplastic anemia. Hematology. 2018;23(5):291–8.
47. Lee SE, Yahng SA, Cho BS, et al. Impact of pretransplant red cell transfusion on outcome after allogeneic stem cell transplantation in adult patients with severe aplastic anemia. Bone Marrow Transplant. 2016;51(10):1323–9.
48. Champlin RE, Horowitz MM, van Bekkum DW, et al. Graft failure following bone marrow transplantation for severe aplastic anemia: risk factors and treatment results. Blood. 1989;73(2):606–13.
49. Storb R, Blume KG, O'Donnell MR, et al. Cyclophosphamide and antithymocyte globulin to condition patients with aplastic anemia for allogeneic marrow transplantations: the experience in four centers. Biol Blood Marrow Transplant. 2001;7(1):39–44.
50. Srinivasan R, Takahashi Y, McCoy JP, et al. Overcoming graft rejection in heavily transfused and Allo-immunised patients with bone marrow failure syndromes using fludarabine-based haematopoietic cell transplantation. Br J Haematol. 2006;133(3):305–14.
51. Liu L, Miao M, He H, et al. Severe aplastic anemia patients with infection who received an allogeneic hematopoietic stem cell transplantation had a better chance: long-term outcomes of a multicenter study. Front Immunol. 2022;13:955095.
52. Storb R, Longton G, Anasetti C, et al. Changing trends in marrow transplantation for aplastic anemia. Bone Marrow Transplant. 1992;10(Suppl 1):45–52.
53. Territo MC. Autologous bone marrow repopulation following high dose cyclophosphamide and allogeneic marrow transplantation in aplastic anaemia. Br J Haematol. 1977;36(3):305–12.
54. Champlin RE, Perez WS, Passweg JR, et al. Bone marrow transplantation for severe aplastic anemia: a randomized controlled study of conditioning regimens. Blood. 2007;109(10):4582–5.
55. Gale RP, Ho W, Feig S, et al. Prevention of graft rejection following bone marrow transplantation. Blood. 1981;57(1):9–12.
56. McCann SR, Bacigalupo A, Gluckman E, et al. Graft rejection and second bone marrow transplants for acquired aplastic anaemia: a report from the Aplastic Anaemia Working Party of the European Bone Marrow Transplant Group. Bone Marrow Transplant. 1994;13(3):233–7.
57. Gluckman E, Horowitz MM, Champlin RE, et al. Bone marrow transplantation for severe aplastic anemia: influence of conditioning and graft-versus-host disease prophylaxis regimens on outcome. Blood. 1992;79(1):269–75.
58. Storb R, Etzioni R, Anasetti C, et al. Cyclophosphamide combined with antithymocyte globulin in preparation for allogeneic marrow transplants in patients with aplastic anemia. Blood. 1994;84(3):941–9.
59. Storb R, Thomas ED, Buckner CD, et al. Allogeneic marrow grafting for treatment of aplastic anemia: a follow-up on long-term survivors. Blood. 1976;48(4):485–90.
60. Storb R, Thomas ED, Buckner CD, et al. Allogeneic marrow grafting for treatment of aplastic anemia. Blood. 1974;43(2):157–80.
61. Zaidi U, Fatima M, Samad SA, et al. Fludarabine/cyclophosphamide conditioning regimen in aplastic anemia patients receiving matched-sibling donor transplant is non-inferior to ATG/cyclophosphamide: a single-center experience from Pakistan. Stem Cells Int. 2022;2022:1442613.

62. Salamonowicz-Bodzioch M, Rosa M, Fraczkiewicz J, et al. Fludarabine-cyclophosphamide-based conditioning with antithymocyte globulin Serotherapy is associated with durable engraftment and manageable infections in children with severe aplastic anemia. J Clin Med. 2021;10(19)
63. El Fakih R, Alhayli S, Ahmed SO, et al. Full dose cyclophosphamide with the addition of Fludarabine for matched sibling transplants in severe aplastic anemia. Transplant Cell Ther. 2021;27(10):851.e1–6.
64. Al-Zahrani H, Nassar A, Al-Mohareb F, et al. Fludarabine-based conditioning chemotherapy for allogeneic hematopoietic stem cell transplantation in acquired severe aplastic anemia. Biol Blood Marrow Transplant. 2011;17(5):717–22.
65. Kim H, Lee JH, Joo YD, et al. A randomized comparison of cyclophosphamide vs. reduced dose cyclophosphamide plus fludarabine for allogeneic hematopoietic cell transplantation in patients with aplastic anemia and hypoplastic myelodysplastic syndrome. Ann Hematol. 2012;91(9):1459–69.
66. Iftikhar R, Chaudhry QUN, Satti TM, et al. Comparison of conventional cyclophosphamide versus Fludarabine-based conditioning in high-risk aplastic anemia patients undergoing matched-related donor transplantation. Clin Hematol Int. 2020;2(2):82–91.
67. Maury S, Bacigalupo A, Anderlini P, et al. Improved outcome of patients older than 30 years receiving HLA-identical sibling hematopoietic stem cell transplantation for severe acquired aplastic anemia using fludarabine-based conditioning: a comparison with conventional conditioning regimen. Haematologica. 2009;94(9):1312–5.
68. Marsh JC, Gupta V, Lim Z, et al. Alemtuzumab with fludarabine and cyclophosphamide reduces chronic graft-versus-host disease after allogeneic stem cell transplantation for acquired aplastic anemia. Blood. 2011;118(8):2351–7.
69. Marsh JC, Pearce RM, Koh MB, et al. Retrospective study of alemtuzumab vs ATG-based conditioning without irradiation for unrelated and matched sibling donor transplants in acquired severe aplastic anemia: a study from the British Society for Blood and Marrow Transplantation. Bone Marrow Transplant. 2014;49(1):42–8.
70. Bejanyan N, Kim S, Hebert KM, et al. Choice of conditioning regimens for bone marrow transplantation in severe aplastic anemia. Blood Adv. 2019;3(20):3123–31.
71. Kekre N, Zhang Y, Zhang MJ, et al. Effect of antithymocyte globulin source on outcomes of bone marrow transplantation for severe aplastic anemia. Haematologica. 2017;102(7):1291–8.
72. Bacigalupo A. Antithymocyte globulin and transplants for aplastic anemia. Haematologica. 2017;102(7):1137–8.
73. Kako S, Kanda Y, Onizuka M, et al. Allogeneic hematopoietic stem cell transplantation for aplastic anemia with pre-transplant conditioning using fludarabine, reduced-dose cyclophosphamide, and low-dose thymoglobulin: a KSGCT prospective study. Am J Hematol. 2020;95(3):251–7.
74. Hinterberger W, Rowlings PA, Hinterberger-Fischer M, et al. Results of transplanting bone marrow from genetically identical twins into patients with aplastic anemia. Ann Intern Med. 1997;126(2):116–22.
75. Gerull S, Stern M, Apperley J, et al. Syngeneic transplantation in aplastic anemia: pre-transplant conditioning and peripheral blood are associated with improved engraftment: an observational study on behalf of the Severe Aplastic Anemia and Pediatric Diseases Working Parties of the European Group for Blood and Marrow Transplantation. Haematologica. 2013;98(11):1804–9.
76. Bacigalupo A, Socie G, Schrezenmeier H, et al. Bone marrow versus peripheral blood as the stem cell source for sibling transplants in acquired aplastic anemia: survival advantage for bone marrow in all age groups. Haematologica. 2012;97(8):1142–8.
77. Schrezenmeier H, Passweg JR, Marsh JC, et al. Worse outcome and more chronic GVHD with peripheral blood progenitor cells than bone marrow in HLA-matched sibling donor transplants for young patients with severe acquired aplastic anemia. Blood. 2007;110(4):1397–400.
78. Morton J, Hutchins C, Durrant S. Granulocyte-colony-stimulating factor (G-CSF)-primed allogeneic bone marrow: significantly less graft-versus-host disease and comparable engraftment to G-CSF-mobilized peripheral blood stem cells. Blood. 2001;98(12):3186–91.

79. El Fakih R, Alfraih F, Alhayli S, et al. Frontline-matched sibling donor transplant of aplastic anemia patients using primed versus steady-state bone marrow grafts. Ann Hematol. 2022;101(2):421–8.
80. Locatelli F, Bruno B, Zecca M, et al. Cyclosporin A and short-term methotrexate versus cyclosporin A as graft versus host disease prophylaxis in patients with severe aplastic anemia given allogeneic bone marrow transplantation from an HLA-identical sibling: results of a GITMO/EBMT randomized trial. Blood. 2000;96(5):1690–7.
81. Passweg JR, Socie G, Hinterberger W, et al. Bone marrow transplantation for severe aplastic anemia: has outcome improved? Blood. 1997;90(2):858–64.
82. Gerrie A, Marsh J, Lipton JH, Messner H, Gupta V. Marrow transplantation for severe aplastic anemia with significant renal impairment. Bone Marrow Transplant. 2007;39(5):311–3.
83. Hill RS, Petersen FB, Storb R, et al. Mixed hematologic chimerism after allogeneic marrow transplantation for severe aplastic anemia is associated with a higher risk of graft rejection and a lessened incidence of acute graft-versus-host disease. Blood. 1986;67(3):811–6.
84. Huss R, Deeg HJ, Gooley T, et al. Effect of mixed chimerism on graft-versus-host disease, disease recurrence and survival after HLA-identical marrow transplantation for aplastic anemia or chronic myelogenous leukemia. Bone Marrow Transplant. 1996;18(4):767–76.
85. Bortin MM, Gale RP, Rimm AA. Allogeneic bone marrow transplantation for 144 patients with severe aplastic anemia. JAMA. 1981;245(11):1132–9.
86. Buchbinder D, Nugent DJ, Brazauskas R, et al. Late effects in hematopoietic cell transplant recipients with acquired severe aplastic anemia: a report from the late effects working committee of the center for international blood and marrow transplant research. Biol Blood Marrow Transplant. 2012;18(12):1776–84.
87. Hinterberger-Fischer M, Kier P, Kalhs P, et al. Fertility, pregnancies and offspring complications after bone marrow transplantation. Bone Marrow Transplant. 1991;7(1):5–9.
88. Schmidt H, Ehninger G, Dopfer R, Waller HD. Pregnancy after bone marrow transplantation for severe aplastic anemia. Bone Marrow Transplant. 1987;2(3):329–32.
89. Sanders JE. The impact of marrow transplant preparative regimens on subsequent growth and development. The Seattle Marrow Transplant Team. Semin Hematol. 1991;28(3):244–9.
90. Deeg HJ, Socie G, Schoch G, et al. Malignancies after marrow transplantation for aplastic anemia and fanconi anemia: a joint Seattle and Paris analysis of results in 700 patients. Blood. 1996;87(1):386–92.
91. Witherspoon RP, Storb R, Pepe M, Longton G, Sullivan KM. Cumulative incidence of secondary solid malignant tumors in aplastic anemia patients given marrow grafts after conditioning with chemotherapy alone. Blood. 1992;79(1):289–91.

Open Access This chapter is licensed under the terms of the Creative Commons Attribution 4.0 International License (http://creativecommons.org/licenses/by/4.0/), which permits use, sharing, adaptation, distribution and reproduction in any medium or format, as long as you give appropriate credit to the original author(s) and the source, provide a link to the Creative Commons license and indicate if changes were made.

The images or other third party material in this chapter are included in the chapter's Creative Commons license, unless indicated otherwise in a credit line to the material. If material is not included in the chapter's Creative Commons license and your intended use is not permitted by statutory regulation or exceeds the permitted use, you will need to obtain permission directly from the copyright holder.

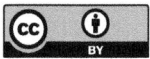

Chapter 11
Unrelated Bone Marrow Transplantation for Acquired Aplastic Anemia

Andrea Bacigalupo and Rainer Storb

Introduction

A program of bone marrow transplantation (BMT) in patients with aplastic anemia (AA) was developed in Seattle in the early seventies, originally from HLA-identical siblings [1]. The outcomes were encouraging for those early days, but problems with rejection and graft versus host disease (GvHD) were immediately evident, especially in patients who were immunized by preceding blood transfusions. The original conditioning regimen included cyclophosphamide (CY 50 mg/kgx4), to which antithymocyte globulin (ATG) was added later [2]; GvHD prophylaxis was methotrexate (MTX) alone, administered on day +1, +3, +11, and then weekly until day +100 [1]. It was in the eighties that cyclosporin (CSA) was added to MTX and proven to be superior to either MTX or CSA alone [3–5]. Unrelated donor transplants were also tested in single patients [6] but became largely employed a decade later, following studies in the canine model [7, 8] and with the availability of volunteer donors through local or international registries [9]. We will discuss specific issues concerning unrelated donor transplants, including (a) selection of patients, (b) choice of the best donor, (c) the conditioning regimen, (d) GvHD prophylaxis, and (e) the stem cell source.

A. Bacigalupo (✉)
Dipartimento di Scienze di Laboratorio ed Ematologiche, Fondazione Policlinico Universitario A. Gemelli IRCCS, Rome, Italy
e-mail: andrea.bacigalupo@unicatt.it

R. Storb
Clinical Research Division, Fred Hutchinson Cancer Center and Division of Hematology and Oncology, University of Washington School of Medicine, Seattle, WA, USA

Selection of Patients

Every patient with a diagnosis of AA should be HLA-typed at diagnosis, together with healthy family members [10]; in the absence of an HLA-identical sibling, the search for an unrelated donor should be started. The choice of whether to proceed with a transplant or immunosuppressive therapy (IST) as the first line depends on the age of the patient and possibly on the severity of the disease: Young patients <40 years of age with severe disease should be considered for early transplantation, with an HLA-identical sibling but also with an HLA-matched unrelated donor [10]. There is no unanimity on whether older patients (>40 years) should be given first-line ATG+CSA and eltrombopag (ACE) [11] or receive an upfront transplant [12]. Several groups are now considering HLA-haploidentical family members also as first-line transplant donors, and this may be considered in young patients, preferably within a clinical trial [13, 14]. Unrelated HLA-matched transplants are now considered the standard of care for AA patients who have failed one course of immunosuppressive therapy, but more and more transplant groups are considering unrelated grafts as the first-line treatment. The upper age limit for unrelated transplantation is a moving target: Until 2015, results were significantly worse in patients over 40 years of age [10] and had not improved with time [15]. But things may be changing, and encouraging outcomes have also been reported in elderly patients with AA [16, 17].

Choice of Unrelated Donor

The technique of HLA typing has significantly improved over the past decades, and we can now identify unrelated donors matched at a high resolution for the HLA A, B, C, DRB1, and DQB1 loci [18], the so-called 8/8 (A, B, C, and DRB1) or 10/10 (A, B, C, DRB1, and DQB1) allele-matched donors. This has resulted in improved outcomes in AA patients [19]. The question is whether, for AA patients, we can accept donors who are less-than-8/8 HLA-matched: In a registry based study of 2010, mortality was 17% for HLA-matched unrelated grafts and 34% for less-than-8/8-matched unrelated grafts [20]; Center for International Blood and Marrow Transplant Research (CIBMTR) study in nonmalignant disorders showed that the outcome of 8/8 HLA-matched unrelated transplants was significantly better than that of HLA-mismatched grafts, the major problem being graft failure [21]. In a multicenter study, Deeg and coworkers also reported superior results with 8/8 HLA-antigen-matched unrelated donors compared to those among less-than-8/8 HLA-antigen-matched donors [22]. HLA-mismatched grafts may be more successful with new transplant platforms, as we will discuss further in this chapter.

Conditioning Regimens

The choice of the optimal conditioning regimen is important: We need to deliver enough immunosuppression to allogeneic engraftment. Myeloablation is probably not important, and long-term toxicity should be kept in mind since AA is a nonmalignant disease. In a trial using a single dose of 5 Gy thoracoabdominal irradiation (TAI), engraftment was very successful, but the cumulative incidence of second tumors at 8 years was 22% [23]. A combination of fludarabine and cyclophosphamide (FC) seems to have gained international approval, given several reports of favorable outcomes [24–28], even when cord blood was used as a stem cell source [29]: The FC regimen combines low toxicity with high immunosuppressive activity.

Doses of cyclophosphamide (CY) ranging from 0 to 150 mg/kg were tested prospectively in combination with fludarabine and low-dose total body irradiation (TBI) [30]: CY at 150 mg/kg was too toxic, and CY at 0 mg/kg resulted in an unacceptably high rejection rate (3/3). A CY dose of either 50 or 100 mg/kg in combination with FLU and low-dose TBI proved to be most effective for the engraftment of unrelated donor transplants [31]. To enhance engraftment, TBI doses ranging from 2 Gy to 10 Gy have been evaluated, and 2 Gy was found to be both well-tolerated and effective for AA patients [32, 33]. Figure 11.1a represents a conditioning regimen, with the combination of CY, FLU, and TBI 2 Gy, together with rabbit ATG, followed by unmanipulated marrow or peripheral blood, if one cannot get marrow, and GvHD prevention with CSA and MTX. The addition of a small dose of anti-CD20 monoclonal antibody will reduce, if not eliminate, the risk of EBV reactivation and lymphoproliferative diseases. Finally, the use of ATG in the conditioning regimen enhances survival in the unrelated donor setting [34]. Also, alemtuzumab can be effectively combined with FLU-CY (Fig. 11.1b) [35]. Of note, however, a CIBMTR study determined that all currently used conditioning regimens resulted in equivalent overall outcomes [36]. While in that study, age remained the most significant predictor of survival, it is unclear whether the adverse effect of age is due to the policy of trying IST first in such patients. Transplanting only after the failure of IST, when patients might have become infected and refractory to transfusions and are suffering from an iron overload, sets the stage for poor transplantation outcomes.

GvHD Prophylaxis

One standard regimen for GvHD prophylaxis includes administering ATG and CSA, 3 mg/kg from day −1, and MTX 10 mg/m^2 on days +1, +3, +6, and +11 [20]. ATG can either be produced in rabbits or horses. A CIBMTR study showed that rabbit ATG is superior to horse ATG in reducing acute and chronic GvHD after HLA-matched sibling grafts as well as in improving survival after unrelated grafts [37]. A conventional dose for rabbit ATG (thymoglobulin) ranges between 5 and 7.5 mg/kg (total dose), administered during 3 days before transplant; for horse ATG

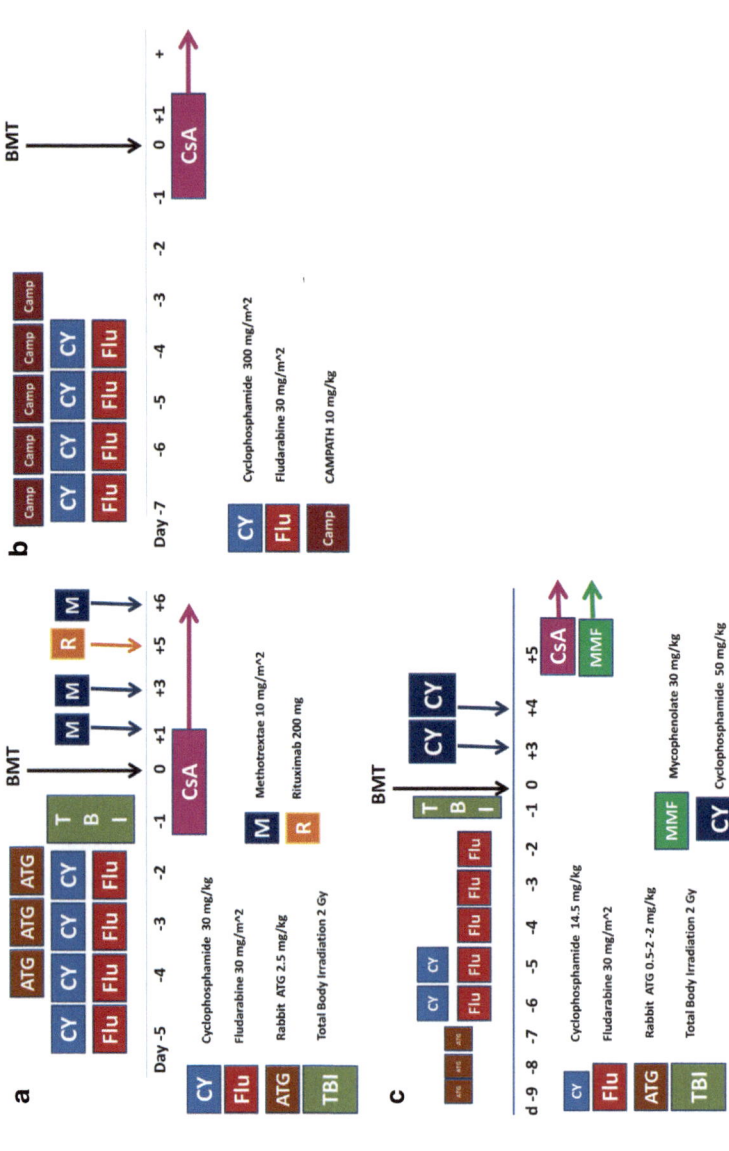

Fig. 11.1 (**a**) A standard platform for unrelated donor transplant, detailed in Ref. [29]: In that study, with cord blood, MTX was omitted. When using marrow or peripheral blood, the combination of CSA and MTX should be used (**b**) The fludarabine, cyclophosphamide, and Campath (FCC) regimen (Ref. [35]), developed in the United Kingdom. This is a radiation-free regimen (**c**) The Baltimore platform, with four drugs preventing GvHD (ATG, PTCY, CSA, and MMF). In the original Baltimore study, this regimen was designed for haploidentical donors. It is now also used in unrelated donor transplants (Ref. [13])

(ATGAM), this converts to a total dose of 120 mg/kg. Alemtuzumab is also used in combination with FC, alongside encouraging the control of acute and chronic GvHD [35]. More recently, high-dose post-transplant cyclophosphamide (PTCY), 50 mg/kg on days +3 and +4, followed by a calcineurin inhibitor (CNI) combined with mycophenolate (MMF) starting on day +5, has been introduced for HLA-haploidentical related grafts [13]. This regimen is outlined in Fig. 11.1c. Given the very encouraging control of GvHD, it is also currently being proposed for unrelated grafts and possibly older HLA-matched sibling transplants [38–40]. If the early results of PTCY are confirmed, we may be encouraged to prefer first-line transplantation for older AA patients rather than trying IST first.

Stem Cell Source

Bone marrow is the preferred stem cell source for patients with AA [41] because the risks of acute and chronic GvHD are minimized compared to peripheral blood–derived grafts [42, 43]. However, it is often difficult to obtain marrow from unrelated donor centers, and peripheral blood has become the most frequently used source of stem cells. It remains to be seen whether GvHD prophylaxis with PTCY or alpha/beta T cell and CD19 cell depletion will enable chronic GvHD-free long-term survival with the use of peripheral blood–derived stem cells in the setting of 8/8 or 7/8 HLA-allele-matched unrelated transplants.

Supportive Care

Supportive care has changed over the past years, including early diagnosis and more effective treatment of bacterial, viral, and fungal infections. Early molecular diagnosis of bloodstream infections has radically improved survival in septic patients. Prophylaxis with oral antibiotics remains the standard in some centers but not in others, out of concern for the emergence of multiresistant bacterial strains. *Pneumocystis jirovecii* and herpes virus prophylaxis should always be standard after an allogeneic hemopoietic stem cell transplantation (HSCT). All blood products, except for the allogeneic graft, are routinely leukocyte-depleted and irradiated at 25 Gy before being transfused. Patients are monitored for cytomegalovirus (CMV) reactivation weekly, by measuring serum CMV copies by PCR, until day +100, and preemptive treatment is started when CMV copies exceed 1000/ml. Recently, letermovir has been approved for CMV prophylaxis, and this has significantly reduced the proportion of patients with CMV reactivation. EBV viremia may be another complication in AA patients since a diagnosis of AA and the use of ATG are risk factors for posttransplant EBV-related lymphoproliferative disorders. Prophylactic use of rituximab 200 mg early after transplantation has been reported to reduce or eliminate the problem of EBV reactivation.

Finding an Appropriately HLA-Matched Unrelated Donor and Treatment Strategies

Maury and coworkers have asked a very simple question: If a patient with AA activates an unrelated donor search, how successful is the search [44]? There were 179 patients, nonresponders to ATG and CSA, who activated a search before ($n = 85$) or after ($n = 94$) the year 2000. An HLA-matched donor was identified for 118 patients. The HLA matching was not up-to-date (class I being low resolution!). However, there was a significant survival advantage for younger patients (<17 years) with a donor (79% versus 53%, $p = 0.001$) and for all ages after the year 2000 (74% versus 47%) [44]. The authors of this "donor versus no-donor" analysis concluded that a transplant is the best option for patients who failed a course of immunosuppressive therapy.

A follow-up question is whether an unrelated HLA-matched transplant should be the first-line therapy [12, 45, 46]. In young patients, the advantages of upfront transplantation, also from an unrelated donor, include reduced early infectious complications, reduced long-term clonal disorders, and excellent survival compared to transplants in patients who had failed IST. A pediatric study showed a 92% 2-year event-free survival for children who underwent unrelated transplantation as the first-line therapy and 87% survival for those who underwent HLA-identical sibling transplantation as the first line ($p = 0.37$). In contrast, 40% survival was observed for patients who were treated with IST ($p = 0.0001$) and 74% survival for patients who underwent unrelated transplantation after the failure of IST ($p = 0.02$). Results were also favorable in terms of neutrophil ($>0.5 \times 10^9/l$) and platelet ($>50 \times 10^9/l$) recovery times. Thus, for young patients, upfront HLA-matched unrelated transplantation appears comparable to HLA-identical sibling BMT. Moreover, it was superior to first-line IST or transplantation after the failure of IST [46]. The latter approach sets the stage for failure because of infections, multiple antibiotic and antifungal use, and detrimental effects from iron overload due to multiple transfusions.

Summary

Bone marrow (or peripheral blood stem cell) transplantation is the only curative option for patients with severe aplastic anemia (AA): This treatment approach establishes normal, long-term hematopoiesis without the risk of clonal evolution. The longest-surviving patients have survived for more than 50 years after transplantation. Gradual but relentless progress in transplantation has been achieved, including the development of new conditioning and GvHD prevention regimens. The coming years will tell us if these changes will also enable early transplantation in older patients with aplastic anemia.

Conflict of Interest The authors have no disclosures.

References

1. Storb R, Thomas ED, Weiden PL, et al. Aplastic anemia treated by allogeneic bone marrow transplantation: a report on 49 new cases from Seattle. Blood. 1976;48(6):817–41.
2. Storb R, Etzioni R, Anasetti C, et al. Cyclophosphamide combined with antithymocyte globulin in preparation for allogeneic marrow transplants in patients with aplastic anemia. Blood. 1994;84(3):941–9.
3. Storb R, Deeg HJ, Whitehead J, et al. Methotrexate and cyclosporine compared with cyclosporine alone for prophylaxis of acute graft versus host disease after marrow transplantation for leukemia. N Engl J Med. 1986;314(12):729–35. https://doi.org/10.1056/NEJM198603203141201.
4. Storb R, Deeg HJ, Farewell V, et al. Marrow transplantation for severe aplastic anemia: methotrexate alone compared with a combination of methotrexate and cyclosporine for prevention of acute graft-versus-host disease. Blood. 1986;68(1):119–25.
5. Locatelli F, Bruno B, Zecca M, Van-Lint MT, McCann S, Arcese W, Dallorso S, Di Bartolomeo P, Fagioli F, Locasciulli A, Lawler M, Bacigalupo A. Cyclosporin A and short-term methotrexate versus cyclosporin A as graft versus host disease prophylaxis in patients with severe aplastic anemia given allogeneic bone marrow transplantation from an HLA-identical sibling: results of a GITMO/EBMT randomized trial. Blood. 2000;96(5):1690–7.
6. Speck B, Zwaan FE, van Rood JJ, Eernisse JG. Allogeneic bone marrow transplantation in a patient with aplastic anemia using a phenotypically HL-A-identifcal unrelated donor. Transplantation. 1973;16(1):24–8.
7. Storb R, Weiden PL, Graham TC, Lerner KG, Thomas ED. Marrow grafts between DLA-identical and homozygous unrelated dogs: evidence for an additional locus involved in graft-versus-host disease. Transplantation. 1977;24(3):165–74.
8. Deeg HJ, Storb R, Shulman HM, Weiden PL, Graham TC, Thomas ED. Engraftment of DLA-nonidentical unrelated canine marrow after high-dose fractionated total body irradiation. Transplantation. 1982;33(4):443–6.
9. Goldman JM. A special report: bone marrow transplants using volunteer donors–recommendations and requirements for a standardized practice throughout the world–1994 update. The WMDA Executive Committee. Blood. 1994;84(9):2833–9.
10. Bacigalupo A. How I treat acquired aplastic anemia. Blood. 2017;129(11):1428–36.
11. Peffault de Latour R, Kulasekararaj A, Iacobelli S, et al. Eltrombopag added to immunosuppression in severe aplastic anemia. N Engl J Med. 2022;386(1):11–23.
12. Georges GE, Doney K, Storb R. Severe aplastic anemia: allogeneic bone marrow transplantation as first-line treatment. Blood Adv. 2018;2(15):2020–8. https://doi.org/10.1182/bloodadvances.2018021162. PMID: 30108110; PMCID: PMC6093726.
13. DeZern AE, Zahurak M, Symons HJ, et al. Alternative donor BMT with posttransplant cyclophosphamide as initial therapy for acquired severe aplastic anemia. Blood. 2023;141(25):3031–8.
14. Liu L, Zhang Y, Jiao W, et al. Comparison of efficacy and health-related quality of life of first-line haploidentical hematopoietic stem cell transplantation with unrelated cord blood infusion and first-line immunosuppressive therapy for acquired severe aplastic anemia. Leukemia. 2020;34(12):3359–69.
15. Giammarco S, Peffault de Latour R, Sica S, et al. Transplant outcome for patients with acquired aplastic anemia over the age of 40: has the outcome improved? Blood. 2018;131(17):1989–92.
16. Storb R. Allogeneic bone marrow transplantation for aplastic anemia. Int J Hematol. 2022;119:220. https://doi.org/10.1007/s12185-022-03506-6.
17. Sheth VS, Potter V, Gandhi SA, et al. Similar outcomes of alemtuzumab-based hematopoietic cell transplantation for SAA patients older or younger than 50 years. Blood Adv. 2019;3(20):3070–9.
18. Petersdorf E. In celebration of Ruggero Cepellini: HLA in transplantation. HLA. 2017;89:71–6.

19. Maury S, Balère-Appert ML, Chir Z, et al. Unrelated stem cell transplantation for severe acquired aplastic anemia: improved outcome in the era of high-resolution HLA matching between donor and recipient. Haematologica. 2007;92(5):589–96.
20. Bacigalupo A, Socie' G, Lanino E, et al. Fludarabine, cyclophosphamide, antithymocyte globulin, with or without low dose total body irradiation, for alternative donor transplants, in acquired severe aplastic anemia: a retrospective study from the EBMT-SAA Working Party. Haematologica. 2010;95(6):976–82.
21. Horan J, Wang T, Haagenson M, et al. Evaluation of HLA matching in unrelated hematopoietic stem cell transplantation for non malignant disorders. Blood. 2012;120(14):2918–24.
22. Deeg HJ, O'Donnell M, Tolar J, et al. Optimization of conditioning for marrow transplantation from unrelated donors for patients with aplastic anemia after failure of immunosuppressive therapy. Blood. 2006;108(5):1485–91.
23. Socié G, Henry-Amar M, Cosset JM, et al. Increased incidence of solid malignant tumors after bone marrow transplantation for severe aplastic anemia. Blood. 1991;78(2):277–9.
24. Okuda S, Terasako K, Oshima K, et al. Fludarabine, cyclophosphamide, anti- thymocyte globulin, and low-dose totalbody irradiation conditioning enables 1-HLA-locus-mismatched hematopoietic stemcell transplantation for very severe aplastic anemia without affecting ovarian function. Am J Hematol. 2009;84(3):167.
25. Koh LP, Koh MB, Ng HY, et al. Allogeneic hematopoietic stem cell transplantation for patients with severe aplastic anemia following non myeloablative conditioning using 200-cGy totalbody irradiation and fludarabine. Biol Blood Marrow Transplant. 2006;12(8):887–90.
26. George B, Mathews V, Viswabandya A, Kavitha ML, Srivastava A, Chandy M. Fludarabine and cyclophosphamide based reduced intensity conditioning (RIC) regimens reduce rejection and improve outcome in Indian patients undergoing allogeneic stem cell transplantation for severe aplastic anemia. Bone Marrow Transplant. 2007;40(1):13–8.
27. ResnickI B, Aker M, Shapira MY, et al. Allogeneic stem cell transplantation for severe acquired aplastic anaemia using a fludarabine-based preparative regimen. Br J Haematol. 2006;133(6):649–54.
28. Srinivasan R, Takahashi Y, McCoy JP, et al. Overcoming graft rejection in heavily transfused and allo-immunised patients with bone marrow failure syndromes using fludarabine-based haematopoietic cell transplantation. Br J Haematol. 2006;133(3):305–9.
29. Peffault de Latour R, Chevret S, Jubert C, et al. Francophone Society of Bone Marrow Transplantation and Cellular Therapy. Unrelated cord blood transplantation in patients with idiopathic refractory severe aplastic anemia: a nationwide phase 2 study. Blood. 2018;132(7):750–4.
30. Tolar J, Deeg HJ, Arai S, Horwitz M, Antin JH, McCarty JM, Adams RH, Ewell M, Leifer ES, Gersten ID, Carter SL, Horowitz MM, Nakamura R, Pulsipher MA, Difronzo NL, Confer DL, Eapen M, Anderlini P. Fludarabine-based conditioning for marrow transplantation from unrelated donors in severe aplastic anemia: early results of a cyclophosphamide dose deescalation study show life-threatening adverse events at predefined cyclophosphamide dose levels. Biol Blood Marrow Transplant. 2012;18(7):1007–11. https://doi.org/10.1016/j.bbmt.2012.04.014. Epub 2012 Apr 27. PMID: 22546497; PMCID: PMC3677744.
31. Anderlini P, Wu J, Gersten I, et al. Cyclophosphamide conditioning in patients with severe aplastic anaemia given unrelated marrow transplantation: a phase 1-2 dose de-escalation study. Lancet Haematol. 2015;2(9):e367–75.
32. Deeg HJ, Amylon ID, Harris RE, et al. Marrow transplants from unrelated donors for patients with aplastic anemia: minimum effective dose of total body irradiation. Biol Blood Marrow Transplant. 2001;7:208–15.
33. Kojima S, Matsuyama T, Kato S, et al. Outcome of 154 patients with severe aplastic anemia who received transplants from unrelated donors: the Japan Marrow Donor Program. Blood. 2002;100:799–803.

34. Bacigalupo A, Socié G, Hamladji RM, et al. Aplastic Anemia Working Party of the European Group for Blood Marrow Transplantation. Current outcome of HLA identical sibling versus unrelated donor transplants in severe aplastic anemia: an EBMT analysis. Haematologica. 2015;100(5):696–702.
35. Marsh JC, Gupta V, Lim Z, et al. Alemtuzumab with fludarabine and cylophosphamide reduces chronic graft-versus-host disease after allogeneic stem cell transplantation for acquired aplastic anemia. Blood. 2011;118(8):2351–7.
36. Bejanyan N, Kim S, Hebert KM, et al. Choice of conditioning regimens for bone marrow transplantation in severe aplastic anemia. Blood Adv. 2019;3(20):3123–31.
37. Kekre N, Zhang Y, Zhan M-J. Effect of antithymocyte globulin source on outcomes of bone marrow transplantation for severe aplastic anemia. Haematologica. 2017;102(7):1291–8.
38. Arcuri LJ, Ribeiro AAF, Hamerschlak N, et al. Posttransplant cyclophosphamide beyond haploidentical transplantation. Ann Hematol. 2023;103:1483–91. https://doi.org/10.1007/s00277-023-05300-8. Epub ahead of print.
39. George B, Pn N, Devasia AJ, Kulkarni U, Korula A, Lakshmi KM, et al. Post-transplant cyclophosphamide as sole graft-versus-host disease prophylaxis is feasible in patients undergoing peripheral blood stem cell transplantation for severe aplastic anemia using matched sibling donors. Biol Blood Marrow Transplant. 2018;24(3):494–500. https://doi.org/10.1016/j.bbmt.2017.10.034. Epub 2017 Oct 31.
40. Kwon M, Bailén R, Pascual-Cascón MJ, et al. Posttransplant cyclophosphamide vs cyclosporin A and methotrexate as GVHD prophylaxis in matched sibling transplantation. Blood Adv. 2019;3(21):3351–9.
41. Bacigalupo A, Socié G, Schrezenmeier H, et al. Aplastic Anemia Working Party of the European Group for Blood and Marrow Transplantation (WPSAA-EBMT). Bone marrow versus peripheral blood as the stem cell source for sibling transplants in acquired aplastic anemia: survival advantage for bone marrow in all age groups. Haematologica. 2012;97(8):1142 8.
42. Lacan C, Lambert J, Forcade E, et al. Bone marrow graft versus peripheral blood graft in haploidentical hematopoietic stem cells transplantation: a retrospective analysis in1344 patients of SFGM-TC registry. J Hematol Oncol. 2024;17(1):2. https://doi.org/10.1186/s13045-023-01515-4. PMID: 38185663; PMCID: PMC10773006.
43. Hayashi H, Iwasaki M, Nakasone H, et al. Impact of stem cell selection between bone marrow and peripheral blood stem cells for unrelated hematopoietic stem cell transplantation for hematologic malignancies: on behalf of the Donor/Source Working Group of the Japanese Society for Transplantation and Cellular Therapy. Cytotherapy. 2023;S1465–3249(23):01122. https://doi.org/10.1016/j.jcyt.2023.11.012. Epub ahead of print.
44. Maury S, Balère-Appert ML, Pollichieni S, et al. Severe Aplastic Anemia Working Party of the European Group for Blood and Marrow Transplantation (EBMT). Outcome of patients activating an unrelated donor search for severe acquired aplastic anemia. Am J Hematol. 2013;88(10):868–73. https://doi.org/10.1002/ajh.23522. Epub 2013 Aug 1.
45. Marsh JCW, Risitano AM, Mufti GJ. The case for upfront HLA-matched unrelated donor hematopoietic stem cell transplantation as a curative option for adult acquired severe aplastic anemia. Biol Blood Marrow Transplant. 2019;25(9):e277–84. https://doi.org/10.1016/j.bbmt.2019.05.012. Epub 2019 May 24.
46. Dufour C, Veys P, Carraro E, et al. Similar outcome of upfront-unrelated and matched sibling stem cell transplantation in idiopathic paediatric aplastic anaemia. A study on behalf of the UK Paediatric BMT Working Party, Paediatric Diseases Working Party and Severe Aplastic Anaemia Working Party of EBMT. Br J Haematol. 2015;171(4):585–94.

Open Access This chapter is licensed under the terms of the Creative Commons Attribution 4.0 International License (http://creativecommons.org/licenses/by/4.0/), which permits use, sharing, adaptation, distribution and reproduction in any medium or format, as long as you give appropriate credit to the original author(s) and the source, provide a link to the Creative Commons license and indicate if changes were made.

The images or other third party material in this chapter are included in the chapter's Creative Commons license, unless indicated otherwise in a credit line to the material. If material is not included in the chapter's Creative Commons license and your intended use is not permitted by statutory regulation or exceeds the permitted use, you will need to obtain permission directly from the copyright holder.

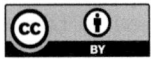

Chapter 12
Haploidentical Donor Bone Marrow Transplantation for Acquired Severe Aplastic Anemia

Amy E. DeZern, Carmem Bonfim, and Andrea Bacigalupo

Introduction

Immunosuppressive therapy (IST) has been the standard frontline treatment for acquired severe aplastic anemia (SAA) for decades, except for patients aged <40 years with a suitable human leukocyte antigen (HLA)-matched-sibling donor (MSD) for bone marrow (BM) transplantation (hematopoietic stem cell transplantation (HSCT)) [1, 2]. Increasingly, the field is moving toward as much HSCT upfront as feasible, and still, patients who do not respond to IST or relapse after it often require HSCT. Utilization of haploidentical donors in both settings is increasingly of value to broaden the donor pool. Successful allogeneic hematopoietic stem cell transplantation (alloHSCT) in SAA not only overcomes the complications of the disease but also eliminates the risk of relapse and secondary clonal disease.

Innovations in HSCT in recent decades have steadily improved the outcomes [3]. Standard platforms exist with the goal of rapid hematopoietic reconstitution, representing a cure in SAA [3]. Long-term historical survival after HSCT is ~90% in patients aged <20 years [4, 5] and 75% in older patients [3, 5]. Due to concerns for morbidity and mortality, HSCT with an unrelated or HLA-haploidentical, related donor has been most commonly used, following the failure of IST in most centers

A. E. DeZern (✉)
Sidney Kimmel Comprehensive Cancer Center, Johns Hopkins University School of Medicine, Baltimore, MD, USA
e-mail: Adezern1@jhmi.edu

C. Bonfim
Division of Pediatric Transplantation and Cellular Therapy, Duke University, Durham, NC, USA

A. Bacigalupo
Dipartimento di Scienze di Laboratorio ed Ematologiche, Fondazione Policlinico Universitario A. Gemelli IRCCS, Rome, Italy
e-mail: andrea.bacigalupo@unicatt.it

[6–12]. However, innovations in recent decades have steadily reduced the morbidity and mortality of adult patients undergoing alternative-donor HSCT [13, 14]. Multicenter clinical trials are ongoing to add to the knowledge of haploidentical HSCT (haplo-HSCT), specifically in SAA.

Results of Haplo-HSCT for SAA

Previous reports of haploidentical HSCT in SAA have produced heterogeneous results depending on the patient population and are also limited by a small sample size (Table 12.1) [8, 9, 19–21, 23–26]. In these small and moderately sized series, rejection has been between 6% and 25%, acute graft-versus-host disease (aGVHD) was between 12% and 30%, chronic GVHD (cGVHD) was between 20% and 40%, and overall survival (OS) was between 60% and 100% [8, 9, 17, 19–21, 23–26]. Limited comparisons can be made across these studies, but some differences between studies may be related to infectious complications, donor-specific antibodies (DSAs), and the amount of patients' previous therapies. Most centers around the world lack horse antithymocyte globulin (ATG), so not only the amount of previous therapies but also the quality of treatment and transfusions can vary widely. Most patients transplanted in developing countries are heavily transfused and have received only rabbit ATG. Nonetheless, in the relapsed and refractory setting, all patients had previously received IST at the time of diagnosis for their SAA, and thus, this may have impacted engraftment more favorably with any of the conditioning regimens. Furthermore, the previous use of multiple lines of therapy could also have contributed to the improved engraftment rates over historical reports [7]. Upfront haploidentical transplant studies are still very early, with limited reports in the literature but extremely favorable responses. Most studies have relatively short follow-up times.

Approaches Using Post-transplant Cyclophosphamide

The first reported use of post-transplant cyclophosphamide (PTCy) for treating SAA was by DeZern et al. with myeloablative conditioning [27]. In a pilot study, Clay et al. [8] reported the use of haplo-HSCT in refractory SAA, using a reduced-intensity conditioning with PTCy and mobilized peripheral blood cells (PBSCs) in eight patients, with successful engraftment in six patients with low acute GVHD and no chronic GVHD. Follow-up was at 14.8 (7.2–44.4) months. Esteves et al. [9] also described haplo-HSCT using the Hopkins regimen (described below) in another small cohort with 16 patients, after the failure of IST or graft failure (GF) following an unrelated-donor or cord blood transplant. Their protocol was similar to Clay et al. [8]. The graft source was the bone marrow in 13 and PBSC in three. The 1-year OS was 67.1% (95% CI: 36.5–86.4%).

Table 12.1 Reports about haploidentical HSCT in SAA

Location	Date	N	Pre-BMT therapy	Median age (range)	Conditioning regimen	Graft source	GVHD prophylaxis	Engraftment	Overall survival	Median follow-up	Acute GVHD	Chronic GVHD
Studies utilizing post-transplant cyclophosphamide as GVHD prophylaxis												
Brazil [9]	2010–2014	16	All R/R to IST; no IBMFS included	17 (5–39)	RIC: Flu, CY, TBI (200–600 cGy)	BM 13 PB 3	PTCy +3,4 MMF to D35 CSA/Tacro	15/16; Secondary graft loss 2/16	67.1%	355 days	13% grade II–IV	20% limited
United Kingdom [8]	Prior to 2014	8	4 R/R to IST; 4 failed to engraft after previous BMT	32 (19–57)	RIC: Flu, CY, TBI (200 cGy)	PB (G-CSF-mobilized)	PTCy +3,4 MMF to D35 CSA/Tacro	6/8	75%	14.8 months (7.2–44.4)	1 grade II aGVHD	0
Baltimore[a] [13, 15, 16]	2011–2023	31	R/R and upfront	30 (11–69)	RIC: rATG, Flu, CY, TBI (200 cGy; later augmented to 400 cGy)	BM	PTCy +3,4 MMF to D35 Tacro	100%	100%	21 months (3–64)	2 grade I–II aGVHD	2 mild
United States (BMT CTN)	2015–2020	32	R/R	25 (10–52)	RIC: rATG, Flu, CY, TBI (200 cGy)	BM	PTCy +3,4 MMF to D35 Tacro	77%	88%	24 months (12–29, IQR)	16%	1 moderate; others mild
Studies NOT utilizing post-transplant cyclophosphamide as GVHD prophylaxis												
China [17]	2007–2010	26	All R/R to IST; no IBMFS included	25.4 (18–41)	RIC: rATG, Flu, CY	BM +PB	CSA to D180 MMF to D90 MTX D+1,3, 6, 11	92.4%	84.6%	1313.2 days (738–2005)	12% grade II–IV	4% extensive

(continued)

Table 12.1 (continued)

Location	Date	N	Pre-BMT therapy	Median age (range)	Conditioning regimen	Graft source	GVHD prophylaxis	Engraftment	Overall survival	Median follow-up	Acute GVHD	Chronic GVHD
China [18]	2012–2015	89	None	22 (4–51)	RIC: Bu, CY, rATG	BM+PB	CSA to 1 yr MMF to D60 MTX D+1, 3, 6, 11	98.9%	86.1%	22.6 (7.1–47.6)	30.3% grade II–IV	3.4% extensive
China[a] [19]	2012–2015	101	All R/R to IST; no IBMFS included	19 (2–45)	RIC: Bu, CY, rATG	BM+PB	CSA to 1 yr; MMF to D60; MTX D+1, 3, 6, 11	100% of 97 who survived to day 28	89%	18.3 months (3–43.6)	33.7% grade II–IV	10% extensive
Studies in pediatric patients												
China [20]	2002–2013	36	All R/R to first-line tx (only 33% had ATG)	5 0.5–14	RIC (three regimens)	PBSCs in 34 1 BM 1UC (matching 3–5/6)	MTX + CSA or Tacro or MMF	34/36	86.1% at 5 years	42 months (20–157)	11 with grade II; 2 with grade III	7 limited 1 extensive
China [21]	2010–2013	17	All R/R to first-line tx (only five had ATG)	10 (4–19)	RIC: Bu, Flu; or CY; ATG or ALG	BM+PB	CSA+MTX+basiliximab	17/17 myeloid 16/17 platelet (one secondary)	71.6%	362 (36–1321) days	12 with grade I–II; 1 with grade III–IV	4 limited
China[a] [22]	2007–2015	52	29 pts. R/R (only 15 had ATG) 23 pts upfront	9 (2–17)	RIC: Bu, CY, rATG	BM+PB	CSA to 1 yr MMF to D60 MTX D+1, 3, 6, 11	96.2%	84.5%	744.5 (100–3294) days	39.2% grade I–II; 13.7 grade III–IV	34.2% (1 extensive)

Peripheral blood stem cell source

India [23]	2012–2014	10	50% failed IST	35 (6–46)	Flu, CY, rATG, melphalan,	PB	Sirolimus (in 5/10), PTCy, MMF to D35, CSA	90%	60%	2 years	1 patient	2 patients
India [24]	2015–2016	10	50% failed IST	12 (4–21)	Flu, CY, rATG, melphalan,	PB	Sirolimus, abatacept, PTCy,	90%	88.9%	NR but >1 year for 8 pts	1 patient grade II–IV	1 patient off IST by 1 year

BMT bone marrow transplant, *R/R* relapsed or refractory, *IBMFS* inherited bone marrow failure syndrome, *IST* immunosuppressive therapy, *GVHD* graft-versus-host disease, *RIC* reduced-intensity conditioning, *rATG* rabbit antithymocyte globulin, *BM* bone marrow, *PB* peripheral blood, *G-CSF* granulocyte colony-stimulating factor, *cGy* centigray, *BU* busulfan, *Flu* fludarabine, *CY* cyclophosphamide, *CSA* cyclosporine, *MTX* methotrexate, *MMF* mycophenolate mofetil, *UCB* umbilical cord blood, *Tacro* tacrolimus, *PTCy* post-transplant cyclophosphamide at 50 mg/kg per dose

aProspective study

More recently, DeZern et al. [15] reported on a prospective phase 2 trial of PTCy for refractory SAA, in which 16 patients (median age 30 years, range 11–69) underwent transplants from 13 haploidentical and three unrelated donors. The conditioning consisted of rabbit antithymocyte globulin (ATG) 4.5 mg/kg (over 3 days), fludarabine (Flu) 30 mg/m^2 over 5 days, Cy 14.5 Mg/kg for 2 days, and total body irradiation (TBI) 200 cGy. The graft source was the bone marrow, with a target yield of 4×10^8 nucleated cells/kg recipient ideal weight. For GVHD prophylaxis, PTCy 50 mg/kg/day IV on days +3 and +4 was administered, along with mycophenolate mofetil (MMF) on days +5 through 35 and tacrolimus from day +5 through 1 year. Granulocyte colony-stimulating factor (G-CSF) was given from day +5 until the absolute neutrophil count was more than 1.5×10^9/l for 3 days. There was no graft failure, and mild GVHD was seen in only two patients. The patients' clonality was eliminated, and excellent performance status was noted in all patients post-transfusion. This study is limited by the small sample size and relatively short follow-up. This is very similar to what was seen in Brazil using the same regimen, though they did have two patients with secondary graft loss and one primary graft failure [9]. However, this PTCy protocol is simple to adopt, and if the results remain reproducible, then it may become the protocol of choice. Currently, this is being studied at the national level in the United States by the Bone Marrow Transplant Clinical Trials Network (NCT02918292).

The Brazilian group updated their experience in 2020, showing the impact of CD34 cell dose and conditioning regimen on outcomes after haploidentical donor HSCT with PTCy for relapsed/refractory severe aplastic anemia (Arcuri et al. [28]; paper attached). In this study, a total of 87 patients underwent haplo-PTCy between 2010 and 2019 with a median age of 14 years (range 1–69), most of them heavily transfused. The majority (63%) received the conventional reduced-intensity conditioning (RIC) regimen from the Johns Hopkins (JH) group, and the remaining received an augmented preparatory regimen with a higher dose of pretransplant cyclophosphamide and/or a higher dose of TBI. Most grafts were from the bone marrow (93%). Primary graft failure occurred in 15%, and secondary GF or poor graft function occurred in 5%. The incidences of acute and chronic GVHD were low, but cytomegalovirus (CMV) reactivation was high (62%). Two-year OS and event-free survival (EFS) were 79% and 70%, respectively. EFS was higher for patients who received augmented Flu/Cy/TBI (HR, 0.28; $p = 0.02$) and those who received higher bone marrow CD34 cell doses ($>3.2 \times 10*6$/kg) (HR, 0.29; $p = 0.004$). Maybe, we could add this to the table (not only the 2015 publication with only 16 patients).

Larger Reports and Other Strategies, Including Upfront Haploidentical Transplant

In a prospective, multicenter study of haplo-HSCT for SAA refractory to IST, Xu et al. [19] analyzed the outcomes of 101 patients. Conditioning was with IV busulfan 6.4 mg/kg, Cy 200 mg/kg, and rabbit ATG 10 mg/kg. The graft source was combined with G-CSF-stimulated bone marrow and PBSC. GVHD prophylaxis was with cyclosporine (CSA), MMF, and short-term methotrexate (MTX). These were compared with 48 patients who had matched related donor (MRD) HSCTs. Recipients from haplo-HSCTs had more grade II–IV acute GVHD (33.7 versus 4.2%, $P < 0.001$) and more chronic GVHD (22.4 versus 6.6%, $p = 0.014$) at 1 year but similar 3-year OS (89.0 versus 91.0%, $p = 0.555$) and failure-free survival (FFS) (86.8 versus 80.3%, $p = 0.659$) compared to MRD transplants [19].

Jaiswal et al. [23] looked at a TBI-sparing regimen in ten patients (median 35 years, 6–46 years), including horse ATG at 15 mg/kg from day −8 to day −6, fludarabine 30 mg/m^2/day for 5 days, and cyclophosphamide 15 mg/kg/day for 2 days with melphalan 120 mg/m^2, followed by PBSCs and PTCy. This protocol was modified with the introduction of sirolimus on day −7 [23]. Six of the ten patients were alive, with the latter five having received the day—7 sirolimus. The authors hypothesized that the early recovery of regulatory T cells in this small cohort might be indicative of a tolerance induction mechanism that could have resulted from synergism between PTCy and sirolimus [23]. Additionally, this group used this same platform and added T cell co-stimulation blockade with abatacept, suggesting a further role in transplant tolerance with this approach [24].

Xu et al. [22] reported on 52 children who received haplo-HSCT, with 29 receiving it as salvage and the remaining 23 receiving it as their upfront therapy, using a protocol described in a previous paper [19]. Primary engraftment was achieved in 51. The cumulative incidence of aGVHD grade II–IV was 39.2% and that of cGVHD was 34.2%, respectively. The 3-year OS and FFS rates were 84.5% and 82.7%, respectively [22].

Upfront haplo-HSCT in 158 SAA patients was reported by Xu et al. [18] based on the Chinese transplant registry. Haplo-HSCTs were performed in 89 patients with a similar protocol [19]. For 69 MRD transplants, conditioning included either Cy+ATG or Cy+Flu+ATG. Haplo-HSCT recipients had increased grade II–IV aGVHD (30.3 versus 1.5%, $p < 0.001$) and cGVHD (30.6 versus 4.4%, $p < 0.001$) at 1 year but similar extensive cGVHD (3.4 versus 0%, $p = 0.426$) compared to related transplants. The 3-year OS rates were 86.1 and 91.3% ($p = 0.358$), whereas the 3-year FFS rates were 85.0 and 89.8% ($p = 0.413$) in the haplo-HSCT and MRD cohorts, respectively [18].

Conditioning for Haploidentical Transplant for Aplastic Anemia

Reduced-intensity conditioning or nonmyeloablative (NMA) conditioning is likely sufficient to balance engraftment and toxicities in this setting. It has been previously shown that TBI-based conditioning regimens reduced the risk of graft rejection but increased GVHD and other late effects [29]. It has recently been demonstrated that when using a haploidentical donor upfront, the TBI dose should be augmented to

400 cGy to ensure adequate engraftment [13]. Standard ATG-based conditioning regimens are employed to aid in engraftment but have also been associated with up to a 30% incidence of cGVHD [30, 31]. Fludarabine has been used in conditioning for patients with both acquired and constitutional aplastic anemia with good results [32–35]. We favor this approach in T-cell-replete allografts. The Brazilian experience also upgraded the conditioning, both in the Cy dose (55) and the TBI dose (4 Gy) [28, 36]. Also, for haplo-transplants, Cy 25* × 2 and TBI 4 Gy are recommended doses in the conditioning.

Additionally, as described above, both T-cell-depleted and T-cell-replete haploidentical strategies have been reported for multiple relapsed SAA patients lacking a matched donor [15, 23, 37]. Im and colleagues describe 21 patients who underwent fludarabine, cyclophosphamide, 400 cGy TBI, and ATG conditioning, followed by either CD3/19- or DC3 alpha-beta / CD19 depleted grafts. OS was reported as 94% at 3 years, without cases of chronic GVHD [38]. T-replete haploidentical approaches have been taken by Wang (17 children, full-intensity conditioning, and four-agent GVHD prophylaxis: OS 71% at 1 year and 20% chronic GVHD) [21] and Gao (26 adults, reduced-intensity conditioning with three-agent GVHD prophylaxis: OS 82% at 2 years and GVHD 40%) [17]. Data are increasingly available for a reduced-intensity approach, followed by T-replete haploidentical transplant and PTCy described above as optimal GVHD prophylaxis as above, with OS approaching 90% and low GVHD rates [8, 9, 15].

A recent publication from Gong et al. reports transplanting 71 patients (86% using haploidentical donors and 14% using unrelated donors) with an ATG- and TBI-free regimen comprising cyclophosphamide, fludarabine, and low-dose busulfan, followed by G-CSF-mobilized peripheral blood stem cells, PTCy, short-term methotrexate, and cyclosporine. The cohort was quite young, with a median age of 16. They included treatment-naïve (TN) ($n = 38$) and relapsed or refractory (R/R) ($n = 33$) patients. The authors report a low incidence of graft failure, grade II–IV GVHD, and moderate-to-severe chronic GVHD, with similar rates between TN and R/R patients. With a median follow-up of 3.5 years, the overall survival and event-free survival were higher for the TN when compared to the R/R group (100% versus 84%; $p = 0.13$ and 86.8% versus 75.8%; $p = 0.25$, respectively). Altogether, 94% of the patients are alive (91.3% in the TN and 89.3% in the R/R) [39].

Donor Selection

Stem Cell Choice

This is an area where data are lacking in a comparative fashion in most malignant diseases for all donor sources. However, to make recommendations for stem cell source in haploidentical transplants in SAA, we can extrapolate from the matched-sibling data. The European Society for Blood and Marrow Transplantation (EBMT) reviewed outcomes in nearly 700 patients with SAA receiving transplants from

HLA-matched siblings. In patients younger than 20 years of age, rates of chronic GVHD (relative risk 2.82; $p = 0.002$) and overall mortality (relative risk 2.04; $p = 0.024$) were higher after transplantation of peripheral blood progenitor cell grafts than after transplantation of bone marrow. In younger patients, the 5-year survival was 85% after marrow transplants but only 73% after PBSC. These data suggest that bone marrow grafts are preferable in this age group [40, 41], but this has not been looked at systematically in haploidentical donors. Most centers in the United States and Brazil favor bone marrow grafts to avoid excessive GVHD in a nonmalignant disease; however, in the United Kingdom, they have successfully used PBSC without increased rates of GVHD [8, 36]. In China, many transplants of this nature follow another procedure to optimize cell counts. Haploidentical donors are treated with subcutaneous granulocyte colony-stimulating factor (G-CSF). Marrow grafts are then collected on day 1, with a target mononuclear cell (MNC) count of $2–4 \times 10^8$/kg of recipient body weight. Peripheral blood stem cells were also collected by apheresis. The target MNC count from BM and PB was $6–8 \times 10^8$/kg of recipient body weight. If the MNC count was not sufficient, additional PBSCs were collected on the following day [19]. BM remains the preferred stem cell source, as long as at least 3×10^8 are collected.

Choice of the Best Haploidentical Donor

In the current system, there are likely multiple potential haploidentical donor options. These can be first-degree relatives of the patient, including biological parents, siblings or half-siblings, or children with two, three, or four mismatches using DNA-based typing. A unidirectional mismatch in either the graft-versus-host or host-versus-graft direction is considered a mismatch. The donor and recipient are recommended to be identical at a minimum of one allele (at high-resolution DNA-based typing) at the following genetic loci: HLA-A, -B, -C, and DRB1 for haplo-matching. There is nothing in AA that is unique compared to hematologic malignancies, which suggests a nonstandard approach to the choice of donor to an AA patient. When more than one donor is available, the donor with the lowest number of HLA allele mismatches will be chosen unless there is HLA crossmatch incompatibility or a medical reason to select otherwise. In cases where there is more than one donor with the least degree of mismatch, donors will be selected based on the most favorable combination of HLA compatibility in crossmatch testing and ABO compatibility. Prioritization is given to the lowest number of mismatches in the host-versus-graft direction to minimize the risk of graft rejection. If there is more than one donor with the least amount of host-versus-graft (HVG) allele mismatches, the suggested prioritization in order of importance includes ABO compatibility, CMV status (use a seronegative donor for a seronegative recipient or a seropositive donor for a seropositive recipient), younger age, lighter weight (this rule applies down to the age of 18; however, children may also be used as donors, if appropriate), and sex of the donor (if everything else is equal, males are preferred over nulliparous females over multiparous females) [42]. Youth (likely age less than 40 years) is increasingly valued when it comes to the choice of any donor, and this may begin to take greater priority here as well [43].

The Challenge of Anti-HLA Antibodies

Donor-specific anti-HLA antibodies have been implicated in graft rejection in solid organ transplantation for many years. More recently, their role in HSCT has been better defined [44]. Results in multiple retrospective reviews have suggested that DSA is associated with a higher rate of graft rejection in patients undergoing HSCT [45], including those from a haploidentical donor [46]. Given that all efforts should be made to optimize engraftment rates in haplo-HSCT for AA, DSA should always be evaluated. Certainly, anti-HLA sensitization can be evaluated in HSCT for AA with haplo-donors, but the haplo-donor without DSA should be chosen where possible [28, 36, 47, 48]. For the Brazilian group, the presence of DSA before HSCT was associated with lower EFS (HR, 3.92; $p = 0.01$). For countries with limited resources, these tests are also very expensive but need to be done when doing haplo-PTCy transplant [49]. It is also much more frequent to find DSA in patients with bone marrow failures compared to malignant diseases.

Graft-Versus-Host Disease Prophylaxis

PTCy is becoming the standard in this arena, as discussed above. Additionally, it is customary for other oral IST for GVHD to continue post-transplant through day 180 or even 1 year in SAA [50], even with PTCy. This often includes mycophenolate mofetil as well as cyclosporine or a calcineurin inhibitor (tacrolimus or sirolimus). The majority of the more favorable results (seen in Table 12.1) utilize this approach. Methotrexate remains commonly used as well. Levels of the calcineurin inhibitors are routinely monitored to maintain a therapeutic goal. Anecdotal reports of loss of chimerism when this is not done in AA are common.

Systematic Reviews

A recent systematic review and meta-analysis of studies related to haploidentical stem cell transplantation in idiopathic AA investigated the rates of successful engraftment, acute graft-versus-host disease (aGVHD), chronic GVHD (cGVHD), treatment related mortality (TRM), and post-transplant viral infections (including cytomegalovirus [CMV]) in patients with AA. The effects of reduced-intensity conditioning (RIC) and nonmyeloablative (NMA) conditioning, as well as various

GVHD prophylaxis regimens on these outcomes, were evaluated. In total, 15 studies were identified (577 patients, 58.9% males), and successful engraftment was observed in 97.3% of patients (95% CI, 95.9–98.7), while grade II–IV aGVHD and cGVHD were reported in 26.6% and 25.0%, respectively. The pooled incidence of TRM was 6.7% per year (95% CI, 4.0–9.4). RIC regimens were associated with higher proportions of successful engraftment (97.7% versus 91.7%, $p = 0.03$) and aGVHD (29.5% versus 18.7%, $p = 0.008$) when compared with NMA regimens, with no differences in cGVHD or mortality incidence. When compared with methotrexate-containing regimens and other regimens, post-transplant cyclophosphamide–containing regimens reduced the rates of aGVHD (28.6%, 27.8%, and 12.8%, respectively, $p = 0.02$) [51].

Another contemporary meta-analysis also evaluated MSD, unrelated donor (URD), haplos, and IST up to June 2022 of 25 studies, comprising 2252 patients. This group did not show a difference between haplo- and MRD-HSCT in the 1-, 2-, and 3-year overall survival (OS), failure-free survival (FFS), and engraftment. However, haplos had higher incidences of II–IV acute graft-versus-host disease (aGVHD), chronic GVHD (cGVHD), and cytomegalovirus infection. There were no differences in the 3- and 5-year OS, 3-year FFS, platelet engraftment, graft failure (GF), II–IV grade of aGVHD, and complication between haplo- and URD-HSCT; however, haplo had a lower incidence of cGVHD. Compared with IST, haplo had a higher 3-year FFS and 3- and 6-month response rates. However, there were no differences in the 3- and 5-year OS and 12-month response rates between haplo and IST [52].

Yet another recent meta-analysis of retrospective studies found a pooled 5-year OS in favor of upfront alternative-donor HSCT over IST [53]. However, graft-versus-host disease (GVHD), graft rejection, treatment-related mortality (TRM), and infertility remain further areas for study. Further development of alternative donor options is under evaluation. There are promising results in haplo- [54, 55] as well as URD-HSCT [56, 57], with URD or haplos possibly moving earlier in the algorithm, given recent promising data and some upfront trials [13, 58].

Conclusion and Future of Alternative Transplants in Aplastic Anemia

In conclusion, haplo-HSCT is now a safe and potentially curative option for treating SAA patients who are refractory to IST, have relapsed after IST, or have acquired a secondary clonal disorder myelodysplastic syndromes/paroxysmal nocturnal hemoglobinuria (MDS/PNH) after IST. Current strategies (including PTCy as GVHD prophylaxis) have increased the availability of haplo-HSCT to patients previously considered transplant-ineligible because they lack a suitable donor or were too high risk for HSCT due to the risk of GVHD. Ongoing investigations seek to increase this option for these patients through the development of further novel therapeutic strategies to optimize haplo-HSCT, both in the treatment-refractory setting as well as the upfront setting. Furthermore, haploidentical transplants are attractive due to the low cost and early availability of a donor, although issues of donor-specific antibodies may be potentially problematic [42, 59]. The current results suggest that haplo-HSCT should be strongly considered for refractory SAA patients. Upfront haplo-HSCT is increasingly utilized and may be very useful for SAA patients lacking an MSD or matched unrelated donor (MUD), who want to consider minimizing the risk of clonal evolution post-IST.

References

1. Scheinberg P, Nunez O, Weinstein B, et al. Horse versus rabbit antithymocyte globulin in acquired aplastic anemia. Comparative Study Randomized Controlled Trial Research Support, N.I.H., Intramural. N Engl J Med. 2011;365(5):430–8. https://doi.org/10.1056/NEJMoa1103975.
2. Townsley DM, Scheinberg P, Winkler T, et al. Eltrombopag added to standard immunosuppression for aplastic anemia. N Engl J Med. 2017;376(16):1540–50. https://doi.org/10.1056/NEJMoa1613878.
3. DeZern AE, Brodsky RA. Combining PTCy and ATG for GvHD prophylaxis in non-malignant diseases. Blood Rev. 2022;62:101016. https://doi.org/10.1016/j.blre.2022.101016.
4. Storb R, Blume KG, O'Donnell MR, et al. Cyclophosphamide and antithymocyte globulin to condition patients with aplastic anemia for allogeneic marrow transplantations: the experience in four centers. Biol Blood Marrow Transplant. 2001;7(1):39–44. https://doi.org/10.1053/bbmt.2001.v7.pm11215697.
5. Simione AJ, das Neves HR, da Silva CC, da Silva Sabaini PM, Geraldo BL, Pasquini M, Vigorito AC, Ammi M, Colturato V, Nabhan S, Seber A. Current use and outcomes of hematopoietic stem cell transplantation: Brazilian summary slides. J Bone Marrow Transplant Cell Ther. 2022;3(2):171.
6. Bacigalupo A, Sica S. Alternative donor transplants for severe aplastic anemia: current experience. Semin Hematol. 2016;53(2):115–9. https://doi.org/10.1053/j.seminhematol.2016.01.002.
7. Ciceri F, Lupo-Stanghellini MT, Korthof ET. Haploidentical transplantation in patients with acquired aplastic anemia. Bone Marrow Transplant. 2013;48(2):183–5. https://doi.org/10.1038/bmt.2012.231.
8. Clay J, Kulasekararaj AG, Potter V, et al. Nonmyeloablative peripheral blood haploidentical stem cell transplantation for refractory severe aplastic anemia. Research Support, Non-U.S. Gov't. Biol Blood Marrow Transplant. 2014;20(11):1711–6. https://doi.org/10.1016/j.bbmt.2014.06.028.
9. Esteves I, Bonfim C, Pasquini R, et al. Haploidentical BMT and post-transplant Cy for severe aplastic anemia: a multicenter retrospective study. Bone Marrow Transplant. 2015;50(5):685–9. https://doi.org/10.1038/bmt.2015.20.
10. Fureder W, Valent P. Treatment of refractory or relapsed acquired aplastic anemia: review of established and experimental approaches. Leuk Lymphoma. 2011;52(8):1435–45. https://doi.org/10.3109/10428194.2011.568646.
11. DeZern AE, Brodsky RA. Haploidentical donor bone marrow transplantation for severe aplastic anemia. Hematol Oncol Clin North Am. 2018;32(4):629–42. https://doi.org/10.1016/j.hoc.2018.04.001.
12. Bacigalupo A, Giammarco S. Haploidentical donor transplants for severe aplastic anemia. Semin Hematol. 2019;56(3):190–3. https://doi.org/10.1053/j.seminhematol.2019.03.004.
13. DeZern A, Zahurak ML, Symons HJ, et al. Alternative donor BMT with post-transplant cyclophosphamide as initial therapy for acquired severe aplastic anemia. Blood. 2023;141:3031–8. https://doi.org/10.1182/blood.2023020435.

14. DeZern AE, Zahurak M, Jones RJ, Brodsky RA. Uniform conditioning regardless of donor in bone marrow transplantation for severe aplastic anemia. Haematologica. 2023;109:657. https://doi.org/10.3324/haematol.2023.284022.
15. DeZern AE, Zahurak M, Symons H, Cooke K, Jones RJ, Brodsky RA. Alternative donor transplantation with high-dose post-transplantation cyclophosphamide for refractory severe aplastic anemia. Biol Blood Marrow Transplant. 2017;23(3):498–504. https://doi.org/10.1016/j.bbmt.2016.12.628.
16. DeZern AE, Zahurak ML, Symons HJ, et al. Haploidentical BMT for severe aplastic anemia with intensive GVHD prophylaxis including posttransplant cyclophosphamide. Blood Adv. 2020;4(8):1770–9. https://doi.org/10.1182/bloodadvances.2020001729.
17. Gao L, Li Y, Zhang Y, et al. Long-term outcome of HLA-haploidentical hematopoietic SCT without in vitro T-cell depletion for adult severe aplastic anemia after modified conditioning and supportive therapy. Bone Marrow Transplant. 2014;49(4):519–24. https://doi.org/10.1038/bmt.2013.224.
18. Xu LP, Jin S, Wang SQ, et al. Upfront haploidentical transplant for acquired severe aplastic anemia: registry-based comparison with matched related transplant. J Hematol Oncol. 2017;10(1):25. https://doi.org/10.1186/s13045-017-0398-y.
19. Xu LP, Wang SQ, Wu DP, et al. Haplo-identical transplantation for acquired severe aplastic anaemia in a multicentre prospective study. Br J Haematol. 2016;175:265–74. https://doi.org/10.1111/bjh.14225.
20. Zhu H, Luo RM, Luan Z, et al. Unmanipulated haploidentical haematopoietic stem cell transplantation for children with severe aplastic anaemia. Br J Haematol. 2016;174:799–805. https://doi.org/10.1111/bjh.14110.
21. Wang Z, Zheng X, Yan H, Li D, Wang H. Good outcome of haploidentical hematopoietic SCT as a salvage therapy in children and adolescents with acquired severe aplastic anemia. Bone Marrow Transplant. 2014;49(12):1481–5. https://doi.org/10.1038/bmt.2014.187.
22. Xu LP, Zhang XH, Wang FR, et al. Haploidentical transplantation for pediatric patients with acquired severe aplastic anemia. Bone Marrow Transplant. 2017;52(3):381–7. https://doi.org/10.1038/bmt.2016.281.
23. Jaiswal SR, Chatterjee S, Mukherjee S, Ray K, Chakrabarti S. Pre-transplant sirolimus might improve the outcome of haploidentical peripheral blood stem cell transplantation with post-transplant cyclophosphamide for patients with severe aplastic anemia. Bone Marrow Transplant. 2015;50(6):873–5. https://doi.org/10.1038/bmt.2015.50.
24. Jaiswal SR, Bhakuni P, Zaman S, et al. T cell costimulation blockade promotes transplantation tolerance in combination with sirolimus and post-transplantation cyclophosphamide for haploidentical transplantation in children with severe aplastic anemia. Transpl Immunol. 2017;43:54–9. https://doi.org/10.1016/j.trim.2017.07.004.
25. Zhang Y, Guo Z, Liu XD, et al. Comparison of haploidentical hematopoietic stem cell transplantation and immunosuppressive therapy for the treatment of acquired severe aplastic anemia in pediatric patients. Am J Ther. 2016;24:e196–201. https://doi.org/10.1097/MJT.0000000000000366.
26. Sarmiento M, Ramirez PA. Unmanipulated haploidentical hematopoietic cell transplantation with post-transplant cyclophosphamide in a patient with paroxysmal nocturnal hemoglobinuria and secondary aplastic anemia. Bone Marrow Transplant. 2016;51(2):316–8. https://doi.org/10.1038/bmt.2015.251.
27. Dezern AE, Luznik L, Fuchs EJ, Jones RJ, Brodsky RA. Post-transplantation cyclophosphamide for GVHD prophylaxis in severe aplastic anemia. Case reports letter. Bone Marrow Transplant. 2011;46(7):1012–3. https://doi.org/10.1038/bmt.2010.213.
28. Arcuri LJ, Nabhan SK, Cunha R, et al. Impact of CD34 cell dose and conditioning regimen on outcomes after haploidentical donor hematopoietic stem cell transplantation with post-transplantation cyclophosphamide for relapsed/refractory severe aplastic anemia. Biol Blood Marrow Transplant. 2020;26(12):2311–7. https://doi.org/10.1016/j.bbmt.2020.09.007.

29. Sanders JE, Woolfrey AE, Carpenter PA, et al. Late effects among pediatric patients followed for nearly 4 decades after transplantation for severe aplastic anemia. Evaluation Studies Research Support, N.I.H., Extramural. Blood. 2011;118(5):1421–8. https://doi.org/10.1182/blood-2011-02-334953.
30. Konopacki J, Porcher R, Robin M, et al. Long-term follow up after allogeneic stem cell transplantation in patients with severe aplastic anemia after cyclophosphamide plus antithymocyte globulin conditioning. Research Support, Non-U.S. Gov't. Haematologica. 2012;97(5):710–6. https://doi.org/10.3324/haematol.2011.050096.
31. Champlin RE, Perez WS, Passweg JR, et al. Bone marrow transplantation for severe aplastic anemia: a randomized controlled study of conditioning regimens. Blood. 2007;109(10):4582–5. NOT IN FILE.
32. Kharfan-Dabaja MA, Otrock ZK, Bacigalupo A, Mahfouz RA, Geara F, Bazarbachi A. A reduced intensity conditioning regimen of fludarabine, cyclophosphamide, antithymocyte globulin, plus 2 Gy TBI facilitates successful hematopoietic cell engraftment in an adult with dyskeratosis congenita. Bone Marrow Transplant. 2012;47(9):1254–5. https://doi.org/10.1038/bmt.2011.257.
33. Dietz AC, Orchard PJ, Baker KS, et al. Disease-specific hematopoietic cell transplantation: nonmyeloablative conditioning regimen for dyskeratosis congenita. Bone Marrow Transplant. 2011;46(1):98–104. NOT IN FILE.
34. Marsh JC, Gupta V, Lim Z, et al. Alemtuzumab with fludarabine and cyclophosphamide reduces chronic graft-versus-host disease after allogeneic stem cell transplantation for acquired aplastic anemia. Clinical Trial Multicenter Study. Blood. 2011;118(8):2351–7. https://doi.org/10.1182/blood-2010-12-327536.
35. Wang SB, Li L, Pan XH, et al. Engraftment of heavily transfused patients with severe aplastic anemia with a fludarabine-based regimen. Clin Transplant. 2013;27(2):E109–15. https://doi.org/10.1111/ctr.12061.
36. Arcuri LJ, Nabhan SK, Loth G, et al. A case series of post-transplantation cyclophosphamide in unrelated donor hematopoietic cell transplantation for aplastic anemia. Biol Blood Marrow Transplant. 2020;26(9):e222–6. https://doi.org/10.1016/j.bbmt.2020.05.023.
37. Gupta N, Choudhary D, Sharma SK, Khandelwal V, Dhamija M. Haploidentical hematopoietic SCT for acquired severe aplastic anemia using post-transplant high-dose CY. Bone Marrow Transplant. 2015;50(1):155–6. https://doi.org/10.1038/bmt.2014.222.
38. Im HJ, Koh KN, Seo JJ. Haploidentical hematopoietic stem cell transplantation in children and adolescents with acquired severe aplastic anemia. Korean J Pediatr. 2015;58(6):199–205. https://doi.org/10.3345/kjp.2015.58.6.199.
39. Gong S, Chen C, Chen K, et al. Alternative transplantation with post-transplantation cyclophosphamide in aplastic anemia: a retrospective report from the BMF-WG of Hunan Province, China. Transplant Cell Ther. 2023;29(1):48 e1–7. https://doi.org/10.1016/j.jtct.2022.10.006.
40. Schrezenmeier H, Passweg JR, Marsh JC, et al. Worse outcome and more chronic GVHD with peripheral blood progenitor cells than bone marrow in HLA-matched sibling donor transplants for young patients with severe acquired aplastic anemia. Research Support, N.I.H., Extramural. Blood. 2007;110(4):1397–400. https://doi.org/10.1182/blood-2007-03-081596.
41. Bacigalupo A, Socie G, Schrezenmeier H, et al. Bone marrow versus peripheral blood as the stem cell source for sibling transplants in acquired aplastic anemia: survival advantage for bone marrow in all age groups. Research Support, Non-U.S. Gov't. Haematologica. 2012;97(8):1142–8. https://doi.org/10.3324/haematol.2011.054841.
42. McCurdy SR, Fuchs EJ. Selecting the best haploidentical donor. Semin Hematol. 2016;53(4):246–51. https://doi.org/10.1053/j.seminhematol.2016.08.001.
43. Kollman C, Spellman SR, Zhang MJ, et al. The effect of donor characteristics on survival after unrelated donor transplantation for hematologic malignancy. Blood. 2016;127(2):260–7. https://doi.org/10.1182/blood-2015-08-663823.
44. Morin-Zorman S, Loiseau P, Taupin JL, Caillat-Zucman S. Donor-specific anti-HLA antibodies in allogeneic hematopoietic stem cell transplantation. Front Immunol. 2016;7:307. https://doi.org/10.3389/fimmu.2016.00307.

45. Ciurea SO, Thall PF, Wang X, et al. Donor-specific anti-HLA abs and graft failure in matched unrelated donor hematopoietic stem cell transplantation. Blood. 2011;118(22):5957–64. https://doi.org/10.1182/blood-2011-06-362111.
46. Ciurea SO, Thall PF, Milton DR, et al. Complement-binding donor-specific anti-HLA antibodies and risk of primary graft failure in hematopoietic stem cell transplantation. Biol Blood Marrow Transplant. 2015;21(8):1392–8. https://doi.org/10.1016/j.bbmt.2015.05.001.
47. Gladstone DE, Zachary AA, Fuchs EJ, et al. Partially mismatched transplantation and human leukocyte antigen donor-specific antibodies. Biol Blood Marrow Transplant. 2013;19(4):647–52. https://doi.org/10.1016/j.bbmt.2013.01.016.
48. Leffell MS, Jones RJ, Gladstone DE. Donor HLA-specific abs: to BMT or not to BMT? Bone Marrow Transplant. 2015;50(6):751–8. https://doi.org/10.1038/bmt.2014.331.
49. Lima ACM, Bonfim C, Getz J, et al. Untreated donor-specific HLA antibodies are associated with graft failure and poor survival after Haploidentical transplantation with post-transplantation cyclophosphamide in pediatric patients with nonmalignant disorders. Transplant Cell Ther. 2022;28(10):698 e1–698 e11. https://doi.org/10.1016/j.jtct.2022.07.019.
50. Bacigalupo A, Brand R, Oneto R, et al. Treatment of acquired severe aplastic anemia: bone marrow transplantation compared with immunosuppressive therapy–The European Group for Blood and Marrow Transplantation experience. Comparative Study Research Support, Non-U.S. Gov't Review. Semin Hematol. 2000;37(1):69–80.
51. ElGohary G, El Fakih R, de Latour R, et al. Haploidentical hematopoietic stem cell transplantation in aplastic anemia: a systematic review and meta-analysis of clinical outcome on behalf of the severe aplastic anemia working party of the European group for blood and marrow transplantation (SAAWP of EBMT). Bone Marrow Transplant. 2020;55(10):1906–17. https://doi.org/10.1038/s41409-020-0897-2.
52. Zhao J, Ma L, Zheng M, Su L, Guo X. Meta-analysis of the results of haploidentical transplantation in the treatment of aplastic anemia. Ann Hematol. 2023;102:2565–87. https://doi.org/10.1007/s00277-023-05339-7.
53. Alotaibi H, Aljurf M, de Latour R, et al. Upfront alternative donor transplant versus immunosuppressive therapy in patients with severe aplastic anemia who lack a fully HLA-matched related donor: systematic review and meta-analysis of retrospective studies, on behalf of the Severe Aplastic Anemia Working Party of the European Group for Blood and Marrow Transplantation. Transplant Cell Ther. 2022;28(2):105 e1–7. https://doi.org/10.1016/j.jtct.2021.10.006.
54. Im HJ, Koh KN, Choi ES, et al. Excellent outcome of haploidentical hematopoietic stem cell transplantation in children and adolescents with acquired severe aplastic anemia. Biol Blood Marrow Transplant. 2013;19(5):754–9. https://doi.org/10.1016/j.bbmt.2013.01.023.
55. Xu LP, Liu KY, Liu DH, et al. A novel protocol for haploidentical hematopoietic SCT without in vitro T-cell depletion in the treatment of severe acquired aplastic anemia. Research Support, Non-U.S. Gov't. Bone Marrow Transplant. 2012;47(12):1507–12. https://doi.org/10.1038/bmt.2012.79.
56. Yamamoto H, Kato D, Uchida N, et al. Successful sustained engraftment after reduced-intensity umbilical cord blood transplantation for adult patients with severe aplastic anemia. Blood. 2011;117(11):3240–2. https://doi.org/10.1182/blood-2010-08-295832.
57. Peffault de Latour R, Rocha V, Socie G. Cord blood transplantation in aplastic anemia. Bone Marrow Transplant. 2013;48(2):201–2. https://doi.org/10.1038/bmt.2012.252.
58. Pulsipher MA, Lehmann LE, Bertuch AA, et al. A study assessing the feasibility of randomization of pediatric and young adult patients between matched unrelated donor bone marrow transplantation and immune-suppressive therapy for newly diagnosed severe aplastic anemia: a joint pilot trial of the North American Pediatric Aplastic Anemia Consortium and the Pediatric Transplantation and Cellular Therapy Consortium. Pediatr Blood Cancer. 2020;67(10):e28444. https://doi.org/10.1002/pbc.28444.
59. Ciurea SO, Champlin RE. Donor selection in T cell-replete haploidentical hematopoietic stem cell transplantation: knowns, unknowns, and controversies. Biol Blood Marrow Transplant. 2013;19(2):180–4. https://doi.org/10.1016/j.bbmt.2012.08.007.

Open Access This chapter is licensed under the terms of the Creative Commons Attribution 4.0 International License (http://creativecommons.org/licenses/by/4.0/), which permits use, sharing, adaptation, distribution and reproduction in any medium or format, as long as you give appropriate credit to the original author(s) and the source, provide a link to the Creative Commons license and indicate if changes were made.

The images or other third party material in this chapter are included in the chapter's Creative Commons license, unless indicated otherwise in a credit line to the material. If material is not included in the chapter's Creative Commons license and your intended use is not permitted by statutory regulation or exceeds the permitted use, you will need to obtain permission directly from the copyright holder.

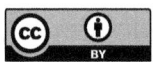

Chapter 13
Umbilical Cord Blood Transplantation for Patients with Idiopathic and Inherited Bone Marrow Failure Disorders

Simona Pagliuca and Arthur Sterin

Introduction

Allogeneic hematopoietic cell transplantation (HCT) represents the backbone for the treatment algorithm for idiopathic and inherited bone marrow failure (BMF) disorders. For most of these disease subcategories, post-HCT survival rates continue to improve, especially for patients undergoing alternative donor transplants. The refinement of human leukocyte antigen (HLA)–matching techniques and of conditioning regimen toxicities and graft versus host disease (GvHD) prophylaxis has tremendously accelerated this improvement. The easy worldwide access to umbilical cord blood (UCB) units has expanded the accessibility to transplant for many patients without a suitable bone marrow (BM) or peripheral blood (PB) donor. Although the rates of its utilization in the past decades have been reduced by the rapid expansion of haploidentical donor transplants, this graft source remains a valid option in both pediatric and adult BMF settings [1]. For BMF, as for other nonmalignant disorders, transplant platforms have always been conceived to drastically decrease transplant- and disease-related toxicities with the aim to avoid deleterious graft versus host (GvH) reactions and facilitate the engraftment. In this chapter, we will discuss the current status of the art of umbilical cord blood transplantation (UCBT) in the BMF setting, offering a fresh and up-to-date overview of the specific indications and disease-related issues.

S. Pagliuca (✉)
Department of Hematology, Nancy University Hospital, and UMR 7365, University of Lorraine, Vandoeuvre-lès-Nancy, France

A. Sterin
Service D'hématologie Immunologie Oncologie Pédiatrique, CHU de Marseille, France

© The Author(s) 2026
M. Aljurf et al. (eds.), *Textbook of Bone Marrow Failure*,
https://doi.org/10.1007/978-3-032-02386-5_13

UCBT in BMF: History and Proof of Concept

BMF disorders represent the first historical indication of UCBT, contributing to its development and expansion. The first UCBT was, in fact, performed in 1988 on a 5-year-old boy diagnosed with a BMF secondary to Fanconi anemia (FA) [2]. The conception of this procedure, realized in Saint Louis Hospital (Paris, France) by Eliane Gluckman's team, was the fruit of an international collaboration with the Rockefeller (New York, USA), and the Indiana (Indianapolis, USA) universities, where the teams, led by Arleen D. Auerbach and Hal E. Broxemeyer, respectively, were investigating methods for prenatal diagnosis in FA and isolation and cryopreservation of hematopoietic progenitors in UCB [3, 4]. Indeed, the first patient was transplanted with cryopreserved UCB issued from his unaffected HLA-identical sister. After receiving conditioning with low-dose cyclophosphamide (Cy) and limited-field thoracoabdominal irradiation, he recovered with a full, functional hematopoiesis, without developing any major complication and maintaining a complete immunological and hematological reconstitution 35 years after transplant [5, 6]. This was the first proof of concept that a single UCB from a newborn is capable of a definitive and long-lasting repopulation of the hematopoietic compartment in an allogeneic recipient. This first successful story was the praeludium to the rapid spread of UCB banks across the world and of the growth of UCBT numbers and indications. The advantages of this procedure appeared immediately clear: higher donor availability, faster recruitment and shorter transplant delay, absence of risk for the donor, and more versatile logistics, with no risk of donor refusal and lower incidence of GvHD despite HLA disparities, because of the lower T cell content and lower risk of donor–recipient pathogen transmission. Thus, since the late 1990s, a number of studies reported the outcomes of UCBT in BMF and other disorders, with many efforts from Eurocord and other international transplant consortia to collect data and boost the knowledge around the use of this graft source in an allogeneic setting [6–10].

Disease-Specific Aspects

While recognizing the rapid propagation of UCB use, with incredible determination in identifying determinants of success and failure of the procedure, it is important to consider that most of the knowledge related to the application of UCBT in the BMF setting comes from retrospective and registry-based data. This feature, combined with the rarity of each specific disorder, makes it very difficult to draw guidelines and recommendations concerning the design of transplant platforms, still characterized by a huge variability, depending on the experience of each transplant center. Moreover, very different outcomes have been observed in patients receiving a related HLA-identical versus an unrelated, often mismatched, HLA UCB unit. While UCB from matched related siblings represents a very unique setting, providing exceptional results (comparable to those obtained with the first "N-of-1 trial") [2] across populations of BMF patients, the availability of such a precious source of hematopoietic stem cells (HSC) is precluded for most of the patients, and most of the evidence has been produced in an unrelated setting, where outcomes are less favorable. For this reason, today, in most of the inherited and acquired BMF disorders, (unrelated) UCBT remains a therapeutic option only in selected eligible patients, after failure of other treatment strategies.

In this section, we will first discuss each disease-related specificity, referring, when not otherwise specified, to the "more classical" unrelated UCBT procedure. In the last paragraph, we will provide an overview of the current knowledge on the particular situation of related HLA-matched UCBT.

Idiopathic Aplastic Anemia

Outcomes of patients with idiopathic, severe aplastic anemia (SAA) without an HLA-matched related donor (MRD) have been largely improved during the past years thanks to the effectiveness of new upfront immunosuppressive treatment combinations [11] and the application of alternative donor transplant strategies in refractory settings [12–15]. In this context, the feasibility of UCBT has been shown not only through registry-based retrospective analyses but also through prospective trials. While in historical reports, a high incidence of graft failure and low survival probabilities undermined the trust in the procedure [7], since the mid-2000s the experience became more encouraging [16–21]. In these retrospective series, survival outcomes ranged between 30% and 70%, with better results associated with >7/8 HLA matching, a total cell dose of >3.9 × 10^7/kg of fludarabine (Flu), low-dose total body irradiation (TBI)–based conditioning regimens, and younger (less than 40) recipient age [19–21]. Major pitfalls of the procedure in refractory SAA were the risks of graft failure and severe infections [19, 20]. A phase II prospective trial conducted in France between 2011 and 2015 assessed the outcomes of unrelated UCBT in 26 young refractory SAA patients (median age 16) after a Flu-Cy/low-dose TBI conditioning regimen associated with an in vivo T cell depletion (see box below) [22]. With impressive survival rates (>80% at 1 year) and a treatment-related mortality (TRM) of 11%, this transplant platform has become the reference in Europe (as per Severe Aplastic Anemia Working Party (SAAWP) recommendations) for patients receiving a single- or double-unit UCBT in the context of refractory SAA [23]. Other conditioning regimens and GvHD prophylaxes have also been demonstrated to be effective in inducing engraftment and long-term survival. A recent multicenter trial from China compared outcomes of upfront intensive immunosuppressive therapy (IST) versus single-unit unrelated UCBT conditioned with a highly immunosuppressive regimen (based on rabbit antithymocyte globulin (ATG), cyclophosphamide, and cyclosporine) [24]. This study, including 123 patients (median age 44), showed the superiority in terms of the overall response rate (ORR) and event-free survival (EFS) of the UCBT. Upfront UCBT has been sometimes proposed for pediatric patients as a possible alternative strategy to IST in the absence of a matched donor, showing interesting results [25]; however, given the lack of prospective data, the concerns related to the possible morbidity and mortality of alternative donor procedures and considering the high rates of success of current IST regimens [11, 26], this indication remains highly experimental. A retrospective comparison between haploidentical transplants and UCBT from the Japanese Society showed similar response, survival, and GvHD rates but better failure-free survival (FFS) in a haploidentical group [27].

Unrelated UCBT in SAA: Practical Recommendations

In general, for eligible patients with SAA, an unrelated UCBT should be considered only in the absence of a suitable BM donor and after the failure of intensive immunosuppression, including the administration of eltrombopag (at least in the adult population). To avoid the risk of graft failure due to an allogeneic immunization, donor-specific antibodies should be screened before transplantation [28–30]. One or two UCB units, each with less than two of six HLA mismatches, may be used to reach at least 4×10^7 cryopreserved nucleated cells/kg of the recipient. Particular attention should also be paid to patient cytomegalovirus (CMV) serostatus since CMV seronegativity is generally easier to manage. However, most of the data on the negative impact of CMV on UCBT come from a pre-letermovir era, and it is possible that this risk factor is now mitigated by the primary prophylaxis [31]. In addition to that, the importance of infection prevention and high-quality supportive care platforms is a key element for the success of this type of procedure, which should only be performed in experienced transplant centers. Other disease-specific considerations in idiopathic SAA concern the risk for long-term complications, including clonal myeloid evolution. In general, in SAA patients receiving an allogeneic HCT, the risk of secondary myeloid neoplasms is abolished across studies, with reassuring long-term data [32]. However, it is important to point out that most of the series addressed this issue after an MRD or matched unrelated donor (MUD) transplant, with scarce or no data for alternative donor platforms, for which long-term outcome data are still warranted.

> **Recommended Conditioning Regimen for Unrelated UCBT in SAA (from APCORD Trial and SAAWP)**
> Flu 30 mg/m²/d (D-6 to D-3), Cy 30 mg/kg/d (D-6 to D-3), ATG 2.5 mg/kg/d (D-4 to D-3), and TBI 2 Gy (D-1); GvHD prophylaxis: CsA alone (from 3 mg/kg D-1)

Fanconi Anemia

Past decades have seen a great improvement of outcomes in patients diagnosed with FA due to a better understanding of the molecular basis of the disease, the underlying genomic instability, and the development of strategies to control long-term complications, such as clonal evolution and solid cancer occurrence [33–36]. Allogeneic HCT is, at the moment, the only strategy able to correct the hematopoietic dysfunctions developed by these patients, ranging from progressive BMF to myelodysplastic syndrome (MDS)/acute myeloid leukemia (AML) [35]. Intensive research work has been done to advance transplant procedures in order to ameliorate the prognosis of this disease. Besides more accurate molecular testing and HLA typing, along with better supportive care, the design of less intensive conditioning regimens (including lower radiation and chemotherapy doses, incorporation of Flu, and the application of in vivo and/or ex vivo T cell depletion), as well as a better screening for post-HCT complications, was able to drastically decrease TRM and GvHD rates, enhancing engraftment and survival probabilities [35, 37–43].

Concerning the role of unrelated UCBT in this disease, most of the results come from historical retrospective studies, providing heterogeneous results. European Society for Blood and Marrow Transplantation (EBMT) provided an analysis of unrelated HLA-mismatched UCBT in 93 FA patients transplanted between 1994 and 2005, showing probabilities of survival at 2 years of about 40%, with a high incidence of acute (32%) and chronic (16%) GvHD [44]. Here, as in other UCBT series, Flu, high cellularity, and negative recipient CMV serology were associated with more favorable outcomes [44]. Similar results were reported by other historical smaller series characterized by a high incidence of graft failure and alloreactive and infectious complications [42, 45]. A more recent study analyzing the outcomes of alternative donor HCT in 130 FA patients (31 receiving a UCB) showed better survival probabilities, higher engraftment, and a lower incidence of acute and chronic GvHD in patients receiving Flu/TBI 3 Gy–based conditioning regimens, with even comparable results with BM [46]. The same group reported the outcomes of 21 FA patients transplanted for overt acute myeloid leukemia (AML)/myelodysplastic syndrome (MDS) evolution, with five receiving an unrelated UCBT with reduced-intensity conditioning (RIC) regimens (only two alive at the last reported follow-up) [47].

If Flu administration seems to improve the results of the procedure, the presence of more than one HLA disparity is associated with an unacceptable rate of failure and GvHD [44, 48]. For this reason, for this particular setting of patients, the current indication for UCBT is the administration of only one unit, with no more than one mismatch [23]. Thus, UCBT, using a specific disease-adapted conditioning regimen, is indicated in FA patients who lack an HLA-matched unrelated BM donor. A recent survey from Eurocord, evaluating long-term outcomes of UCBT in a large pediatric population, demonstrated the crucial role of HLA matching even upon graft cellularity, pointing toward this important prerequisite in the selection of UCB unit [49].

Unrelated UCBT in FA: Practical Recommendations

Despite all the improvements, unrelated UCBT in FA is still associated with unsatisfactory outcomes and a high rate of toxicity as compared to other graft sources. However, whenever an allogeneic HCT indication is considered and a suitable HLA-matched BM donor is missing, this procedure remains the only curative option, especially for young patients. HLA matching, along with the presence of alloreactive donor-specific antibodies and total cell doses, remains a crucial parameter to consider. For patients with a BMF indication, low-intensity conditioning regimens, Flu and low-dose Cy and TBI-based, associated with in vivo T cell depletion, are recommended, based on the current evidence. For patients diagnosed with an AML or MDS, many concerns are related to the type of pre-HCT cytoreduction and transplant procedures, which should proceed as for FA patients without clonal evolution due to the excessive toxicity in case of more intensive regimens [35]. Some groups have proposed sequential strategies, with acceptable results in patients receiving HLA-related or unrelated BM transplants, but at the moment of this manuscript writing, these procedures are not reproducible in the context of UCBT [50, 51].

Post-UCBT, long-term follow-up recommendations for FA are the same as for other stem cell sources, with further considerations related to the delayed immune reconstitution and risk of infection. FA patients are at an increased risk of post-HCT malignancies: The German Fanconi Anemia Registry reports about 30% of the incidence of solid malignancy by the age of 50 [52], and a fourfold higher rate of squamous cell carcinomas has been observed as compared to FA patients not receiving an allogeneic HCT [53]. Although in FA, there is a natural propensity to tumor development, chronic GvHD is an accelerator factor, especially for oral and neck carcinoma [38, 54]. Generally speaking, for all FA patients, regardless of the stem cell source, a regular screening for malignancies should be part of a long-term patient care program, with systematic evaluations proposed every 6 months by gynecologists and stomatologists to allow early cancer detection and promptly intervene with surgery [35]. Special attention to oral hygiene and limited alcohol consumption and smoking are mandatory. Screening for post-HCT endocrine dysfunctions (including hypothyroidism, diabetes, metabolic syndromes, and growth hormone deficiency) is also warranted and demands a comprehensive follow-up by pediatric endocrinologists [35, 55, 56].

> **Recommended Conditioning Regimen for FA in Unrelated UCBT (Eurocord)**
> Flu 30 mg/m^2/d (D-6 to D-3), Cy 10 mg/kg/d (D-6 to D-3), ATG 2.5 mg/kg/d (D-3 to D-2), and TBI 2 Gy (D-2); GvHD prophylaxis: CsA (3 mg/kg from D-1) and MMF (30 mg/kg from D+1)

Telomere Diseases

Telomere diseases, and in particular dyskeratosis congenita (DC), are rare, multisystem, heterogeneous disorders, characterized by a disruption of the telomere machinery, leading to the alteration of cell cycle regulation, with an impact on several organs and systems; impaired hepatic, lung, and hematopoietic functions; and cancer predisposition. BMF is a possible manifestation at all ages, and at least one single lineage cytopenia has been described in 50%–90% of patients after the age of 40 [57, 58]. HCT is the only curative strategy to definitely correct the underlying hematological deficiency; however, this approach is unable to solve the dysfunction of the other tissues and may, in contrast, accelerate it. As the disease is rare and associated with high mortality rates, no prospective studies have been conducted, and most of the evidence available has been produced by retrospective registry analyses or single-center experiences.

Historically, transplant regimens for DC patients were based on myeloablative chemotherapy, with disastrous outcomes [59]. The transition to RIC regimens has shown improved results but still with unsatisfactory late morbidity and mortality [60–64]. In previous series, early deaths were related to infection, graft failure, and hemorrhage, whereas late mortality >1 year was mostly attributed to pulmonary, liver, and vascular complications [60–64].

The first successful UCBT in DC was performed in 2002 from an HLA-identical sibling donor, using a fludarabine-based non-myeloablative conditioning regimen [65].

A large study cohort of DC patients ($N = 94$) reports the results of several transplant procedures (13% UCBT), showing lower survival probabilities for UCBT as compared to BM and peripheral blood stem cell (PBSC) (3-year overall survival (OS) 49% versus 68% and 72%, respectively) [64]. In another large study of 64 patients with inherited BMF, including eight cases of DC, receiving a UCBT, the only survivor was transplanted from an HLA-identical donor, while outcomes were very dismal in an unrelated setting [11].

Unrelated UCBT in Telomere Disorders: Practical Recommendations

Although it is not possible to draw recommendations, given the lack of prospective data and the small case series analyzed in retrospective setting, the goal of transplant procedures should be the same as for other inherited BMF and cancer-predisposing disorders to reduce (and avoid) early toxicity and long-term complications as much as possible. In this view, close clinico-biological monitoring is mandatory, leading to an early detection of solid cancers, chronic infections, pulmonary and liver dysfunctions, and endocrinological complications. Particular attention, as in FA and other cancer-predisposing disorders, should be devoted to avoiding chronic infections and GvHD, which are sources of tissue inflammation and transformation. Given the high incidence of lung and liver complications in telomere disorders, it is mandatory to adapt posttransplant follow-up to this specificity, with routine radiologic, functional, and if necessary, histological assessments. Unrelated UCB should be considered a transplant source only in the absence of any other therapeutic option, bearing in mind the high toxicity and mortality rate associated with the procedure. Given the lack of prospective data and large retrospective studies, it is not possible to recommend a specific conditioning regimen. It is important to note that telomere disorders may be highly responsive to androgen-based therapy, which should always be considered a non-transplant alternative if a matched related sibling donor is not available [26, 66–69].

Shwachman–Diamond Syndrome

Shwachman–Diamond syndrome (SDS) is a rare inherited disorder, associated with a dysfunction of the ribosome assembly machinery, leading to bone marrow dysfunction, skeletal abnormalities, short stature, exocrine pancreatic insufficiency, and predisposition to solid and hematological malignancies. HCT is a curable option for patients developing SDS-associated BMF (before overt AML or MDS), and as in other BMF syndromes, the use of reduced-intensity conditioning regimens and the limitation of total body irradiation have contributed to improving the results of the transplant procedure over time. The few (retrospective) studies on the outcomes of UCBT in SDS have demonstrated variable results, emphasizing the complexity and challenges associated with this treatment approach [70]. A large retrospective analysis by the SAAWP of the EBMT reported on the outcomes of 74 patients with SDS treated with HCT between 1988 and 2016 (70% BM, 19% PBSC, and 11% UCBT). Univariable analyses did not show any difference in terms of long-term outcomes based on the graft source and the type of donor (5-year OS: 63.3%, non-relapse mortality: 19.8%, CI of graft failure: 15%, and acute and chronic GvHD: 55 and 20%, respectively, for the whole population); however, the number of UCBT was very low ($N = 8$), precluding further in-depth analyses [71]. Unfortunately, other studies reporting specifically on outcomes of unrelated UCBT in this syndrome are too fragmented [72, 73], with only two patients reported by the Eurocord experience, making any formal statement of conclusion on the procedure [72] impossible.

One important finding across transplant studies is that, as in other inherited BMF, the evolution to MDS is associated with a high risk of mortality and toxicity [70].

It is also noteworthy to highlight that while HCT offers a potential cure for the hematologic aspects of SDS, it does not address all aspects of the syndrome, such as pancreatic dysfunction, which may continue to affect the patient's quality of life even after the underlying BMF syndrome is resolved.

Diamond–Blackfan Anemia

Diamond–Blackfan anemia (DBA) is a rare inherited BMF syndrome, characterized by an ineffective erythropoiesis, typically leading to severe anemia, often detected in infancy. This condition can present with various congenital abnormalities, including growth retardation, craniofacial deformities, and limb abnormalities [74]. DBA is caused by mutations in genes that encode ribosomal proteins, which are crucial components for ribosome function and cellular protein synthesis. The exact pathophysiology involves defective ribosome biogenesis, triggering p53-mediated apoptosis of erythroid progenitor cells. Treatment options are limited and typically include corticosteroids, which are effective in about 80% of cases; blood transfusions for those who are steroid-resistant; and allogeneic HCT in severe cases. Long-term management focuses on monitoring for complications such as iron overload from repeated transfusions and an increased risk of cancer [74].

Single successful cases concerning the use of unrelated UCBT in DBA are reported across the literature since the late 1990s [73, 75, 76]. Eurocord reported 21 patients receiving UCBT (13 related and eight unrelated) for this syndrome in Bizzetto's study [72]. Of note, while all DBA patients who received a related graft were alive, with a median follow-up of 65 months, in the unrelated context, only three survivors were censored at the last follow-up (median 31 months). If outcomes of unrelated UCBT were less interesting than those of related UCBT, age at transplant <5 years and UCB unit richness >6.7 × 10^7/kg were shown as factors associated with better OS in an unrelated context. In this series, conditioning regimens were extremely variable, precluding the possibility of extending recommendations.

Other Inherited BMF Disorders

Congenital amegakaryocytic thrombocytopenia (CAMT) is a rare hematopoietic disorder characterized by severe thrombocytopenia and the potential for progression to aplastic anemia or MDS, related to mutations in the MPL gene, coding for the thrombopoietin receptor, essential for megakaryocyte and platelet production. Due to the absence of effective long-term treatments and the severe risk of bleeding complications, allogeneic HCT is the only curative therapy. A few experiences have reported the use of UCB as a stem cell source, with interesting results. A series from Duke University was reported in 2015, describing five consecutive patients with CAMT who received a myeloablative conditioning (MAC) regimen and partially HLA-mismatched, unrelated UCBT, showing an excellent neutrophil engraftment (median time of 19 days in all patients) but very slow platelet recovery (median >50 days) and low rates of acute and chronic GvHD (one patient). In this series, at a median follow-up of 14 years, all patients were alive with a sustained donor cell engraftment [77]. Eurocord reported 16 patients in Bizzetto's study, three receiving a related and 13 receiving an unrelated UCBT [72]. Of this last group, four died within 2 months after transplantation, and the others are alive, with a median follow-up of 65 months (range: 25–121 months). The Center for International Blood and Marrow Transplant Research (CIBMTR) recently published a series of 86 CAMT patients (median age of 3 years) transplanted between 2000 and 2018, of whom 53 (62%) received BM and 26 (29%) received a single or double UCB. Although no adjustment was made based on the graft source, graft failure-free survival showed no difference according to the donor type, which, instead, influenced OS (reduced in case of mismatched donor, hazard ratio 3.52 [1.05–11.85]) [78]. Based on these few retrospective evidences, it is impossible to draw recommendations or guidelines, but UCBT needs to be acknowledged as a possible transplant strategy in the absence of other more suitable donors, able to rescue the hematological disease phenotype of this syndrome.

Congenital neutropenia (CN) is a rare group of disorders characterized by a marked decrease in neutrophil counts, leading to an augmented susceptibility to infections. Various forms can be considered, including severe congenital neutropenia (Kostmann syndrome) and cyclic neutropenia, each with distinct genetic etiologies and clinical manifestations. Mutations in genes such as ELANE, which encodes neutrophil elastase, are commonly implicated [79, 80]. Management strategies focus on preventing infections through the use of granulocyte colony-stimulating factor (G-CSF) to stimulate neutrophil production, and in severe cases or those with mutations predisposing to leukemia, HCT may be considered. Early diagnosis and tailored treatment are critical for improving outcomes and quality of life for patients with CN. UCBT, in this setting, may offer a potential cure in the absence of a suitable donor; however, as for the previously described BMF syndromes, only anecdotical cases are referenced in the literature. Eurocord experience reported the outcomes of UCBT in 16 patients with severe congenital neutropenia (SCN) (one receiving a related and the other 15 receiving unrelated grafts). In this series, three patients were transplanted for secondary leukemia or MDS. The others were transplanted because of a lack of response to G-CSF. Overall, 11 were reported as alive at a median follow-up of 41 months (range: 4–142 months) [72].

Special Situations: Matched-Related UCBT for BMF

Outcomes of UCBT derived from an HLA-identical sibling donor have been variously reported in the literature across several malignant and nonmalignant disorders, in particular for pediatric populations, featuring very interesting results, with a low rate of acute and chronic GvHD, high engraftment, and long-term survival [81–87]. These results were magnified in patients with nonmalignant diseases, and in BMF, very high survival probabilities and low toxicity were observed despite heterogeneous conditioning regimens and GvHD prophylaxes. Besides the historical literature, Eurocord reported more recently, in collaboration with the SAAWP and the cellular therapy and immunobiology working party (CTIWP) of the EBMT, the outcomes of 117 children and young adults (median age of 6 years) diagnosed with acquired and inherited BMF, receiving such a transplant modality (82 transplanted with a single UCB unit and 35 with a mixed BM+UCB graft) [88]. The cumulative incidence (CI) of neutrophil recovery was 89%, with a median engraftment time of 21 days. While the probability of long-term survival (almost 8 years) was 88%, the CIs of acute and chronic GvHD were 15% and 14%, respectively. In this cohort, secondary malignancies were observed only in one patient (osteosarcoma, in the context of a DBA diagnosis), while other types of late complications described were mostly endocrinological [88].

This and the previous quoted studies confirmed that UCBT from a matched related donor could be a valid option for patients with BMF lacking a suitable BM donor due to the excellent survival outcomes and the low risk of toxicity and graft failure. This possibility may give rise to the question as to whether we should collect in a family, whereby an individual is affected, cord blood from HLA-identical-related newborns. However, it is important to note that family-directed cord blood banking is not so promoted, and in contrast to the well-developed public banking systems for allogeneic use, only a few countries have centralized programs for family-directed UCB storage [89].

Conclusive Remarks

The use of UCB as a stem cell source is particularly attractive due to its ready availability, reduced risk of transmitting infections, and the lower stringency required for HLA matching, which decreases the incidence and severity of GvHD, compared to other stem cell sources. Its use in BMF syndromes can be considered in case of the absence of matched related or unrelated donors and possibly after considering other alternative donors (mismatched unrelated and haploidentical), in case of the failure of other non-transplant approaches (i.e., androgens for DC, steroids for DBA, etc.) or evidence of clonal evolution. If related HLA-matched UCBT procedures have shown excellent results across the spectrum of BMF and are now more and more considered in transplant centers as add-ons of BM grafts when available, a more cautious evaluation should be addressed regarding the consideration of unrelated UCB units, carefully paying attention to the aspects of patient selection, optimization of conditioning regimens, and effective management of transplantation-related complications, which can significantly improve outcomes and quality of life for affected individuals.

References

1. Passweg JR, Baldomero H, Chabannon C, et al. Hematopoietic cell transplantation and cellular therapy survey of the EBMT: monitoring of activities and trends over 30 years. Bone Marrow Transplant. 2021;56:1651.
2. Gluckman E, Broxmeyer HA, Auerbach AD, et al. Hematopoietic reconstitution in a patient with Fanconi's anemia by means of umbilical-cord blood from an HLA-identical sibling. N Engl J Med. 1989;321(17):1174–8.
3. Auerbach AD, Liu Q, Ghosh R, et al. Prenatal identification of potential donors for umbilical cord blood transplantation for Fanconi anemia. Transfusion. 1990;30(8):682–7.
4. Broxmeyer HE, Douglas GW, Hangoc G, et al. Human umbilical cord blood as a potential source of transplantable hematopoietic stem/progenitor cells. Proc Natl Acad Sci USA. 1989;86(10):3828–32.
5. Ballen KK, Gluckman E, Broxmeyer HE. Umbilical cord blood transplantation: the first 25 years and beyond. Blood. 2013;122(4):491–8.
6. Wagner JE, Gluckman E. Umbilical cord blood transplantation: the first 20 years. Semin Hematol. 2010;47(1):3–12.
7. Gluckman E, Rocha V, Boyer-Chammard A, et al. Outcome of cord-blood transplantation from related and unrelated donors. Eurocord Transplant Group and the European Blood and Marrow Transplantation Group. N Engl J Med. 1997;337(6):373–81.
8. Gluckman E, Rocha V. Cord blood transplantation: state of the art. Haematologica. 2009;94(4):451–4.
9. Wagner John E, Steinbuch M, Kernan Nancy A, Broxmayer Hal E, Gluckman E. Allogeneic sibling umbilical-cord-blood transplantation in children with malignant and non-malignant disease. Lancet. 1995;346(8969):214–9.
10. Rocha V, Gluckman E, Eurocord and European Blood and Marrow Transplant Group. Clinical use of umbilical cord blood hematopoietic stem cells. Biol Blood Marrow Transplant. 2006;12(1 Suppl 1):34–41.
11. Peffault de Latour R, Kulasekararaj A, Iacobelli S, et al. Eltrombopag added to immunosuppression in severe aplastic anemia. N Engl J Med. 2022;386(1):11–23.
12. Prata PH, Eikema D-J, Afansyev B, et al. Haploidentical transplantation and posttransplant cyclophosphamide for treating aplastic anemia patients: a report from the EBMT Severe Aplastic Anemia Working Party. Bone Marrow Transplant. 2020;55(6):1050–8.
13. DeZern AE, Zahurak M, Symons HJ, et al. Alternative donor BMT with posttransplant cyclophosphamide as initial therapy for acquired severe aplastic anemia. Blood. 2023;141(25):3031–8.
14. DeZern AE, Brodsky RA. Combining PTCy and ATG for GvHD prophylaxis in non-malignant diseases. Blood Rev. 2023;62:101016.
15. DeZern AE, Eapen M, Wu J, et al. Haploidentical bone marrow transplantation in patients with relapsed or refractory severe aplastic anaemia in the USA (BMT CTN 1502): a multicentre, single-arm, phase 2 trial. Lancet Haematol. 2022;9(9):e660–9.
16. Ochi T, Onishi Y, Nasu K, et al. Umbilical cord blood transplantation using reduced-intensity conditioning without antithymocyte globulin in adult patients with severe aplastic anemia. Biol Blood Marrow Transplant. 2019;25(2):e55–9.
17. Lau FY, Wong R, Chui CH, Cheng G. Successful engraftment in two adult patients with severe aplastic anemia using nonmyeloablative conditioning followed by unrelated HLA-mismatched cord blood transplantation. J Hematother Stem Cell Res. 2001;10(2):309–11.
18. Mao P, Zhu Z, Wang H, et al. Sustained and stable hematopoietic donor-recipient mixed chimerism after unrelated cord blood transplantation for adult patients with severe aplastic anemia. Eur J Haematol. 2005;75(5):430–5.
19. Yoshimi A, Kojima S, Taniguchi S, et al. Unrelated cord blood transplantation for severe aplastic anemia. Biol Blood Marrow Transplant. 2008;14(9):1057–63.

20. Peffault de Latour R, Purtill D, Ruggeri A, et al. Influence of nucleated cell dose on overall survival of unrelated cord blood transplantation for patients with severe acquired aplastic anemia: a study by eurocord and the aplastic anemia working party of the European group for blood and marrow transplantation. Biol Blood Marrow Transplant. 2011;17(1):78–85.
21. Kuwatsuka Y, Kanda J, Yamazaki H, et al. A comparison of outcomes for cord blood transplantation and unrelated bone marrow transplantation in adult aplastic anemia. Biol Blood Marrow Transplant. 2016;22(10):1836–43.
22. Peffault de Latour R, Chevret S, Jubert C, et al. Unrelated cord blood transplantation in patients with idiopathic refractory severe aplastic anemia: a nationwide phase 2 study. Blood. 2018;132(7):750–4.
23. Peffault de Latour R. Transplantation for bone marrow failure: current issues. Hematology. 2016;2016(1):90–8.
24. Zhou F, Zhang F, Zhang L, et al. A multicentre trial of intensive immunosuppressive therapy combined with umbilical cord blood for the treatment of severe aplastic anaemia. Ann Hematol. 2022;101(8):1785–94.
25. Zhao X, Lv W, Song K, et al. Upfront umbilical cord blood transplantation versus immunosuppressive therapy for pediatric patients with idiopathic severe aplastic anemia. Transplant Cell Ther. 2024;60:442-e1. S2666636724001659.
26. Pagliuca S, Kulasekararaj AG, Eikema D-J, et al. Current use of androgens in bone marrow failure disorders: a report from the Severe Aplastic Anemia Working Party of the European Society of Blood and Marrow Transplantation. Haematologica. 2023;109:765.
27. Onishi Y, Mori T, Yamazaki H, et al. Comparison of Haploidentical stem cell transplantation with post-transplantation cyclophosphamide versus umbilical cord blood transplantation in adult patients with aplastic anemia. Transplant Cell Ther. 2023;29(12):766.e1–8.
28. Yamamoto H, Uchida N, Matsuno N, et al. Anti-HLA antibodies other than against HLA-A, -B, -DRB1 adversely affect engraftment and nonrelapse mortality in HLA-mismatched single cord blood transplantation: possible implications of unrecognized donor-specific antibodies. Biol Blood Marrow Transplant. 2014;20(10):1634–40.
29. Morin-Zorman S, Loiseau P, Taupin J-L, Caillat-Zucman S. Donor-specific anti-HLA antibodies in allogeneic hematopoietic stem cell transplantation. Front Immunol. 2016;7:307.
30. van Besien K. Advances in umbilical cord blood transplant: a summary of the 11th international cord blood symposium, San Francisco, 6–8 June 2013. Leuk Lymphoma. 2014;55(8):1735–8.
31. Rivera Franco MM, Rafii H, Volt F, et al. Use of letermovir in umbilical cord blood transplantation based on risk scores. Blood Adv. 2023;7(16):4315–8.
32. Gurnari C, Pagliuca S, Prata PH, et al. Clinical and molecular determinants of clonal evolution in aplastic anemia and paroxysmal nocturnal hemoglobinuria. J Clin Oncol. 2023;41:132–42.
33. Sebert M, Gachet S, Leblanc T, et al. Clonal hematopoiesis driven by chromosome 1q/MDM4 trisomy defines a canonical route toward leukemia in Fanconi anemia. Cell Stem Cell. 2023;30(2):153–170.e9.
34. Bluteau O, Sebert M, Leblanc T, et al. A landscape of germ line mutations in a cohort of inherited bone marrow failure patients. Blood. 2018;131(7):717–32.
35. Peffault de Latour R, Soulier J. How I treat MDS and AML in Fanconi anemia. Blood. 2016;127(24):2971–9.
36. Kutler DI, Singh B, Satagopan J, et al. A 20-year perspective on the International Fanconi Anemia Registry (IFAR). Blood. 2003;101(4):1249–56.
37. Benajiba L, Salvado C, Dalle J-H, et al. HLA-matched related-donor HSCT in Fanconi anemia patients conditioned with cyclophosphamide and fludarabine. Blood. 2015;125(2):417–8.
38. Peffault de Latour R, Porcher R, Dalle J-H, et al. Allogeneic hematopoietic stem cell transplantation in Fanconi anemia: the European Group for Blood and Marrow Transplantation experience. Blood. 2013;122(26):4279–86.
39. Eyrich M, Winkler B, Schlegel PG. Stem cell transplantation in Fanconi anemia – recent advances with alternative donors. Monogr Hum Genet. 2007;15:173–82.

40. Kapelushnik J, Or R, Slavin S, Nagler A. A fludarabine-based protocol for bone marrow transplantation in Fanconi's anemia. Bone Marrow Transplant. 1997;20(12):1109–10.
41. Bitan M, Or R, Shapira MY, et al. Fludarabine-based reduced intensity conditioning for stem cell transplantation of Fanconi anemia patients from fully matched related and unrelated donors. Biol Blood Marrow Transplant. 2006;12(7):712–8.
42. Ruggeri A, Peffault de Latour R, Rocha V, et al. Double cord blood transplantation in patients with high risk bone marrow failure syndromes. Br J Haematol. 2008;143(3):404–8.
43. Pagliuca S, Ruggeri A, Peffault de Latour R. Cord blood transplantation for bone marrow failure syndromes: state of art. Stem Cell Investig. 2019;6:39.
44. Gluckman E, Rocha V, Ionescu I, et al. Results of unrelated cord blood transplant in fanconi anemia patients: risk factor analysis for engraftment and survival. Biol Blood Marrow Transplant. 2007;13(9):1073–82.
45. Ayas M, Al-Seraihi A, El-Solh H, et al. The Saudi experience in fludarabine-based conditioning regimens in patients with Fanconi anemia undergoing stem cell transplantation: excellent outcome in recipients of matched related stem cells but not in recipients of unrelated cord blood stem cells. Biol Blood Marrow Transplant. 2012;18(4):627–32.
46. MacMillan ML, DeFor TE, Young J-AH, et al. Alternative donor hematopoietic cell transplantation for Fanconi anemia. Blood. 2015;125(24):3798–804.
47. Mitchell R, Wagner JE, Hirsch B, et al. Haematopoietic cell transplantation for acute leukaemia and advanced myelodysplastic syndrome in F anconi anaemia. Br J Haematol. 2014;164(3):384–95.
48. Sauter C, Barker JN. Unrelated donor umbilical cord blood transplantation for the treatment of hematologic malignancies. Curr Opin Hematol. 2008;15(6):568–75.
49. Kurtzberg J, Troy JD, Page KM, et al. Unrelated donor cord blood transplantation in children: lessons learned over 3 decades. Stem Cells Transl Med. 2023;12(1):26–38.
50. Talbot A, Peffault de Latour R, Raffoux E, et al. Sequential treatment for allogeneic hematopoietic stem cell transplantation in Fanconi anemia with acute myeloid leukemia. Haematologica. 2014;99(10):e199–200.
51. Mehta PA, Ileri T, Harris RE, et al. Chemotherapy for myeloid malignancy in children with Fanconi anemia. Pediatr Blood Cancer. 2007;48(7):668–72.
52. Rosenberg PS, Alter BP, Ebell W. Cancer risks in Fanconi anemia: findings from the German Fanconi Anemia Registry. Haematologica. 2008;93(4):511–7.
53. Rosenberg PS, Socié G, Alter BP, Gluckman E. Risk of head and neck squamous cell cancer and death in patients with Fanconi anemia who did and did not receive transplants. Blood. 2005;105(1):67–73.
54. Deeg HJ, Socie G. Malignancies after hematopoietic stem cell transplantation: many questions, some answers. Blood. 1998;91(6):1833–44.
55. Sanders JE. Endocrine complications of high-dose therapy with stem cell transplantation. Pediatr Transplant. 2004;8(s5):39–50.
56. Sanders JE. Growth and development after hematopoietic cell transplant in children. Bone Marrow Transplant. 2008;41(2):223–7.
57. Alter BP, Giri N, Savage SA, et al. Malignancies and survival patterns in the National Cancer Institute inherited bone marrow failure syndromes cohort study. Br J Haematol. 2010;150(2):179–88.
58. Alter BP, Giri N, Savage SA, Rosenberg PS. Cancer in the National Cancer Institute inherited bone marrow failure syndrome cohort after fifteen years of follow-up. Haematologica. 2018;103(1):30–9.
59. Langston AA, Sanders JE, Deeg HJ, et al. Allogeneic marrow transplantation for aplastic anaemia associated with dyskeratosis congenita. Br J Haematol. 1996;92(3):758–65.
60. Imai J, Suzuki T, Yoshikawa M, et al. Fatal hemorrhagic gastrointestinal angioectasia after bone marrow transplantation for dyskeratosis congenita. Intern Med. 2016;55(23):3441–4.

61. Amarasinghe K, Dalley C, Dokal I, et al. Late death after unrelated-BMT for dyskeratosis congenita following conditioning with alemtuzumab, fludarabine and melphalan. Bone Marrow Transplant. 2007;40(9):913–4.
62. Nishio N, Takahashi Y, Ohashi H, et al. Reduced-intensity conditioning for alternative donor hematopoietic stem cell transplantation in patients with dyskeratosis congenita. Pediatr Transplant. 2011;15(2):161–6.
63. Bhoopalan SV, Wlodarski M, Reiss U, Triplett B, Sharma A. Reduced-intensity conditioning-based hematopoietic cell transplantation for dyskeratosis congenita: single-center experience and literature review. Pediatr Blood Cancer. 2021;68(10):e29177.
64. Fioredda F, Iacobelli S, Korthof ET, et al. Outcome of haematopoietic stem cell transplantation in dyskeratosis congenita. Br J Haematol. 2018;183(1):110–8.
65. Nobili B, Rossi G, De Stefano P, et al. Successful umbilical cord blood transplantation in a child with dyskeratosis congenita after a fludarabine-based reduced-intensity conditioning regimen. Br J Haematol. 2002;119(2):573–4.
66. Savage SA, Niewisch MR. Dyskeratosis congenita and related telomere biology disorders. In: GeneReviews®. Seattle: University of Washington; 1993.
67. Townsley DM, Dumitriu B, Liu D, et al. Danazol treatment for telomere diseases. N Engl J Med. 2016;374(20):1922–31.
68. Townsley DM, Winkler T. Nontransplant therapy for bone marrow failure. Hematology Am Soc Hematol Educ Program. 2016;2016(1):83–9.
69. Clé DV, Catto LFB, Gutierrez-Rodrigues F, et al. Effects of nandrolone decanoate on telomere length and clinical outcome in patients with telomeropathies: a prospective trial. Haematologica. 2023;108(5):1300–12.
70. Cesaro S, Donadieu J, Cipolli M, et al. Stem cell transplantation in patients affected by Shwachman-diamond syndrome: expert consensus and recommendations from the EBMT severe aplastic Anaemia Working Party. Transplant Cell Ther. 2022;28(10):637–49.
71. Cesaro S, Pillon M, Sauer M, et al. Long-term outcome after allogeneic hematopoietic stem cell transplantation for Shwachman–Diamond syndrome: a retrospective analysis and a review of the literature by the Severe Aplastic Anemia Working Party of the European Society for Blood and Marrow Transplantation (SAAWP-EBMT). Bone Marrow Transplant. 2020;55(9):1796–809.
72. Bizzetto R, Bonfim C, Rocha V, et al. Outcomes after related and unrelated umbilical cord blood transplantation for hereditary bone marrow failure syndromes other than Fanconi anemia. Haematologica. 2011;96(1):134–41.
73. Vibhakar R, Radhi M, Rumelhart S, Tatman D, Goldman F. Successful unrelated umbilical cord blood transplantation in children with Shwachman-Diamond syndrome. Bone Marrow Transplant. 2005;36(10):855–61.
74. Da Costa L, Leblanc T, Mohandas N. Diamond-Blackfan anemia. Blood. 2020;136(11):1262–73.
75. Shaw PH, Haut PR, Olszewski M, Kletzel M. Hematopoietic stem-cell transplantation using unrelated cord-blood versus matched sibling marrow in pediatric bone marrow failure syndrome: one center's experience. Pediatr Transplant. 1999;3(4):315–21.
76. Bonno M, Azuma E, Nakano T, et al. Successful hematopoietic reconstitution by transplantation of umbilical cord blood cells in a transfusion-dependent child with Diamond-Blackfan anemia. Bone Marrow Transplant. 1997;19(1):83–5.
77. Mahadeo KM, Tewari P, Parikh SH, et al. Durable engraftment and correction of hematological abnormalities in children with congenital amegakaryocytic thrombocytopenia following myeloablative umbilical cord blood transplantation. Pediatr Transplant. 2015;19(7):753–7.
78. Cancio M, Hebert K, Kim S, et al. Outcomes in hematopoietic stem cell transplantation for congenital amegakaryocytic thrombocytopenia. Transplant Cell Ther. 2022;28(2):101.e1–6.
79. Skokowa J, Dale DC, Touw IP, Zeidler C, Welte K. Severe congenital neutropenias. Nat Rev Dis Primers. 2017;3:17032.

80. Donadieu J, Bellanné-Chantelot C. Genetics of severe congenital neutropenia as a gateway to personalized therapy. Hematology Am Soc Hematol Educ Program. 2022;2022(1):658–65.
81. Rocha V, Wagner JE, Sobocinski KA, et al. Graft-versus-host disease in children who have received a cord-blood or bone marrow transplant from an HLA-identical sibling. Eurocord and International Bone Marrow Transplant Registry Working Committee on alternative donor and stem cell sources. N Engl J Med. 2000;342(25):1846–54.
82. Rocha V, Chastang C, Souillet G, et al. Related cord blood transplants: the Eurocord experience from 78 transplants. Eurocord Transplant group. Bone Marrow Transplant. 1998;21(Suppl 3):S59–62.
83. Grewal SS, Kahn JP, MacMillan ML, Ramsay NKC, Wagner JE. Successful hematopoietic stem cell transplantation for Fanconi anemia from an unaffected HLA-genotype-identical sibling selected using preimplantation genetic diagnosis. Blood. 2004;103(3):1147–51.
84. Reed W, Walters M, Trachtenberg E, Smith R, Lubin BH. Sibling donor cord blood banking for children with sickle cell disease. Pediatr Pathol Mol Med. 2001;20(2):167–74.
85. de Vries ACH, Bredius RGM, Lankester AC, et al. HLA-identical umbilical cord blood transplantation from a sibling donor in juvenile myelomonocytic leukemia. Haematologica. 2009;94(2):302–4.
86. Kuskonmaz B, Gocer S, Ersoy-Ewans S, et al. Hyperacute graft-vs.-host disease after related HLA-identical umbilical cord blood transplantation. Pediatr Transplant. 2007;11(7):818–20.
87. Soni S, Boulad F, Cowan MJ, et al. Combined umbilical cord blood and bone marrow from HLA-identical sibling donors for hematopoietic stem cell transplantation in children with hemoglobinopathies. Pediatr Blood Cancer. 2014;61(9):1690–4.
88. Pagliuca S, Peffault de Latour R, Volt F, et al. Long-term outcomes of cord blood transplantation from an HLA-identical sibling for patients with bone marrow failure syndromes: a report from Eurocord, cord blood committee and severe aplastic anemia Working Party of the European Society for Blood and Marrow Transplantation. Biol Blood Marrow Transplant. 2017;23(11):1939–48.
89. Gluckman E, Ruggeri A, Rocha V, et al. Family-directed umbilical cord blood banking. Haematologica. 2011;96(11):1700–7.

Open Access This chapter is licensed under the terms of the Creative Commons Attribution 4.0 International License (http://creativecommons.org/licenses/by/4.0/), which permits use, sharing, adaptation, distribution and reproduction in any medium or format, as long as you give appropriate credit to the original author(s) and the source, provide a link to the Creative Commons license and indicate if changes were made.

The images or other third party material in this chapter are included in the chapter's Creative Commons license, unless indicated otherwise in a credit line to the material. If material is not included in the chapter's Creative Commons license and your intended use is not permitted by statutory regulation or exceeds the permitted use, you will need to obtain permission directly from the copyright holder.

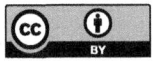

Part VI
Paroxysmal Nocturnal Hemoglobinuria (PNH) and Bone Marrow Failure

Chapter 14
Paroxysmal Nocturnal Hemoglobinuria: Bone Marrow Failure and Beyond

Antonio M. Risitano, Camilla Frieri, Pedro H. Prata, and Régis Peffault de Latour

Introduction

The diagnosis of aplastic anemia (AA) is defined by the association of pancytopenia with persistent and unexplained reduced marrow hematopoietic cellularity in the absence of dysplastic features. There are thus no specific biological markers, and the diagnosis is reached by the exclusion of other reasonable entities. The diagnosis of idiopathic AA (IAA) can be difficult, basically due to the overlapping morphological characteristics with other bone marrow failure (BMF) disorders, especially Fanconi anemia [1–3]. In this context, the detection of a paroxysmal nocturnal hemoglobinuria (PNH) clone is helpful since it is generally the signature of an autoimmune-mediated process, eliminating a constitutional disorder per se. However, the presence of a PNH clone in the context of BMF is confusing most of the time for hematologist colleagues, especially when the question of a specific treatment of PNH (i.e., treatment with a complement inhibitor, with the aim of controlling hemolysis and preventing thromboembolisms) arises. Indeed, the diagnosis of classic PNH is based on additional clinical manifestations (i.e., overt hemolysis), which do not often occur in the context of BMF, where usually the diagnosis of an AA/PNH syndrome (here, hemolysis is still present) or of subclinical PNH and intermediate PNH (these two subcategories are less well-defined and may generate

---

A. M. Risitano (✉) · C. Frieri
Hematology and Hematopoietic Transplant Unit, Azienda Ospedaliera di Rilievo Nazionale San Giuseppe Moscati, Avellino, Italy
e-mail: amrisita@unina.it

P. H. Prata
Hematology and Cellular Therapy Department, CHU de Limoges, France

R. Peffault de Latour
Hematology and Transplant Unit, Saint-Louis Hospital, AP-HP and Université Paris Cité, Paris, France

confusion in the daily practice [4, 5]). Here, we will start discussing the pathophysiology of this particular disease, aiming to describe a unifying interpretation that may account for the pleiotropic disease presentation leading to distinct clinical manifestations. This paper will successively address the significance of a PNH clone in the context of bone marrow failure and the treatment approach for each of the clinical presentations mentioned above.

Pathophysiology of BMF in PNH

As discussed below, bone marrow failure is one of the three typical manifestations of PNH, the other two being complement-mediated hemolysis and thrombophilia. Indeed, PNH patients are not only anemic since they often exhibit cytopenias involving other blood lineages, which result from an impaired production from the bone marrow rather than from increased turnover (as for erythrocytes). The impairment of the bone marrow in PNH is confirmed by in vitro studies showing reduced numbers of lineage-committed hematopoietic progenitors (CFU-E, BFU-E, CFU-GM, and CFU-GEMM) [6, 7] and also a contraction of the best in vitro surrogate for hematopoietic stem cells (HSCs), the so-called long-term culture-initiating cells (LTC-ICs) [7]. Thus, in PNH, the underlying bone marrow disorder is not only qualitative (i.e., the production of mature blood cells lacking from their surface all GPI-linked proteins, which eventually accounts for hemolysis and thrombophilia) but also quantitative. This bone marrow failure (BMF) represents a bridge between PNH and the most typical acquired BMF, idiopathic aplastic anemia (IAA). Clinically, many PNH patients develop mild-to-severe cytopenia (up to frank IAA) during their disease course [5, 8], and many IAA patients harbor PNH cell populations (and may even develop clinical PNH) [9–12]. The association between these diseases has been well-known for almost half a century, with the initial description by Dr. Lewis and Sir Dacie [13, 14], and even the pathogenic similarities induced investigators to consider AA and PNH the two faces of the same medal rather than two distinct diseases [14]. Several pieces of evidence suggest that an immune-mediated pathophysiology plays a role in BMF in PNH, and it is eventually involved even in the expansion of the *PIGA*-mutated hematopoiesis, which is needed to develop the clinical disease; all these aspects are discussed below in more detail.

Derangement of the Immune System

The immune-mediated pathophysiology of bone marrow failure is well-established in IAA: A plethora of in vitro and ex vivo data demonstrates that an immune-mediated attack on normal hematopoiesis may damage HSCs and hematopoietic progenitors [15, 16]. While it is still unknown what the target antigens are and why such a response eludes the physiological control of self-reactive immunity, the key role of preferentially expanded clonal T cells has been documented [17]. Because of the clinical overlap between IAA and PNH, several investigators have searched for evidence of antigen-driven immune responses even in PNH. Indeed, the oligoclonality of the T cell pool was initially reported by Karadimitris et al. [18] and subsequently confirmed by other groups [17, 19]. As for IAA, highly homologous TCR-beta sequences were found in different PNH patients, consistent with an antigen-driven public immune response [20]. Interestingly, in contrast with AA, in PNH, these homologous TCRs were shared among patients, irrespective of their human leukocyte antigen (HLA) background, possibly suggesting that the driving antigen may be non-peptidic (i.e., non-HLA restricted), such as glycolipids [20]. And among glycolipids, an obvious candidate antigen could be the glycosylphosphatidylinositol (GPI) anchor itself, which is lacking on PNH cells due to the pathogenic *PIGA* mutation. Notably, this hypothesis is supported by the observation that GPI-specific T cells were found, albeit at a very low frequency, both in PNH and AA patients [21, 22]. As in IAA, these clonal T cell populations often exhibit an effector, cytotoxic phenotype, characterized by the expression of CD8 and CD57, with a possible imbalance of the activating and inhibitory surface receptors [23]. In a few cases, these T cell clonal expansions may functionally resemble those seen in large granular lymphocytes [24, 25].

The Dual Pathophysiology Theory

The immunological abnormalities found in PNH patients are crucial not only because they support an immune-mediated BMF, such as in IAA, but also because they may shed light upon the key pathogenic event in PNH, namely the expansion of the aberrant, *PIGA*-mutated HSCs. Indeed, while it is well-accepted that a somatic mutation in HSCs is necessary to develop PNH, several observations support the concept that the mutation itself is not sufficient to cause the disease [26]. Indeed, if it is true that a *PIGA* mutation (or very rarely, inactivating mutations of other genes involved in the same pathway) is found in all PNH patients, on the other hand, the same mutation can be detected even in subjects without PNH. A few blood cells with the PNH phenotype (namely, a complete or partial deficiency in all GPI-linked proteins) and harboring inactivating *PIGA* mutations may be found even in normal individuals, even if at a very low frequency (ranging between ten and 50 cells per million) [27]. Thus, at least in these subjects, a *PIGA* mutation was not sufficient to cause PNH, possibly because it arose in blood cells without self-renewal capability (i.e., not in an HSC). This observation was also confirmed in the animal model; indeed, in all the sophisticated attempts aiming to generate a mouse model of PNH, the *PIGA*-mutated hematopoiesis usually disappears over time, eventually suggesting that other mechanisms are required to sustain the expansion of PNH-like hematopoiesis [28–30]. The possibility that such additional factors exist comes again from clinical observation in PNH patients; indeed, it is well-known that the same PNH patient may harbor distinct PNH clones with different

PIGA mutations [31, 32]. Thus, it is conceivable that a *PIGA* mutation simply confers a biological phenotype (the GPI anchor deficiency) that eventually requires additional, *PIGA*-independent factors/events for further clonal expansion, necessary for developing PNH as a disease. In fact, the expansion of distinct clones carrying the same, albeit molecularly heterogeneous, functional defect does not seem to fit with a random process, as also supported by the observation that in case of relapse of PNH, clones harboring *PIGA* mutations different from those identified at diagnosis can be found [33].

To reconcile all these observations, in 1989, Rotoli and Luzzatto drafted the theory of the "dual pathophysiology" of PNH [26], which is also known as the "relative advantage" [34] or "escape" theory [16]. According to this theory, a *PIGA* mutation is required but not sufficient to promote the expansion of GPI-deficient hematopoiesis because it does not confer any intrinsic proliferation advantage on normal hematopoiesis [27]. Then, additional events may occur, which eventually promote the expansion of PNH HSCs over normal ones; this second event is likely an immune-mediated attack on hematopoiesis, similar to that causing IAA. However, such an immune attack for some reasons (a putative antigen, which is absent on PNH cells, such as the GPI anchor, or the intrinsic resistance of PNH cells to T-cell-mediated immune attack, possibly due to functionally impaired immune synapsis as a consequence of GPI deficiency) may spare PNH HSCs, eventually resulting in their relative expansion over normal, damaged hematopoiesis; thus, PNH hematopoiesis may finally limit the development of clinical bone marrow failure but, on the other hand, results in PNH with its typical clinical phenotype [16, 26, 34]. This scenario is supported by the immune derangement discussed above and even more by the gene expression profile data on PNH and non-PNH CD34+ cells isolated from PNH patients. In this study, while PNH (GPI-deficient) CD34+ cells showed a gene expression profile almost indistinguishable from healthy individuals, phenotypically normal (GPI-positive) CD34+ cells harbored diffuse abnormalities, with the overexpression of genes involved in apoptosis and immune activity, paralleling the findings seen in CD34+ cells of AA patients [35]. These data strongly support the presence of an immune-mediated extrinsic, sublethal damage, which selectively pertains to normal HSCs in PNH patients and, apparently, spares PNH HSCs [35]. Thus, PNH hematopoiesis eventually expands as a result of this persistent selective pressure; the reasons accounting for the escape of PNH HSC are still unknown. It has been hypothesized that the antigen targeted by the immune attack may be absent on PNH cells; quite recently, GPI-specific, clonal, CD8+ T cells have been found in several PNH patients, possibly suggesting that the GPI anchor itself (thus, a glycolipid antigen presented via C1d rather than via HLA molecules) may be the target of the autoimmune process causing BMF in PNH patients (and even the expansion of PNH HSCs, eventually causing the clinical phenotype of PNH) [21]. Clinically speaking, this scenario also accounts for the relatively frequent expansion of PNH hematopoiesis in IAA patients who have received immunosuppressive treatments (ISTs); in this context, the improvement of peripheral blood counts should be interpreted as the development of clinical PNH instead of as a response to immunosuppression (which would rather lead to re-expansion of normal, non-PNH hematopoiesis).

The Role of Somatic Mutations

The presence of an immune-mediated attack sparing PNH hematopoiesis reconciles with most of the observations described above; however, a definitive proof of this pathogenic mechanism is still lacking, eventually giving rise to an alternative hypothesis. Indeed, the selective advantage of the PNH HSCs may result from secondary genetic events, which may confer an absolute growth advantage. Even if the demonstration that the *PIGA* mutation does not confer any intrinsic genetic susceptibility [27] argued against this hypothesis, recent data may now change this view. A few cases of PNH patients harboring well-defined mutations in the 3' of the HMGA2 gene have been reported [36]; however, even if HMGA2 overexpression may lead to proliferative advantage, this mutation has not been found in larger series of patients. More recently, the availability of next-generation sequencing techniques allowed the identification of additional somatic mutations in several PNH patients [37]. Notably, even if mutations were not recurrent, they may also affect genes involved in the pathophysiology of myeloid neoplasm, such as TET2, SUZ12, U2AF1, and JAK2 [37]. The definition of the hierarchical clonal architecture of hematopoiesis in PNH patients defines a complex scenario where accessory genetic events may occur before or after the *PIGA* mutation, similar to stepwise clonal evolution seen in hematological malignancies [37]. However, in contrast to *PIGA*, these additional mutations remain patient-specific, and further canonical mutational patterns have not been identified, eventually suggesting that these additional mutations should not play a specific role in PNH pathophysiology, even if they can still affect the fitness of specific stem cells, with possible clinical implications.

These data have to be interpreted in the context of our novel understanding of clonal hematopoiesis, and they have clearly demonstrated that some of these somatic mutations do not necessarily imply an obvious transformation to myeloid cancers, nor any increased risk of malignant transformation [38, 39]. Indeed, these mutations have also been found in IAA, and their pathogenic meaning remains elusive [40]; even if, in the context of PNH pathophysiology, they might account for selective clonal expansion, eventually, arguing against the need for an immune-mediated selection, further investigations are needed to define their possible pathogenic role.

PNH Clone(s) in Patients with BMF

PNH Disease Subcategories

PNH is characterized by a unique triad of clinical features: intravascular hemolysis, thromboembolic events, and cytopenia [4, 5, 8, 41]. However, not all three manifestations are present in all the patients, and the individual presentation of each patient may greatly vary according to the most dominant signs and symptoms. Thus, many investigators have tried to classify PNH according to the most typical clinical presentations; however, distinct categories are hard to define for a disease with such an unpredictable presentation and evolution.

The most adopted classification of PNH was proposed by the International PNH Interest Group (IPIG) in 2005 [4], whereby PNH patients are grouped according to the presence of hemolysis and an underlying bone marrow disorder. Accordingly, three distinct subtypes are identified: i.e., classic PNH, characterized by hemolysis without other marrow disorder (i.e., hemolytic PNH patients without relevant cytopenia); (ii) PNH in the setting of another bone marrow disorder, characterized by hemolysis associated with an underlying marrow disorder, usually AA or myelodysplastic syndromes (MDS) (i.e., hemolytic PNH patients with cytopenia; AA or MDS may be concomitant or may have preceded PNH); and (iii) subclinical PNH, characterized by the presence of PNH cells in the absence of any clinical or laboratory signs of hemolysis, in the setting of other hematological disorders (i.e., AA or MDS patients with GPI-AP deficient cells but not clinical PNH). This classification has generated some confusion in the past for different reasons: (i) PNH is a bone marrow disorder per se; thus, it always emerges in the context "of another bone marrow disorder"; (ii) this additional "bone marrow disorder" is always exclusively an immune-mediated BMF, which should be classified as AA (association between PNH and MDS is quite rare and may also be due to the misdiagnosis of MDS, albeit evolution to MDS and other myeloid malignancy is a well-defined event in the context of AA and more rarely PNH; association with other bone marrow disorders is even more rare, even if anecdotic cases of PNH and myeloproliferative neoplasms have been reported); and (iii) The definition of subclinical PNH remains quite arbitrary (and it is an oxymoron since, semantically speaking, PNH includes hemoglobinuria/hemolysis); while it seems appropriate for the presence of clearly detectable PNH clones (cutoff remains arbitrary, 1% versus 0.1% versus 0.03%, depending on the sensitivity and specificity of the assay in individual labs) in the absence of clinically meaningful hemolysis (or thrombosis), it should not be used outside this context (which is rather clinically relevant for the implications discussed above). Furthermore, this classification does not completely take into account that, in addition to the pathogenic role of an underlying bone marrow disorder, most PNH patients have cytopenia as a clinical consequence of such bone marrow failure. In fact, a recent registry study [5] made the point that many PNH patients do not fit into either one of the two major categories, and a fourth subgroup has been included (defined as "intermediate PNH," characterized by hemolysis and mild cytopenia not qualifying for the diagnosis of AA or typical classic PNH). However, even this classification seems to fail the goal of identifying patient subgroups with distinct clinical outcomes, mainly because of the overlapping form of the disease (evolution from an aplastic form to a hemolytic form, and vice versa, during evolution) [5]. Some other groups have used a different classification [42] in the past, where the category of AA/PNH patients is restricted to those with concomitant severe AA and clinically meaningful hemolysis, who require more intensive care and are supposed to have a worse prognosis. According to this classification, classic PNH patients are further grouped into hyperplastic and hypoplastic (based on peripheral counts and bone marrow analysis), and AA/PNH patients are only those with severe marrow failure and concomitant clinically relevant hemolysis, whereas subclinical PNH patients are characterized by small PNH clone(s) (even with minimal signs of hemolysis) associated with either AA or thromboembolic disease. This latter condition is very rare and includes a few patients in whom thromboembolic disease can be found in the absence of hemolysis. This rare condition may also be described as "myeloid PNH" or "white PNH" and seems to imply the possibility that the expansion of a GPI-deficient hematopoiesis may be restricted to specific blood lineages (i.e., mutations occurring in committed progenitors or *PIGA*-mutated HSCs, which preferentially contribute to myelopoiesis or megakaryocytopoiesis), eventually driving the subsequent clinical phenotype (thrombophilia would be explained directly by GPI-deficient platelets, which are unable to control complement activation on their surface).

While disease subcategories are now under revision by the IPIG, at the moment, we may identify a spectrum of at least four categories that cover the clinical overlap between PNH and AA: (1) classic PNH, (2) intermediate PNH, (3) AA/PNH, and (4) subclinical PNH (in the context of AA). For clinical purposes, it seems reasonable to consider each disease (aplastic anemia with subclinical PNH, AA/PNH syndrome, and hemolytic PNH) separately, which helps in discussing treatment indications and management with the assumption that it is the specific disease presentation(s) that drives the therapeutic decision(s) (see below).

The Clinical Relevance of a PNH Clone in the Context of BMF

Pathophysiology

As described before, the presence of a PNH clone is detectable due to an underlying ongoing autoimmune process in the bone marrow. The diagnosis of aplastic anemia (AA) is defined by the association of pancytopenia with persistent and unexplained reduced marrow hematopoietic cellularity, with no major dysplastic features. There are thus no specific biological markers, and the diagnosis is reached by the exclusion of other reasonable entities. The diagnosis is thus difficult, particularly to eliminate a constitutional disorder, especially in young patients. The presence of a significant PNH clone (1% or more but even less in dedicated research labs) is in favor of an underlying autoimmune process and, thus, an idiopathic aplastic anemia. A PNH clone is diagnosed in 30%–40% of patients with idiopathic AA at diagnosis or during evolution [9–12]. This justifies testing all patients with aplastic anemia for PNH, at least once a year or in the presence of clinical signs of hemolysis (abdominal pain, nausea, or red urine).

Risk of Thrombosis

This represents the third typical manifestation of PNH, with thrombosis developing in about 40% of all patients; accordingly, PNH is the medical condition with the highest risk of thrombosis. While the pathophysiology of thrombosis occurrence in PNH is still not clear, its presentation is quite unique because it mostly occurs at venous sites, which is unusual for other non-PNH-related thrombosis. Intra-abdominal veins are the most frequent sites, followed by cerebral and limb veins; other possible sites include the dermal veins, the lungs—with pulmonary embolus—and the arteries—leading to arterial thrombosis. Thrombotic disease may be life-threatening and is the main cause of death for PNH patients [5, 8]. Typical severe presentations of thrombotic PNH include hepatic venous (Budd–Chiari syndrome) [43], portal, mesenteric, and renal vein thrombosis. Usually, patients are asymptomatic until clinical manifestations appear, especially pain; other signs and symptoms are specific according to the vessel involved (e.g., ascites, varices, and splenomegaly in hepatic/portal thrombosis or stroke in cerebral venous thrombosis). According to most series, they generally develop in patients with large clones and massive hemolysis [44, 45] but may also complicate a significant number of patients with BMF and a PNH clone (i.e., a 10-year cumulative incidence of thrombosis of 30% in those patients [5]). This is the reason why patients with BMF and a PNH clone are exposed to a higher risk of thrombosis and should be explored quickly in case they have symptoms that might be related to this complication (headache or abdominal pain).

Evolution to Classic PNH

Hemolysis is the most typical manifestation of PNH, which, by definition, affects all patients with clinical PNH (i.e., classic PNH, intermediate PNH, and AA/PNH all harbor hemolysis by definition). However, the extent of (chronic) intravascular hemolysis varies among patients, according to the size of the PNH clone(s), the type of PNH erythrocytes (type II versus type III), and possibly, the level of complement activation (which may vary according to specific medical conditions or patient-specific features). Furthermore, in addition to the chronic hemolysis, hemolysis should be evaluated in terms of (risk of) acute events (the so-called paroxysms that give the name to the disease)and the frequency and severity of hemolytic crises. Thus, patients with BMF and a PNH clone generally have a low level of hemolysis or no hemolysis and do not classically suffer from clinical signs of intravascular hemolysis. However, 20% of patients diagnosed with PNH in the context of BMF will further develop a typical, classic, highly hemolytic PNH [5]. This is the reason why such patients should be monitored carefully at the clinical level (hemoglobinuria, abdominal pain, or fatigue). At the biological level, the typical biochemical marker of hemolysis is the increase in lactate dehydrogenase (LDH), which may be as high as tenfold the upper normal value; additional intra-erythrocytary components may also increase, such as aminotransferases (especially the alanine one). As in other hemolytic disorders, unconjugated bilirubin levels may increase, even up to frank jaundice; compensatory erythropoiesis is usually demonstrated by very high reticulocyte counts, even if the latter value is rarely present in patients with BMF. Clinical and biological follow-up of patients with BMF and a PNH clone should thus include this particular follow-up.

Treatment

The management of marrow failure in PNH patients is the same as for AA patients and represents the main challenge for physicians dealing with the treatment of this condition; thus, the main treatment strategies are hematopoietic stem cell transplantation (HSCT) and immunosuppressive treatment (IST) [46]. Indeed, in addition to supportive strategies, such as anti-infectious, antithrombotic, and antihemorrhagic prophylaxis and/or treatment, etiologic therapies can also be attempted. However, as discussed above, PNH is more than simply BMF; thus, treatment decisions should take into account additional clinical presentations (namely, hemolysis) or specific clinical risks (thrombophilia), which may justify more elaborate treatment strategies [47]. In the absence of intravascular hemolysis (normal LDH), there is no reason to consider a treatment algorithm other than the one applied to patients with idiopathic aplastic anemia with a PNH clone (please see specific sections of this handbook). Indeed, several reports have suggested that the presence of a PNH population may even increase the chance of response to standard IST [11, 48]. Conversely, patients with BMF and a PNH clone with a significant level of intravascular hemolysis (LDH more than twice the normal) might be more challenging to manage since an additional, concomitant treatment with complement inhibitors might be considered to mitigate the symptoms, signs, and clinical consequences of hemolysis.

Treatment of Bone Marrow Failure in PNH

Immunosuppressive Therapy

According to the pathogenic mechanisms and the dual hypothesis described above, an immune-mediated inhibition of hematopoiesis is postulated in PNH, similar to that demonstrated in AA. Thus, immunosuppressive strategies have been reasonably utilized in PNH patients, even if large prospective studies specifically looking at patients with classic PNH are lacking. Cyclosporine A (CsA) has led to some improvement in a few series [49, 50]. More intensive regimens (as those recommended in severe AA) using the antithymocyte globulin (ATG) associated with high-dose prednisone and cyclosporin A have also been exploited; however, the available results are quite heterogeneous [51, 52]. On the other hand, the literature contains plenty of data about AA patients harboring PNH clones, who have received standard IST (ATG + CsA). In all these studies, the presence of PNH clone does not preclude the possible hematological response to IST; rather, in some studies, the PNH clone emerged as a predicting factor positively associated with the probability of response to IST [11, 48, 53, 54]. These data were recently confirmed with the most recent IST regimen, the so-called triple therapy, which adds the thrombopoietin-mimetic agent eltrombopag on top of standard ATG and CsA. Even if, in the two major studies, the PNH clone was not associated with statistically higher response rates (at least in multivariable analysis), AA patients with a PNH clone showed at least the same likelihood of hematological response, without any specific risk of additional adverse events [55, 56]. In this context, the concern of a possible increased risk of thromboembolisms associated with eltrombopag was not confirmed, possibly extending the recommendation for triple therapy (see AA chapter) to all AA adult patients, even in the presence of a PNH clone. Of course, specific risk mitigation strategies may be exploited, depending on the clinical presentations: Indeed, while patients with subclinical PNH may not require specific interventions, in patients with clinical PNH due to overt hemolysis or thrombosis, a concomitant treatment with complement inhibitors may be considered (see below).

Alternative immunosuppressive agents, such as the anti-CD52 monoclonal antibody alemtuzumab [57], may be alternative options (as salvage treatment); in the setting of alemtuzumab-based treatment, there is no concern over the potential selection risk of PNH hematopoiesis, given that the GPI-linked CD52 is not expressed on HSCs [57]. Cyclophosphamide has been suggested by some [58] but has never been reproduced and is potentially toxic (for a review, see [59]). Regardless of the specific immunosuppressive regimen, when this etiological treatment leads to an improvement of the underlying bone marrow impairment, usually normal (non-PNH) hematopoiesis may be restored, possibly resulting in a progressive dilution (or even extinction) of the PNH clone.

Hematopoietic Stem Cell Transplantation

The only curative strategy for PNH is allogeneic hematopoietic stem cell transplantation (HSCT); HSCT has been exploited since the late 1980s and has proven effective in eradicating the abnormal PNH clone, possibly leading to a definitive cure of PNH, even if morbidity and mortality remain major limitations. All young PNH patients with bone marrow failure should be considered for transplantation if they have an HLA-matched donor [1] or even if they have an unrelated donor (later in their disease course). Indeed, marrow failure of PNH patients has to be treated as aplastic anemia by either immunosuppression or allogeneic stem cell transplantation, regardless of the presence of the PNH clone(s) [46]. Most reports in the literature refer to single cases or small series from single institutions [60–62]. The International Bone Marrow Transplant Registry reported 57 consecutive stem cell transplantations (SCTs) performed for PNH patients (16 AA/PNH) between 1978 and 1995 [63], showing a 2-year survival of 56% in 48 HLA-identical sibling transplants (the median follow-up was 44 months). The incidence of grade II or more severe acute graft-versus-host disease (GvHD) was 34% and that of chronic GvHD was 33%; graft failure ($n = 7$) and infections ($n = 3$) were the most common causes of treatment failure. Another retrospective study from the Italian Transplant Group (GITMO) on 26 PNH patients (four AA/PNH) transplanted between 1998 and 2006 showed a 57% survival rate at 10 years. Acute and chronic GvHD were 42% (grade III–IV: 12%) and 50% (extensive: 16%), respectively [64]. The largest study published so far was the report of the European Society for Blood and Marrow Transplantation (EBMT) experience in 2012 [65]. The characteristics and overall survival (OS) of 211 patients transplanted for PNH in 83 EBMT centers from 1978 to 2007 were analyzed. The three main indications for HSCT were aplastic anemia ($n = 100$, 48%), severe recurrent hemolytic crisis ($n = 64$, 30%), and thrombosis ($n = 47$, 22%). Engraftment failed in 14 (7%) of the 202 transplanted patients, for whom there was documentation on this aspect. Eighty-five patients developed acute GvHD, leading to a CIF of grade II–IV acute GvHD of 40% (95% CI 34–47%). Fifty-seven patients developed chronic GvHD (extensive, $n = 24$), leading to a CIF of 29% (95% CI 23%–36%) at 5 years. After a median (±standard error) follow-up time of 61 ± 6 months, 64 patients had died, and the 5-year OS probability was $68\% \pm 3\%$. Infections and GvHD were the main causes of death. None of the variables investigated for an association with transplant outcome was a statistically significant predictor of survival, except for the indication for HSCT, with the outcome being worse if the indication for HSCT was thromboembolism ($p = 0.03$). The conclusions of this large study were (1) HSCT could no longer be considered a standard of care for PNH patients with thromboembolism when eculizumab is available; (2) regarding the good results of HSCT, in the case of recurrent hemolytic crises, HSCT can be a valuable option for patients living in countries where they cannot afford eculizumab, regardless of the type of donor; and (3) PNH patients with BMF are appropriate candidates for HSCT if they have indications for treatment (i.e., severe aplastic anemia or moderate AA but transfused). The EBMT is currently investigating the outcome of HSCT in the more recent decade, 2010–2020: These data will eventually inform whether all the statements listed above remain valid in the era of complement inhibitors, clarifying the role of HSCT for PNH nowadays. In these settings, these data will also show if there is any room for HSCT from haplo-identical donors, which is becoming popular in the context of patients with AA [66–68].

At the moment, the main indication for HSCT in PNH patients is thus an underlying bone marrow failure; as for AA patients, HSCT may be performed as first-line therapy in the presence of an HLA-identical sibling donor or in case of treatment failure in patients with an HLA-matched unrelated donor [46]. The patient's age largely drives the choice of treatment, given that transplant-related mortality and morbidity increase with age. Refractoriness to transfusions and life-threatening thrombosis were also indications for HSCT in the past, but nowadays, they represent indications to anticomplement treatment, with the exception of countries where complement inhibitors are not available (yet). Poor response to standard anti-C5 therapy (eculizumab) was another indication for HSCT [69], even if in this setting, nowadays, novel complement inhibitors will likely replace HSCT quite quickly (see below) [70].

Because of the retrospective nature of available studies, several aspects about the best way to perform an HSCT in PNH remain open to discussion; however, since the main indication for HSCT is BMF, a lot of information can be drawn from SCTs for AA (please see specific sections of this handbook). The two main open questions concern the HSC source and the conditioning regimens. As for AA, GvHD is the most feared complication after HSCT for PNH, and a plethora of data demonstrates that bone marrow should be preferred over peripheral blood as the stem cell source [71, 72]. Some investigators have pointed out that a "graft versus PNH" effect may be needed to eradicate the PNH clone, especially in non-hypoplastic PNH [73]; however, since PNH is not a cancer, this does not seem to be enough to justify the increased risk of GvHD expected with the use of peripheral blood stem cells. Strategies of GvHD prophylaxis should parallel those used in the context of AA, eventually guided by the donor type and the donor's HLA compatibility (please see specific sections of this handbook). Even for the conditioning regimen (i.e., myeloablative versus reduced-intensity regimens), objective data are lacking, and information can only be drawn from the AA experience (please see specific sections of this handbook). PNH patients transplanted for concomitant AA should follow the same conditioning regimens used for AA (i.e., cyclophosphamide/ATG for sibling transplants and fludarabine-based reduced-intensity conditioning (RIC) for unrelated transplants) (please see specific sections of this handbook). Conversely, there are no specific guidelines for patients transplanted for a non-hypoplastic PNH; based on available data [65], myeloablative conditioning should be recommended, even busulfan-based [61]. However, fludarabine-based reduced-intensity regimens can be considered in older patients or in the presence of relevant comorbidities since they have been proven effective as well [73]. Again, the ongoing EBMT study on HSCT in PNH will inform on the best way to perform a transplant in this condition.

Treatment of Hemolysis

Standard Anti-C5 Treatment (Terminal Complement Inhibitors)

In some patients with AA and a PNH clone, hemolysis may appear even concomitantly to severe cytopenia, and for all patients with clinically meaningful hemolysis, it seems appropriate speaking about clinical PNH (classified as described above). Most of the time, the level of hemolysis is low (less than 1.5 times the normal), and no specific treatment is required. Conversely, in some cases, patients with true AA/

PNH syndrome present with a high level of hemolysis, with, in some cases, clinical signs (abdominal pain or hemoglobinuria) and even thrombosis. There are very few reports in the literature regarding the association [74], and no guidelines can be drawn. The main recommendation is to first treat the most severe presentation (i.e., bone marrow failure or intravascular hemolysis); indeed, sequential treatment should be preferred over concomitant delivery of IST and eculizumab [75, 76], even if the preferred option may vary case by case. Patients who are transfused with platelets or those with low neutrophil count should be primarily treated with HSCT or immunosuppression, irrespective of hemolysis (please see specific sections of this handbook), even if complement inhibitors may be used as a bridge to transplant [77–80]. Eculizumab is the first C5 inhibitor developed for PNH, which dramatically improved survival and all clinical outcomes in patients with hemolytic(and thrombotic) PNH. Eculizumab (as well as its long-acting derivative ravulizumab) has no role in the treatment of bone marrow failure in PNH, being the standard treatment for classic PNH [81, 82]. Indeed, by controlling intravascular hemolysis, eculizumab results in Hb stabilization and transfusion independence in at least half of the PNH patients with severe hemolytic anemia. Furthermore, eculizumab significantly reduced the risk of thromboembolic events [83], eventually impacting the long-term survival of PNH patients [84]. Thus, eculizumab treatment should be considered in case of symptomatic hemolysis, aiming to control the clinical symptomatology and, possibly, improve Hb levels, eventually reducing the need for red blood cell (RBC) transfusions. However, it has to be remarked that, in the context of BMF, the hematological benefit of eculizumab may be limited because anemia of AA/PNH patients may result mostly from impaired erythropoiesis rather than from intravascular hemolysis; reticulocyte count is always very informative to predict the possible benefit from anticomplement treatment in these patients. Nevertheless, the use of anticomplement treatment may be useful to handle the risk of thromboembolic complications, which may occur even in AA/PNH patients [5]; again, the presence of specific risk factors for thrombophilia (e.g., previous thrombotic events, extent of hemolysis, size of PNH population [45], and additional genetic or acquired factors) may guide the therapeutic decision. In all these conditions, the use of eculizumab concomitantly to IST represents a medical challenge; even if the clinical outcome may be excellent [74], this treatment should be handled only in centers with the highest expertise in IST and anticomplement treatment.

It has to be remarked that, nowadays, eculizumab has been flanked by additional anti-C5 monoclonal antibodies, which have extended the pipeline of terminal complement inhibitors. They mainly include the long-acting derivative ravulizumab, which was demonstrated to be non-inferior when compared with eculizumab, keeping the obvious benefit of a more convenient treatment schedule (every 8 weeks instead of every 2 weeks) [85–87]. Another long-acting anti-C5 antibody is crovalimab, which showed similar efficacy in different settings of PNH patients, with the advantage of subcutaneous delivery [88, 89]. In addition to these two long-acting agents, different biosimilars of eculizumab have been developed and are becoming available in different countries. For all these agents, all the statements made for eculizumab remain fully valid: They can be considered for the treatment of hemolytic/thrombotic PNH, even in the context of BMF, with no expected benefit on cytopenias. Since they all act on the same target, C5, there is no rationale to switch from one agent to the other (with the exception of the demonstration of the very rare inherited C5 polymorphism, which precludes the binding of eculizumab, ravulizumab, and their biosimilars) [90, 91].

Novel Proximal Complement Inhibitors

The treatment options of PNH were recently enriched by the introduction of the so-called proximal complement inhibitors [92, 93]. These agents were developed to address the problem of C3-mediated extravascular hemolysis, which may emerge during the treatment of hemolytic PNH with C5 inhibitors [94]. At the moment, three different classes may be identified: (i) C3 inhibitors (compstatin and derivatives), (ii) Factor B inhibitors (iptacopan), and (iii) Factor D inhibitors (danicopan and vemircopan). All these agents seem quite effective in PNH patients with residual anemia despite anti-C5 treatment; however, it has to be remarked that they are effective when such poor hematological response is due to residual hemolysis, mainly extravascular. Indeed, as for any complement inhibitor, proximal complement inhibitors are not indicated when the anemia of a PNH patient is due to BMF. Nevertheless, BMF may appear at any time during the PNH course, even in patients receiving proximal complement inhibitors. For this reason, we briefly summarize the key data with these novel molecules, with some final comments for treating physicians.

Pegcetacoplan is a pegylated version of the peptide C3 inhibitor compstatin, which is given via subcutaneous infusions twice a week. In a phase 3 randomized study enrolling patients with meaningful anemia despite eculizumab treatment, at week 16, pegcetacoplan in monotherapy was superior to eculizumab in terms of change in the hemoglobin level (mean difference between arms of 3.84 g/dL) and transfusion avoidance (85% versus 15%), with obvious benefit in patient-reported outcomes as well [95]. The safety profile was favorable, with no concern about infectious complications; transient reappearance of hemolysis (the so-called breakthrough hemolysis (BTH)) was observed in some patients, possibly requiring specific interventions [96]. These data were confirmed with a longer follow-up of 48 weeks [97]. This agent was approved by the FDA for the treatment of all PNH patients and by the EMA only for patients remaining anemic despite anti-C5 treatment.

Iptacopan is a Factor B inhibitor, which is given orally twice a day. In a phase 3 randomized study enrolling patients with meaningful anemia despite anti-C5 (eculizumab or ravulizumab) treatment, iptacopan in monotherapy was superior to anti-C5 treatment in terms of hemoglobin response, measured both as the proportion of patients achieving a $\geq$2-g/dL hemoglobin increase from baseline in the absence of red blood cell (RBC) transfusions (82.3% versus 2.0%) and as the proportion of patients achieving $\geq$12 g/dL hemoglobin in the absence of RBC transfusions (68.8% versus 1.8%). Iptacopan was also superior to anti-C5 for transfusion avoidance, changes from baseline in hemoglobin, patient-reported fatigue, and the absolute reticulocyte count. Iptacopan was also investigated in a single-arm phase 3 study enrolling previously untreated PNH patients. In this setting, the proportions of patients achieving a ≥2-g/dL hemoglobin increase from baseline and of patients achieving ≥12 g/dL hemoglobin (both in the absence of RBC transfusions) were 92.2% and 62.8%, respectively, with other secondary endpoints paralleling the data observed in poor responder patients. The safety profile was favorable, with no concern about infectious complications and the frequency and severity of BTH events [98]. This agent was recently approved by the FDA for the treatment of all PNH patients and by the EMA only for patients remaining anemic despite anti-C5 treatment.

Danicopan is a Factor D inhibitor, which is given orally thrice a day; it was developed as an add-on therapy to ravulizumab/eculizumab. In a phase 3 randomized study enrolling patients with meaningful anemia despite anti-C5 (eculizumab or ravulizumab) treatment, danicopan as an add-on was superior to placebo at week 12 in terms of hemoglobin gain (2.94 versus 0.5 g/dL), with no safety concern [99]. These data support the use of a combination treatment, including an anti-C5 agent associated with the Factor D inhibitor danicopan. A different Factor D inhibitor named vemircopan, given orally twice a day, was investigated as monotherapy in PNH; however, despite promising phase 2 data [100], its development as monotherapy for PNH has recently been discontinued.

Based on these data, proximal complement inhibitors are now offered to growing numbers of PNH patients, even as the initial treatment or very early in case of inadequate hematological response. Indeed, since these agents are able to prevent C3-mediated extravascular hemolysis while providing the same protection from intravascular hemolysis (even in monotherapy, provided that pharmacokinetics and pharmacodynamics are good enough), they seem to maximize the hematological response in all patient populations. Concomitant BMF was an exclusion criterion in most initial trials; thus, the use of proximal complement inhibitors in the context of BMF has not been systematically investigated. Even if their pattern of efficacy and safety should be largely overlapping with that of anti-C5 agents, it has to be recommended that their use in the presence of BMF should be advised by reference centers, which are familiar not only with PNH but also with the caveats and pitfalls of each individual treatment.

Conclusion

BMF is a common finding in patients with clinical PNH, eventually requiring specific treatment. Even outside clinical PNH, the presence of a PNH population in the context of a BMF syndrome is common, carrying specific pathophysiologic and therapeutic implications. Indeed, a typical immune-mediated aplastic anemia should be suspected, ruling out constitutional forms of BMF. Nevertheless, the management of a BMF associated with a PNH clone may be challenging because specific clinical presentations may appear anytime during the disease course: usually, intravascular hemolysis and, possibly, thromboembolic events. The specific clinical presentation guides the treatment choice in PNH according to the main (and prognostically more severe) manifestation. Indeed, in the presence of severe BMF, patients should be treated as those affected by AA (either IST or HSCT, based on age and donor availability); in contrast, when BMF is clinically less meaningful, other manifestations of PNH may be treated (i.e., complement inhibitors for hemolytic and/or thromboembolic PNH). Sometimes the clinical picture may be more complex because more manifestations may be present at the same time; in these conditions, these different treatment approaches may be considered sequentially or even concomitantly. Nevertheless, these cases remain very challenging and should be handled with the active involvement of reference centers for AA and PNH. This appears even more true nowadays due to the increased treatment options both as management of BMF (triple therapies and thrombopoietin-mimetic agents, in general, as well as HSCT from alternative donors, including haplo-identical donors) and of hemolytic PNH (long-acting terminal complement inhibitors and proximal complement inhibitors), with the ultimate goal of choosing a treatment that may really impact the outcomes of individual patients instead of trying agents/strategies for which the dominant clinical presentation is not expected to be modified substantially.

References

1. Young NS, Calado RT, Scheinberg P. Current concepts in the pathophysiology and treatment of aplastic anemia. Blood. 2006;108:2509–19.
2. Shimamura A. Clinical approach to marrow failure. Hematology Am Soc Hematol Educ Program. 2009;2009:329–37.
3. Young NS. Acquired aplastic anemia. Ann Intern Med. 2002;136:534–46.
4. Parker C, Omine M, Richards S, et al. Diagnosis and management of paroxysmal nocturnal hemoglobinuria. Blood. 2005;106:3699–709.
5. de Latour RP, Mary JY, Salanoubat C, et al. Paroxysmal nocturnal hemoglobinuria: natural history of disease subcategories. Blood. 2008;112:3099–106.
6. Rotoli B, Robledo R, Scarpato N, Luzzatto L. Two populations of erythroid cell progenitors in paroxysmal nocturnal hemoglobinuria. Blood. 1984;64:847–51.
7. Maciejewski JP, Sloand EM, Sato T, Anderson S, Young NS. Impaired hematopoiesis in paroxysmal nocturnal hemoglobinuria/aplastic anemia is not associated with a selective proliferative defect in the glycosylphosphatidylinositol-anchored protein-deficient clone. Blood. 1997;89:1173–81.
8. Hillmen P, Lewis SM, Bessler M, Luzzatto L, Dacie JV. Natural history of paroxysmal nocturnal hemoglobinuria. N Engl J Med. 1995;333:1253–8.
9. Nissen C, Tichelli A, Gratwohl A, et al. High incidence of transiently appearing complement-sensitive bone marrow precursor cells in patients with severe aplastic anemia–a possible role of high endogenous IL-2 in their suppression. Acta Haematol. 1999;101:165–72.
10. Mukhina GL, Buckley JT, Barber JP, Jones RJ, Brodsky RA. Multilineage glycosylphosphatidylinositol anchor-deficient haematopoiesis in untreated aplastic anaemia. Br J Haematol. 2001;115:476–82.

11. Sugimori C, Chuhjo T, Feng X, et al. Minor population of CD55-CD59- blood cells predicts response to immunosuppressive therapy and prognosis in patients with aplastic anemia. Blood. 2006;107:1308–14.
12. Scheinberg P, Marte M, Nunez O, Young NS. Paroxysmal nocturnal hemoglobinuria clones in severe aplastic anemia patients treated with horse anti-thymocyte globulin plus cyclosporine. Haematologica. 2010;95:1075–80.
13. Lewis SM, Dacie JV. The aplastic anaemia–paroxysmal nocturnal haemoglobinuria syndrome. Br J Haematol. 1967;13:236–51.
14. Dameshek W. Riddle: what do aplastic anemia, paroxysmal nocturnal hemoglobinuria (PNH) and "hypoplastic" leukemia have in common? Blood. 1967;30:251–4.
15. Young NS, Maciejewski J. The pathophysiology of acquired aplastic anemia. N Engl J Med. 1997;336:1365–72.
16. Young NS, Maciejewski JP. Genetic and environmental effects in paroxysmal nocturnal hemoglobinuria: this little PIG-A goes "why? Why? Why?". J Clin Invest. 2000;106:637–41.
17. Risitano AM, Maciejewski JP, Green S, Plasilova M, Zeng W, Young NS. In-vivo dominant immune responses in aplastic anaemia: molecular tracking of putatively pathogenetic T-cell clones by TCR beta-CDR3 sequencing. Lancet. 2004;364:355–64.
18. Karadimitris A, Manavalan JS, Thaler HT, et al. Abnormal T-cell repertoire is consistent with immune process underlying the pathogenesis of paroxysmal nocturnal hemoglobinuria. Blood. 2000;96:2613–20.
19. Plasilova M, Risitano AM, O'Keefe CL, et al. Shared and individual specificities of immunodominant cytotoxic T-cell clones in paroxysmal nocturnal hemoglobinuria as determined by molecular analysis. Exp Hematol. 2004;32:261–9.
20. Gargiulo L, Lastraioli S, Cerruti G, et al. Highly homologous T-cell receptor beta sequences support a common target for autoreactive T cells in most patients with paroxysmal nocturnal hemoglobinuria. Blood. 2007;109:5036–42.
21. Gargiulo L, Papaioannou M, Sica M, et al. Glycosylphosphatidylinositol-specific, CD1d-restricted T cells in paroxysmal nocturnal hemoglobinuria. Blood. 2013;121:2753–61.
22. Gargiulo L, Zaimoku Y, Scappini B, et al. Glycosylphosphatidylinositol-specific T cells, IFN-gamma-producing T cells, and pathogenesis of idiopathic aplastic anemia. Blood. 2017;129:388–92.
23. Poggi A, Negrini S, Zocchi MR, et al. Patients with paroxysmal nocturnal hemoglobinuria have a high frequency of peripheral-blood T cells expressing activating isoforms of inhibiting superfamily receptors. Blood. 2005;106:2399–408.
24. Karadimitris A, Li K, Notaro R, et al. Association of clonal T-cell large granular lymphocyte disease and paroxysmal nocturnal haemoglobinuria (PNH): further evidence for a pathogenetic link between T cells, aplastic anaemia and PNH. Br J Haematol. 2001;115:1010–4.
25. Risitano AM, Maciejewski JP, Muranski P, et al. Large granular lymphocyte (LGL)-like clonal expansions in paroxysmal nocturnal hemoglobinuria (PNH) patients. Leukemia. 2005;19:217–22.
26. Rotoli B, Luzzatto L. Paroxysmal nocturnal haemoglobinuria. Baillieres Clin Haematol. 1989;2:113–38.
27. Araten DJ, Nafa K, Pakdeesuwan K, Luzzatto L. Clonal populations of hematopoietic cells with paroxysmal nocturnal hemoglobinuria genotype and phenotype are present in normal individuals. Proc Natl Acad Sci USA. 1999;96:5209–14.
28. Tremml G, Dominguez C, Rosti V, et al. Increased sensitivity to complement and a decreased red blood cell life span in mice mosaic for a nonfunctional Piga gene. Blood. 1999;94:2945–54.
29. Keller P, Payne JL, Tremml G, et al. FES-Cre targets phosphatidylinositol glycan class A (PIGA) inactivation to hematopoietic stem cells in the bone marrow. J Exp Med. 2001;194:581–9.

30. Jasinski M, Keller P, Fujiwara Y, Orkin SH, Bessler M. GATA1-Cre mediates Piga gene inactivation in the erythroid/megakaryocytic lineage and leads to circulating red cells with a partial deficiency in glycosyl phosphatidylinositol-linked proteins (paroxysmal nocturnal hemoglobinuria type II cells). Blood. 2001;98:2248–55.
31. Endo M, Ware RE, Vreeke TM, et al. Molecular basis of the heterogeneity of expression of glycosyl phosphatidylinositol anchored proteins in paroxysmal nocturnal hemoglobinuria. Blood. 1996;87:2546–57.
32. Nishimura J, Inoue N, Wada H, et al. A patient with paroxysmal nocturnal hemoglobinuria bearing four independent PIG-A mutant clones. Blood. 1997;89:3470–6.
33. Nafa K, Bessler M, Castro-Malaspina H, Jhanwar S, Luzzatto L. The spectrum of somatic mutations in the PIG-A gene in paroxysmal nocturnal hemoglobinuria includes large deletions and small duplications. Blood Cells Mol Dis. 1998;24:370–84.
34. Luzzatto L, Bessler M, Rotoli B. Somatic mutations in paroxysmal nocturnal hemoglobinuria: a blessing in disguise? Cell. 1997;88:1–4.
35. Chen G, Zeng W, Maciejewski JP, Kcyvanfar K, Billings EM, Young NS. Differential gene expression in hematopoietic progenitors from paroxysmal nocturnal hemoglobinuria patients reveals an apoptosis/immune response in 'normal' phenotype cells. Leukemia. 2005;19:862–8.
36. Inoue N, Izui-Sarumaru T, Murakami Y, et al. Molecular basis of clonal expansion of hematopoiesis in 2 patients with paroxysmal nocturnal hemoglobinuria (PNH). Blood. 2006;108:4232–6.
37. Shen W, Clemente MJ, Hosono N, et al. Deep sequencing reveals stepwise mutation acquisition in paroxysmal nocturnal hemoglobinuria. J Clin Invest. 2014;124:4529–38.
38. Steensma DP, Bejar R, Jaiswal S, et al. Clonal hematopoiesis of indeterminate potential and its distinction from myelodysplastic syndromes. Blood. 2015;126:9–16.
39. Malcovati L, Cazzola M. The shadowlands of MDS: idiopathic cytopenias of undetermined significance (ICUS) and clonal hematopoiesis of indeterminate potential (CHIP). Hematology Am Soc Hematol Educ Program. 2015;2015:299–307.
40. Yoshizato T, Dumitriu B, Hosokawa K, et al. Somatic mutations and clonal hematopoiesis in aplastic anemia. N Engl J Med. 2015;373:35–47.
41. Dunn DE, Tanawattanacharoen P, Boccuni P, et al. Paroxysmal nocturnal hemoglobinuria cells in patients with bone marrow failure syndromes. Ann Intern Med. 1999;131:401–8.
42. Luzzatto L, Gianfaldoni G, Notaro R. Management of paroxysmal nocturnal haemoglobinuria: a personal view. Br J Haematol. 2011;153:709–20.
43. Hoekstra J, Leebeek FW, Plessier A, et al. Paroxysmal nocturnal hemoglobinuria in Budd-Chiari syndrome: findings from a cohort study. J Hepatol. 2009;51:696–706.
44. Hall C, Richards S, Hillmen P. Primary prophylaxis with warfarin prevents thrombosis in paroxysmal nocturnal hemoglobinuria (PNH). Blood. 2003;102:3587–91.
45. Moyo VM, Mukhina GL, Garrett ES, Brodsky RA. Natural history of paroxysmal nocturnal haemoglobinuria using modern diagnostic assays. Br J Haematol. 2004;126:133–8.
46. Risitano AM. Immunosuppressive therapies in the management of immune-mediated marrow failures in adults: where we stand and where we are going. Br J Haematol. 2010;152:127–40.
47. Brodsky RA. How I treat paroxysmal nocturnal hemoglobinuria. Blood. 2009;113:6522–7.
48. Scheinberg P, Wu CO, Nunez O, Young NS. Predicting response to immunosuppressive therapy and survival in severe aplastic anaemia. Br J Haematol. 2009;144:206–16.
49. Stoppa AM, Vey N, Sainty D, et al. Correction of aplastic anaemia complicating paroxysmal nocturnal haemoglobinuria: absence of eradication of the PNH clone and dependence of response on cyclosporin A administration. Br J Haematol. 1996;93:42–4.
50. van Kamp H, van Imhoff GW, de Wolf JT, Smit JW, Halie MR, Vellenga E. The effect of cyclosporine on haematological parameters in patients with paroxysmal nocturnal haemoglobinuria. Br J Haematol. 1995;89:79–82.
51. Tichelli A, Gratwohl A, Nissen C, Signer E, Stebler Gysi C, Speck B. Morphology in patients with severe aplastic anemia treated with antilymphocyte globulin. Blood. 1992;80:337–45.

52. Sanchez-Valle E, Morales-Polanco MR, Gomez-Morales E, Gutierrez-Alamillo LI, Gutierrez-Espindola G, Pizzuto-Chavez J. Treatment of paroxysmal nocturnal hemoglobinuria with antilymphocyte globulin. Rev Investig Clin. 1993;45:457–61.
53. Yoshida N, Yagasaki H, Takahashi Y, et al. Clinical impact of HLA-DR15, a minor population of paroxysmal nocturnal haemoglobinuria-type cells, and an aplastic anaemia-associated autoantibody in children with acquired aplastic anaemia. Br J Haematol. 2008;142:427–35.
54. Li J, Li X, Cai L, et al. Prognostic value of pre-treatment PNH clone among the patients with aplastic anemia: a meta-analysis. Hematology. 2023;28:2204617.
55. Townsley DM, Scheinberg P, Winkler T, et al. Eltrombopag added to standard immunosuppression for aplastic anemia. N Engl J Med. 2017;376:1540–50.
56. Peffault de Latour R, Kulasekararaj A, Iacobelli S, et al. Eltrombopag added to immunosuppression in severe aplastic anemia. N Engl J Med. 2022;386:11–23.
57. Risitano AM, Selleri C, Serio B, et al. Alemtuzumab is safe and effective as immunosuppressive treatment for aplastic anaemia and single-lineage marrow failure: a pilot study and a survey from the EBMT WPSAA. Br J Haematol. 2009;148:791–6.
58. Brodsky RA, Chen AR, Dorr D, et al. High-dose cyclophosphamide for severe aplastic anemia: long-term follow-up. Blood. 2010;115:2136–41.
59. Peffault de Latour R. Cyclophosphamide in severe aplastic anemia? Blood. 2014;124:2758–60.
60. Bemba M, Guardiola P, Garderet L, et al. Bone marrow transplantation for paroxysmal nocturnal haemoglobinuria. Br J Haematol. 1999;105:366–8.
61. Raiola AM, Van Lint MT, Lamparelli T, et al. Bone marrow transplantation for paroxysmal nocturnal hemoglobinuria. Haematologica. 2000;85:59–62.
62. Saso R, Marsh J, Cevreska L, et al. Bone marrow transplants for paroxysmal nocturnal haemoglobinuria. Br J Haematol. 1999;104:392–6.
63. Matos-Fernandez NA, Abou Mourad YR, Caceres W, Kharfan-Dabaja MA. Current status of allogeneic hematopoietic stem cell transplantation for paroxysmal nocturnal hemoglobinuria. Biol Blood Marrow Transplant. 2009;15:656–61.
64. Santarone S, Bacigalupo A, Risitano AM, et al. Hematopoietic stem cell transplantation for paroxysmal nocturnal hemoglobinuria: long-term results of a retrospective study on behalf of the Gruppo Italiano Trapianto Midollo Osseo (GITMO). Haematologica. 2010;95:983–8.
65. Peffault de Latour R, Schrezenmeier H, Bacigalupo A, et al. Allogeneic stem cell transplantation in paroxysmal nocturnal hemoglobinuria. Haematologica. 2012;97:1666–73.
66. DeZern AE, Brodsky RA. Haploidentical donor bone marrow transplantation for severe aplastic anemia. Hematol Oncol Clin North Am. 2018;32:629–42.
67. DeZern AE, Eapen M, Wu J, et al. Haploidentical bone marrow transplantation in patients with relapsed or refractory severe aplastic anaemia in the USA (BMT CTN 1502): a multicentre, single-arm, phase 2 trial. Lancet Haematol. 2022;9:e660–e9.
68. DeZern AE, Zahurak M, Symons HJ, et al. Alternative donor BMT with posttransplant cyclophosphamide as initial therapy for acquired severe aplastic anemia. Blood. 2023;141:3031–8.
69. Schrezenmeier H, Passweg JR, Marsh JC, et al. Worse outcome and more chronic GVHD with peripheral blood progenitor cells than bone marrow in HLA-matched sibling donor transplants for young patients with severe acquired aplastic anemia. Blood. 2007;110:1397–400.
70. Risitano AM. Dissecting complement blockade for clinic use. Blood. 2015;125:742–4.
71. Bacigalupo A, Socie G, Schrezenmeier H, et al. Bone marrow versus peripheral blood as the stem cell source for sibling transplants in acquired aplastic anemia: survival advantage for bone marrow in all age groups. Haematologica. 2012;97:1142–8.
72. Eapen M, Le Rademacher J, Antin JH, et al. Effect of stem cell source on outcomes after unrelated donor transplantation in severe aplastic anemia. Blood. 2011;118:2618–21.
73. Takahashi Y, McCoy JP Jr, Carvallo C, et al. In vitro and in vivo evidence of PNH cell sensitivity to immune attack after nonmyeloablative allogeneic hematopoietic cell transplantation. Blood. 2004;103:1383–90.

74. Marotta S, Pagliuca S, Risitano AM. Hematopoietic stem cell transplantation for aplastic anemia and paroxysmal nocturnal hemoglobinuria: current evidence and recommendations. Expert Rev Hematol. 2014;7:775–89.
75. Pagliuca S, Risitano AM, De Fontbrune FS, et al. Combined intensive immunosuppression and eculizumab for aplastic anemia in the context of hemolytic paroxysmal nocturnal hemoglobinuria: a retrospective analysis. Bone Marrow Transplant. 2018;53:105–7.
76. Griffin M, Kulasekararaj A, Gandhi S, et al. Concurrent treatment of aplastic anemia/paroxysmal nocturnal hemoglobinuria syndrome with immunosuppressive therapy and eculizumab: a UK experience. Haematologica. 2018;103:e345–e7.
77. DeZern AE, Jones RJ, Brodsky RA. Eculizumab bridging before bone marrow transplant for marrow failure disorders is safe and does not limit engraftment. Biol Blood Marrow Transplant. 2018;24:e26–30.
78. Peffault de Latour R, Hosokawa K, Risitano AM. Hemolytic paroxysmal nocturnal hemoglobinuria: 20 years of medical progress. Semin Hematol. 2022;59:38–46.
79. Vallet N, de Fontbrune FS, Loschi M, et al. Hematopoietic stem cell transplantation for patients with paroxysmal nocturnal hemoglobinuria previously treated with eculizumab: a retrospective study of 21 patients from SFGM-TC centers. Haematologica. 2018;103:e103–e5.
80. Fattizzo B, Ireland R, Dunlop A, et al. Clinical and prognostic significance of small paroxysmal nocturnal hemoglobinuria clones in myelodysplastic syndrome and aplastic anemia. Leukemia. 2021;35:3223–31.
81. Hillmen P, Young NS, Schubert J, et al. The complement inhibitor eculizumab in paroxysmal nocturnal hemoglobinuria. N Engl J Med. 2006;355:1233–43.
82. Brodsky RA, Young NS, Antonioli E, et al. Multicenter phase 3 study of the complement inhibitor eculizumab for the treatment of patients with paroxysmal nocturnal hemoglobinuria. Blood. 2008;111:1840–7.
83. Hillmen P, Muus P, Duhrsen U, et al. Effect of the complement inhibitor eculizumab on thromboembolism in patients with paroxysmal nocturnal hemoglobinuria. Blood. 2007;110:4123–8.
84. Kelly RJ, Hill A, Arnold LM, et al. Long-term treatment with eculizumab in paroxysmal nocturnal hemoglobinuria: sustained efficacy and improved survival. Blood. 2011;117:6786–92.
85. Kulasekararaj AG, Hill A, Rottinghaus ST, et al. Ravulizumab (ALXN1210) vs eculizumab in C5-inhibitor-experienced adult patients with PNH: the 302 study. Blood. 2019;133:540–9.
86. Lee JW, Sicre de Fontbrune F, Wong Lee Lee L, et al. Ravulizumab (ALXN1210) vs eculizumab in adult patients with PNH naive to complement inhibitors: the 301 study. Blood. 2019;133:530–9.
87. Kulasekararaj AG, Griffin M, Langemeijer S, et al. Long-term safety and efficacy of ravulizumab in patients with paroxysmal nocturnal hemoglobinuria: 2-year results from two pivotal phase 3 studies. Eur J Haematol. 2022;109:205–14.
88. Roth A, Nishimura JI, Nagy Z, et al. The complement C5 inhibitor crovalimab in paroxysmal nocturnal hemoglobinuria. Blood. 2020;135:912–20.
89. Roth A, Ichikawa S, Ito Y, et al. Crovalimab treatment in patients with paroxysmal nocturnal haemoglobinuria: long-term results from the phase I/II COMPOSER trial. Eur J Haematol. 2023;111:300–10.
90. Nishimura J, Yamamoto M, Hayashi S, et al. Genetic variants in C5 and poor response to eculizumab. N Engl J Med. 2014;370:632–9.
91. Nishimura JI, Usuki K, Ramos J, et al. Crovalimab for treatment of patients with paroxysmal nocturnal haemoglobinuria and complement C5 polymorphism: subanalysis of the phase 1/2 COMPOSER study. Br J Haematol. 2022;198:e46–50.
92. Risitano AM, Marotta S, Ricci P, et al. Anti-complement treatment for paroxysmal nocturnal hemoglobinuria: time for proximal complement inhibition? A position paper from the SAAWP of the EBMT. Front Immunol. 2019;10:1157.
93. Risitano AM, Frieri C, Urciuoli E, Marano L. The complement alternative pathway in paroxysmal nocturnal hemoglobinuria: from a pathogenic mechanism to a therapeutic target. Immunol Rev. 2023;313:262–78.

94. Risitano AM, Notaro R, Marando L, et al. Complement fraction 3 binding on erythrocytes as additional mechanism of disease in paroxysmal nocturnal hemoglobinuria patients treated by eculizumab. Blood. 2009;113:4094–100.
95. Hillmen P, Szer J, Weitz I, et al. Pegcetacoplan versus Eculizumab in paroxysmal nocturnal hemoglobinuria. N Engl J Med. 2021;384:1028–37.
96. Griffin M, Kelly R, Brindel I, et al. Real-world experience of pegcetacoplan in paroxysmal nocturnal hemoglobinuria. Am J Hematol. 2024;99:816.
97. de Latour RP, Szer J, Weitz IC, et al. Pegcetacoplan versus eculizumab in patients with paroxysmal nocturnal haemoglobinuria (PEGASUS): 48-week follow-up of a randomised, open-label, phase 3, active-comparator, controlled trial. Lancet Haematol. 2022;9:e648–e59.
98. Peffault de Latour R, Röth A, Kulasekararaj AG, Han B, Scheinberg P, Maciejewski JP, Ueda Y, de Castro C, Di Bona E, Fu R, Zhang L, Griffin M, Langemeijer SMC, Panse J, Schrezenmeier H, Barcellini W, Mauad VAQ, Schafhausen P, Tavitian S, Beggiato E, Chew LP, Gaya A, Huang W-H, Jang JH, Kitawaki T, Kutlar A, Notaro R, Pullarkat V, Schubert J, Terriou L, Uchiyama M, Lee LW, Yap E-S, Sicre de Fontbrune F, Marano L, Alashkar F, Gandhi S, Trikha R, Yang C, Liu H, Kelly RJ, Höchsmann B, Kerloeguen C, Banerjee P, Levitch R, Kumar R, Wang Z, Thorburn C, Maitra S, Li S, Verles A, Dahlke M, Risitano AM. Oral Iptacopan Monotherapy in Paroxysmal Nocturnal Hemoglobinuria. N Engl J Med. 2024;390:994–1008.
99. Lee JW, Griffin M, Kim JS, et al. Addition of danicopan to ravulizumab or eculizumab in patients with paroxysmal nocturnal haemoglobinuria and clinically significant extravascular haemolysis (ALPHA): a double-blind, randomised, phase 3 trial. Lancet Haematol. 2023;10:e955–e65.
100. Browett PJ, Kulasekararaj A, Notaro R, Ogawa M, Risitano A, Yu J, Lee JW. Vemircopan (ALXN2050) monotherapy in paroxysmal nocturnal hemoglobinuria: interim data from a phase 2 open-label proof-of-concept study. Blood. 2022;140:717–9.

Open Access This chapter is licensed under the terms of the Creative Commons Attribution 4.0 International License (http://creativecommons.org/licenses/by/4.0/), which permits use, sharing, adaptation, distribution and reproduction in any medium or format, as long as you give appropriate credit to the original author(s) and the source, provide a link to the Creative Commons license and indicate if changes were made.

The images or other third party material in this chapter are included in the chapter's Creative Commons license, unless indicated otherwise in a credit line to the material. If material is not included in the chapter's Creative Commons license and your intended use is not permitted by statutory regulation or exceeds the permitted use, you will need to obtain permission directly from the copyright holder.

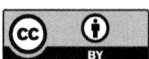

Part VII
Constitutional Bone Marrow Failure Syndromes

Chapter 15
Constitutional Bone Marrow Failure due to Immune Dysregulation Disorders

Maurizio Miano, Francesca Tucci, and Alessandro Aiuti

Introduction

The diagnostic workup of patients affected with bone marrow failure (BMF) has traditionally included the search for classical forms of constitutional marrow failure syndromes [7, 52] (such as Fanconi anemia and telomere biology disorders), which require specific follow-up and treatment, particularly when hematopoietic stem cell transplantation (HSCT) is required. Although their pathogenesis is clearly defined and does not directly involve the immune system, this can be impaired as a consequence of the reduced production of lymphocytes. Sometimes, the scenario can be even more complicated since the immune dysregulation secondary to lymphocytopenia can be the first or the only sign of the disease [1, 16, 33].

On the other hand, the involvement of the bone marrow (BM) in the setting of immune-dysregulation syndromes has also been reported: The impairment of B cell compartment can lead to the production of autoantibodies against erythropoietin, resulting in pure red cell aplasia (PRCA), anti-reticulocytes, or even earlier erythroid precursors in the setting of AHIA [53]. Moreover, it is well-known that cytokines such as tumor necrosis factor (TNF)-α and IFN-γ play an inhibitory role in marrow precursors' growth [25], and therefore, any hyperinflammatory condition leading to higher levels of such cytokines may play a role in this regard. In the past few years, the increasing knowledge of primary immunodeficiencies (PIDs) and, in particular, the primary immunoregulatory disorders (PIRDs) has highlighted the important role of autoimmunity and inflammation in the impairment of the bone marrow. These congenital disorders are characterized by incomplete genetic

---

M. Miano (✉)
Hematology Unit, IRCCS Istituto Giannina Gaslini, Genoa, Italy
e-mail: mauriziomiano@gaslini.org

F. Tucci · A. Aiuti
Pediatric Immunohematology and Bone Marrow Transplantation Unit, San Raffaele Telethon Institute for Gene Therapy (SR-Tiget), IRCCS San Raffaele Scientific Institute, Milan, Italy

© The Author(s) 2026
M. Aljurf et al. (eds.), *Textbook of Bone Marrow Failure*,
https://doi.org/10.1007/978-3-032-02386-5_15

penetrance, different ages of disease onset, and heterogeneous clinical phenotypes, mainly characterized by autoimmunity, lymphoproliferation, inflammation, and immunodeficiency. For these reasons, the diagnosis is often difficult. A recent cohort of children affected with BMF and genetically screened for classical constitutional BMF and immunodeficiencies has shown that in 17% of cases, the disorder was secondary to immune-dysregulation syndromes [42]. Other cases of BMF have also been occasionally reported in patients with cytotoxic T-lymphocyte-associated protein 4 (CTLA4) or NFKB1 haplo-insufficiencies [32, 54, 57] and gain-of-function mutations on toll-like receptor 8 (TLR8) [3, 12, 13] or signal transducer and activator of transcription 1 (STAT1) genes [51, 63]. The pathogenesis of BMF in this setting of disorders depends on different mechanisms related to the impaired pathway and, in most cases, is still under investigation.

This complex scenario should also take into consideration other rare congenital disorders secondary to molecular defects, which cause the concomitant impairment of both marrow precursor growth and the immune system [6], as in the case of deficiencies of *GATA2* or adenosine deaminase 2 (ADA2) (deficiency of adenosine deaminase 2 (DADA2)) [34, 45, 47] or in DNA double-strand break (DBS) repair disorders [2, 15]. In such rare cases, cytopenia can be secondary to both destruction and reduced production of marrow precursors.

On the basis of these considerations, a specific diagnostic workup investigating any potential sign of immune dysregulation should be offered to patients with BMF, especially children. Immunologic screening should include lymphocyte subsets (including double-negative T cells and $CD21^{low}$ B cells), serum Ig levels, IgG subclasses, autoantibody screening, vaccine titer evaluation, C3, C4, CH50, and if available, ALPS biomarkers (vitamin B12, IL-10, IL-18, and sFas).

In addition, genetic studies by next-generation sequencing panels, also including the genes related to immune-dysregulation syndromes, or by whole exome sequencing (WES)/whole genome sequencing (WGS) should be performed. In fact, an early identification of such disorders may be crucial not only to identify potential targeted treatments [42] but also to screen the best donor and the most adequate conditioning regimen when HSCT is required, as in the setting of any other congenital disease [28, 29, 39–41].

DNA Double-Strand Break Repair Disorders

DNA double-strand break repair disorders are a group of heterogeneous syndromes characterized by defects in the nonhomologous end joining (NHEJ) mechanisms, which are essential to repair DNA double-strand breaks (DSBs) [30]. This system is made of a number of key components, which are crucial not only to prevent mutagenesis and apoptosis but also to perform VDJ recombination, a fundamental mechanism to achieve the diverse T- and B-lymphocyte repertoire. Defects in any of these components lead to a DNA replication impairment, which usually causes carcinogenesis or premature cell death by apoptosis. For these reasons, patients usually show cellular sensitivity to ionizing radiation and chemicals. The impairment of genomic stability is also the cause of physical abnormalities such as microcephaly and "bird-like" facial features as well as growth and neurodevelopmental delay [17]. Moreover, bone marrow precursors' growth is also impaired, and marrow failure is often present. In addition, the concomitant ineffective VDJ recombination leads to an abnormal T cell receptor (TCR) and immunoglobulin function, which, in turn, causes immunodeficiency and immune dysregulation. Patients may have profound T- and B-lymphocytopenia and varying degrees of hypogammaglobulinemia, often associated with a hyper-IgM due to defective isotype class switching, which also relies on programmed DNA-DSB.

Defects in any gene encoding the NHEJ enzymes cause different disorders, all having a similar heterogeneous phenotype, which often includes both BMF and immunodeficiency and may range from mild to severe forms: Nijmegen breakage syndrome (*NBN*), ligase IV deficiency (*LIG4*), and Cernunnos-XLF deficiency (*XLF*) [14, 26, 56]. Interestingly, Cernunnos is the only enzyme not required for VDJ recombination. Nonetheless, patients usually show immunodeficiency, which, in this case, is secondary to premature aging of hematopoietic stem cells, in particular, lymphocytes [5].

Patients should receive supportive therapy for clinical symptoms related to BMF and immunoglobulin substitution when needed. However, the risk of very severe infection and malignancies is high and requires specific follow-up. Excessive exposure to ionizing radiation, such as X-ray and CT scans, should be avoided when possible. The only curative option for BMF and immunodeficiency secondary to these disorders is the HSCT, which might also reduce the long-term risk of developing lymphoid malignancy. Patients with BMF and significant immunodeficiency should be considered for HSCT before the development of significant multiorgan damage [55]. Due to the high radiosensitivity, conditioning regimens should not include irradiation [19], and patients undergoing myeloablative conditioning regimens have been reported with inferior overall survival compared to those who receive reduced-intensity ones [61].

GATA2 Deficiency

In *GATA2* deficiency, hematopoietic stem cell (HSC) disruption leads to peripheral cytopenias and bone marrow (BM) stress. The continuous stress to which the BM is subjected by recurrent infections and by the cytopenias themselves selects clones with a proliferative advantage. Indeed, *GATA2* mutations constitute a major myelodysplastic syndrome (MDS)–predisposition syndrome: Germline *GATA2* mutations are present in about 7% of primary MDS cases in children and adolescents [60].

The *GATA2* gene encodes a chief hematopoietic transcription factor that, through its two zinc fingers (ZFs), can occupy GATA DNA motifs in several thousand genes [24, 36]. The *GATA2* germline mutational landscape involves truncating mutations, presumably resulting in the loss of the second ZF (ZF2) [22]. In addition, missense mutations within ZF2 and noncoding variants in the +9.5-kb regulatory region of *GATA2* are thought to result in haplo-insufficiency [60]. The haplo-insufficiency, caused by a great variety of heterozygous loss-of-function mutations, determines an extensive phenotype, characterized by hematological malignancies; immunodeficiency responsible for mycobacterial, viral, and fungal infections; pulmonary alveolar proteinosis; and lymphedema [60].

The level of expression of *GATA2* relative to other transcription factors is important in gene regulation and cell fate decisions, but how *GATA2* deficiency negatively affects hematopoiesis is only partially understood. Haplo-insufficiency has been demonstrated to induce defects of hematopoiesis in animal models [18]: The production and expansion of murine HSCs is inferior, and a perturbation of the granulocyte-macrophage colony-forming unit compartment was observed [35, 49, 50]. Insufficient *GATA2* appears to allow HSCs to enter the cell cycle and differentiate, depleting self-renewal capacity [20, 27], while overexpression impairs hematopoiesis by blocking differentiation, highlighting *GATA2* as a molecular entry point into the transcriptional program regulating quiescence in human HSC cells [59]. Moreover, as the serum levels of FLT3 ligand correlate inversely with the reduction of CD34$^+$ cells, FLT3 ligand is potentially a marker for monitoring the evolution of BMF [23].

The defect in lympho-myeloid lineages appeared partially due to the expression of aberrant gene programs in stem cells prior to lineage commitment. Wu et al. [62], through single-cell RNA sequencing, observed decreased B progenitor gene expression and preserved erythroid/megakaryocytic gene expression in HSCs, suggesting intrinsic defects in early stem cells and multipotent progenitors, affecting lymphoid differentiation. The apparent defect in myeloid/lymphoid lineages seen in this study and by others [10, 11] may be partly ascribed to a skewed differentiation potential in HSCs.

In *GATA2* syndrome, monocyte, B cell, NK cell, and dendritic cell (DC) populations are profoundly diminished or undetectable [22], highlighting the importance of *GATA2* as an essential regulator of DC differentiation [46]. NK cells are diminished or partially absent with specific loss of the CD56^{bright} subset [23, 37], and T cells are elevated in percentage but sometimes with reduced absolute counts due to overall lymphopenia [44]. CD4$^+$ lymphocytopenia [58] with reduced numbers of naïve T cells and an accumulation of CD8$^+$ TEMRA have also been observed [23]. The function of terminally differentiated cells indicates that viral infections may leave specific adaptive signatures on NK- and T cell phenotypes. While the source of the defect in innate-like T cells in *GATA2* deficiency is unclear, it is possible that the reduction in numbers of antigen-presenting cells could produce a dysregulated increase of invariant T cells, such as TCRγδ and NKT cells [23]. Indeed, those patients with *GATA2* deficiency and rheumatological manifestations have decreased CD4$^+$ helper T cell proportions and a decreased naïve helper T cell sub-compartment. Dendritic cell deficiency was correlated with the depletion of regulatory T cells in patients with *GATA2* deficiency [10], and regulatory T cells play key self-tolerance roles that, when dysregulated, can contribute to autoimmune diseases [4].

The only curative treatment is HSCT, which can restore the function of both hematopoietic and immune systems and prevent lung deterioration. Overall survival and HSCT outcomes were not influenced by the mutational status. However, despite *GATA2* mutations not conferring poor prognosis in childhood MDS, the high risk for progression to advanced disease must guide decision-making toward timely HSCT.

Deficiency of Adenosine Deaminase 2

Deficiency of adenosine deaminase 2 (DADA2) is a recessively inherited inborn error of immunity, caused by biallelic hypomorphic mutations in the ADA2 gene that encodes the adenosine deaminase 2 (ADA2) protein on chromosome 22q11. DADA2 is among the more common monogenic autoinflammatory diseases, and it is characterized by systemic vasculitis, early-onset stroke, BMF, and/or immunodeficiency affecting both children and adults [38]. How defects in a single gene translate into these heterogeneous presentations remains to be answered. However, the role of ADA2 deficiency on different subpopulations of the immune system is predictable due to the high expression of the ADA2 protein in immune cells [31], particularly in the myeloid ones [64, 66], from which it is actively secreted [64] and binds to other immune cell lineages (monocytes, B cells, neutrophils, and NK cells). Moreover, the identification of immune dysregulation in DADA2 patients was demonstrated by in vitro data, which suggested that ADA2 binds to a receptor on the cell surface of T cells to induce T cell-dependent differentiation of monocytes into macrophages [64].

Bone marrow biopsy typically demonstrates hypoplasia of the affected lineages, suggesting a defect in cell production [34, 66]. It is unclear whether HSC loss is a direct consequence of ADA2 deficiency or occurs due to extrinsic factors. Knockdown of ADA2 in the zebrafish model was shown to cause neutropenia, supporting an intrinsic role of ADA2 in normal hematopoiesis [65]. Patients' BM plasma markedly inhibited the growth of progenitor cells obtained from healthy BM donors, suggesting a humoral inhibitory effect and pro-inflammatory modulation [8, 21]. Recently, reduced clonogenic capacity and impaired proliferation of DADA2 mesenchymal stromal cells (MSCs) in BM have been shown, suggesting that defective functions of the stromal BM niche may also contribute to the reduction of HSCs and their multi-lineage differentiation [48].

The severity of the BMF may lead to the indication for HSCT, which represents the only curative option, especially for patients who did not respond to treatments such as tumor necrosis factor inhibitors [9]. Recent gene therapy preclinical studies demonstrate that HSC gene therapy is a promising approach to reestablish stable ADA2 activity and correct the hematologic and inflammatory manifestations in patients with DADA2 [43].

Immunologic Workup
   Lymphocyte subsets: CD3[a], CD4[a], CD19[a], CD16[a], CD56[a], B naïve (CD19+IgD+CD27−), B memory (CD19+CD27+,), and double-negative T cells (CD3+)
   Immunoglobulin serum levels[a, b]
   IgG subclasses (patients >2 years)[b]
   C3, C4, and CH50
   Autoantibodies: antinuclear, anti-extractable nuclear, anti-DNA, antiphospholipid, anti-Sm, anti-TG, and anti-TPO[b]
   ALPS screening: double-negative T cells, vitamin B12, IL-10, IL-18, circulating Fas, and Fas-apoptosis functional test
Radiological Evaluation
   Chest X-ray
   Abdominal sonography (spleen, liver, and lymph nodes)
[a]Mandatory first-line evaluation
[b]Before transfusion/intravenous immunoglobulin (IVIG) administration

References

1. Allenspach EJ, et al. Common variable immunodeficiency as the initial presentation of dyskeratosis congenita. J Allergy Clin Immunol. 2013;132(1):223–6.
2. Al-Marhoobi R, et al. Combined immunodeficiency, hemolytic anemia, and growth retardation secondary to a homozygous mutation in the NHEJ1 gene. J Pediatr Hematol Oncol. 2020;42(4):333–5.
3. Aluri J, et al. Immunodeficiency and bone marrow failure with mosaic and germline TLR8 gain of function. Blood. 2021;137(18):2450–62.
4. Amarnani AA, et al. A panoply of rheumatological manifestations in patients with GATA2 deficiency. Sci Rep. 2020;10(1):8305.
5. Avagyan S, et al. Hematopoietic stem cell dysfunction underlies the progressive lymphocytopenia in XLF/Cernunnos deficiency. Blood. 2014;124(10):1622–5.
6. Bahrami E, et al. Myb-like, SWIRM, and MPN domains 1 (MYSM1) deficiency: genotoxic stress-associated bone marrow failure and developmental aberrations. J Allergy Clin Immunol. 2017;140(4):1112–9.
7. Barone A, et al. Diagnosis and management of acquired aplastic anemia in childhood. Guidelines from the Marrow Failure Study Group of the Pediatric Haemato-Oncology Italian Association (AIEOP). Blood Cells Mol Dis. 2015;55(1):40–7.
8. Barzaghi F, et al. ALPS-like phenotype caused by ADA2 deficiency rescued by allogeneic hematopoietic stem cell transplantation. Front Immunol. 2019;9:2767.
9. Barzaghi F, et al. Case report: consistent disease manifestations with a staggered time course in two identical twins affected by adenosine deaminase 2 deficiency. Front Immunol. 2022;13:910021.
10. Bigley V, Collin M. Dendritic cell, monocyte, B and NK lymphoid deficiency defines the lost lineages of a new GATA-2 dependent myelodysplastic syndrome. Haematologica. 2011;96(8):1081–3.
11. Bigley V, et al. The human syndrome of dendritic cell, monocyte, B and NK lymphoid deficiency. J Exp Med. 2011;208(2):227–34.

12. Bleesing J. Gain-of-function defects in toll-like receptor 8 shed light on the interface between immune system and bone marrow failure disorders. Front Immunol. 2022;13:935321.
13. Boisson B, Casanova JL. TLR8 gain of function: a tall surprise. Blood. 2021;137(18):2420–2.
14. Buck D, et al. Cernunnos, a novel nonhomologous end-joining factor, is mutated in human immunodeficiency with microcephaly. Cell. 2006;124(2):287–99.
15. Carrillo J, et al. Mutations in XLF/NHEJ1/Cernunnos gene results in downregulation of telomerase genes expression and telomere shortening. Hum Mol Genet. 2017;26(10):1900–14.
16. Chianucci B, et al. Autoimmune neutropenia and immune-dysregulation in a patient carrying a TINF2 variant. Int J Mol Sci. 2022;23(23):14535.
17. Chrzanowska KH, et al. Nijmegen breakage syndrome (NBS). Orphanet J Rare Dis. 2012;7:13.
18. Collin M, Dickinson R, Bigley V. Haematopoietic and immune defects associated with GATA2 mutation. Br J Haematol. 2015;169(2):173–87.
19. Cowan MJ, Gennery AR. Radiation-sensitive severe combined immunodeficiency: the arguments for and against conditioning before hematopoietic cell transplantation—what to do? J Allergy Clin Immunol. 2015;136(5):1178–85.
20. de Pater E, et al. Gata2 is required for HSC generation and survival. J Exp Med. 2013;210(13):2843–50.
21. Dell'Orso G, et al. Case report: deficiency of adenosine deaminase 2 presenting with overlapping features of autoimmune lymphoproliferative syndrome and bone marrow failure. Front Immunol. 2021;12:754029.
22. Dickinson RE, et al. Exome sequencing identifies GATA-2 mutation as the cause of dendritic cell, monocyte, B and NK lymphoid deficiency. Blood. 2011;118(10):2656–8.
23. Dickinson RE, et al. The evolution of cellular deficiency in GATA2 mutation. Blood. 2014;123(6):863–74.
24. Dore LC, et al. Chromatin occupancy analysis reveals genome-wide GATA factor switching during hematopoiesis. Blood. 2012;119(16):3724–33.
25. Dufour C, et al. Interferon gamma and tumour necrosis factor alpha are overexpressed in bone marrow T lymphocytes from paediatric patients with aplastic anaemia. Br J Haematol. 2001;115(4):1023–31.
26. Enders A, et al. A severe form of human combined immunodeficiency due to mutations in DNA ligase IV. J Immunol. 2006;176(8):5060–8.
27. Ezoe S, et al. GATA-2/estrogen receptor chimera regulates cytokine-dependent growth of hematopoietic cells through accumulation of p21(WAF1) and p27(Kip1) proteins. Blood. 2002;100(10):3512–20.
28. Fioredda F, et al. Outcome of haematopoietic stem cell transplantation in dyskeratosis congenita. Br J Haematol. 2018;183(1):110–8.
29. Giardino S, et al. Outcome of patients with Fanconi anemia developing myelodysplasia and acute leukemia who received allogeneic hematopoietic stem cell transplantation: a retrospective analysis on behalf of EBMT group. Am J Hematol. 2020;95(7):809–16.
30. Iyama T, Wilson DM 3rd. DNA repair mechanisms in dividing and non-dividing cells. DNA Repair (Amst). 2013;12(8):620–36.
31. Kaljas Y, et al. Human adenosine deaminases ADA1 and ADA2 bind to different subsets of immune cells. Cell Mol Life Sci. 2017;74(3):555–70.
32. Kallen ME, et al. Acquired and germline predisposition to bone marrow failure: diagnostic features and clinical implications. Semin Hematol. 2019;56(1):69–82.
33. Korthof ET, et al. Immunological profile of Fanconi anemia: a multicentric retrospective analysis of 61 patients. Am J Hematol. 2013;88(6):472–6.
34. Lee PY. Vasculopathy, immunodeficiency, and bone marrow failure: the intriguing syndrome caused by deficiency of adenosine deaminase 2. Front Pediatr. 2018;6:282.
35. Ling KW, et al. GATA-2 plays two functionally distinct roles during the ontogeny of hematopoietic stem cells. J Exp Med. 2004;200(7):871–82.
36. Linnemann AK, et al. Genetic framework for GATA factor function in vascular biology. Proc Natl Acad Sci. 2011;108(33):13641–6.

37. Mace EM, et al. Mutations in GATA2 cause human NK cell deficiency with specific loss of the CD56(bright) subset. Blood. 2013;121(14):2669–77.
38. Meyts I, Aksentijevich I. Deficiency of Adenosine Deaminase 2 (DADA2): updates on the phenotype, genetics, pathogenesis, and treatment. J Clin Immunol. 2018;38(5):569–78.
39. Miano M, et al. Unrelated donor marrow transplantation for inborn errors. Bone Marrow Transplant. 1998;21(Suppl 2):S37–41.
40. Miano M, et al. Stem cell transplantation for congenital dyserythropoietic anemia: an analysis from the European Society for Blood and Marrow Transplantation. Haematologica. 2019;104(8):e335–9.
41. Miano M, et al. Stem Cell Transplantation for Diamond-Blackfan Anemia. A retrospective study on behalf of the severe aplastic anemia working party of the European Blood and Marrow Transplantation Group (EBMT). Transplant Cell Ther. 2021;27(3):274.e1–5.
42. Miano M, et al. Genetic screening of children with marrow failure. The role of primary immunodeficiencies. Am J Hematol. 2021;96(9):1077–86.
43. Mortellaro A, et al. Lentiviral-mediated gene therapy for the treatment of adenosine deaminase 2 deficiency. Blood. 2021;138(Supplement 1):2937.
44. Novakova M, et al. Loss of B cells and their precursors is the most constant feature of GATA-2 deficiency in childhood myelodysplastic syndrome. Haematologica. 2016;101(6):707–16.
45. Oleaga-Quintas C, et al. Inherited GATA2 deficiency is dominant by haploinsufficiency and displays incomplete clinical penetrance. J Clin Immunol. 2021;41(3):639–57.
46. Onodera K, et al. GATA2 regulates dendritic cell differentiation. Blood. 2016;128(4):508–18.
47. Pilania RK, et al. Deficiency of human adenosine deaminase type 2 – a diagnostic conundrum for the hematologist. Front Immunol. 2022;13:869570.
48. Rigamonti C, et al. ESGCT 30th annual congress in collaboration with SFTCG and NVGCT Brussels, Belgium October 24–27, 2023 abstracts. Hum Gene Ther. 2024;35(3–4):A1–336.
49. Rodrigues NP, et al. Haploinsufficiency of GATA-2 perturbs adult hematopoietic stem-cell homeostasis. Blood. 2005;106(2):477–84.
50. Rodrigues NP, et al. GATA-2 regulates granulocyte-macrophage progenitor cell function. Blood. 2008;112(13):4862–73.
51. Rosenberg JM, et al. JAK inhibition in a patient with a STAT1 gain-of-function variant reveals STAT1 dysregulation as a common feature of aplastic anemia. Med. 2022;3(1):42–57.e5.
52. Rovo A, et al. Diagnosis of acquired aplastic anemia. Bone Marrow Transplant. 2013;48(2):162–7.
53. Sayour EJ, et al. Bone marrow transplantation for CVID-like humoral immune deficiency associated with red cell aplasia. Pediatr Blood Cancer. 2016;63(10):1856–9.
54. Sklarz T, et al. Aplastic anemia in a patient with CVID due to NFKB1 haploinsufficiency. Cold Spring Harb Mol Case Stud. 2020;6(6):a005769.
55. Slack J, et al. Outcome of hematopoietic cell transplantation for DNA double-strand break repair disorders. J Allergy Clin Immunol. 2018;141(1):322–328 e10.
56. Slatter MA, Gennery AR. Primary immunodeficiencies associated with DNA-repair disorders. Expert Rev Mol Med. 2010;12:e9.
57. Solhaug TS, et al. A family with cytotoxic T-lymphocyte-associated protein 4 haploinsufficiency presenting with aplastic anaemia. BMJ Case Rep. 2022;15(2):e247653.
58. Spinner MA, et al. GATA2 deficiency: a protean disorder of hematopoiesis, lymphatics, and immunity. Blood. 2014;123(6):809–21.
59. Tipping AJ, et al. High GATA-2 expression inhibits human hematopoietic stem and progenitor cell function by effects on cell cycle. Blood. 2009;113(12):2661–72.
60. Wlodarski MW, et al. Prevalence, clinical characteristics, and prognosis of GATA2-related myelodysplastic syndromes in children and adolescents. Blood. 2016;127(11):1387–97; quiz 1518.
61. Wolska-Kusnierz B, Gennery AR. Hematopoietic stem cell transplantation for DNA double strand breakage repair disorders. Front Pediatr. 2019;7:557.

62. Wu Z, et al. Sequencing of RNA in single cells reveals a distinct transcriptome signature of hematopoiesis in GATA2 deficiency. Blood Adv. 2020;4(12):2656–70.
63. Xie Y, et al. Case report: a STAT1 gain-of-function mutation causes a syndrome of combined immunodeficiency, autoimmunity and pure red cell aplasia. Front Immunol. 2022;13:928213.
64. Zavialov AV, et al. Human adenosine deaminase 2 induces differentiation of monocytes into macrophages and stimulates proliferation of T helper cells and macrophages. J Leukoc Biol. 2010;88(2):279–90.
65. Zhou Q, et al. Early-onset stroke and vasculopathy associated with mutations in ADA2. N Engl J Med. 2014;370(10):911–20.
66. Zoccolillo M, et al. Lentiviral correction of enzymatic activity restrains macrophage inflammation in adenosine deaminase 2 deficiency. Blood Adv. 2021;5(16):3174–87.

Open Access This chapter is licensed under the terms of the Creative Commons Attribution 4.0 International License (http://creativecommons.org/licenses/by/4.0/), which permits use, sharing, adaptation, distribution and reproduction in any medium or format, as long as you give appropriate credit to the original author(s) and the source, provide a link to the Creative Commons license and indicate if changes were made.

The images or other third party material in this chapter are included in the chapter's Creative Commons license, unless indicated otherwise in a credit line to the material. If material is not included in the chapter's Creative Commons license and your intended use is not permitted by statutory regulation or exceeds the permitted use, you will need to obtain permission directly from the copyright holder.

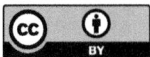

Chapter 16
Fanconi Anemia

Filomena Pierri, Thierry Leblanc, Carlo Dufour, Jean Soulier, Jean-Hugues Dalle, and Régis Peffault de Latour

Introduction

Fanconi anemia (FA) is a rare genetic disorder characterized by physical abnormalities, bone marrow failure (BMF), and increased risk for malignancy (mainly acute myeloid leukemia (AML) and epithelial cancers of the head and neck (head and neck squamous cell carcinoma (HNSCC))) [1].

Pathogenic variants in at least 23 genes have been identified in the FA/ Breast Cancer 1 (BRCA) DNA repair pathway that functions to remove DNA interstrand cross-links. Furthermore, in addition to DNA repair, FA proteins are involved in numerous functions, including aldehyde detoxification, inflammatory cytokine hypersensitivity, cell cycle regulation via the p53/p21 pathway, and oxidative phosphorylation.

F. Pierri
Hematopoietic Stem Cell Transplantation Unit, IRCSS Istituto Giannina Gaslini, Genoa, Italy

T. Leblanc · J.-H. Dalle
Department of Pediatric Hematology and Immunology, Robert Debré Academic Hospital, GHU AP-HP Nord Université Paris Cité, Paris, France

C. Dufour
Hematology Unit, IRCCS Istituto Giannina Gaslini, Genoa, Italy

J. Soulier
Hematology Laboratory, Saint Louis Hospital, APHP, Inserm, Saint Louis Research Institute, Université Paris Cité, Paris, France

R. Peffault de Latour (✉)
Hematology and Transplant Unit, Saint-Louis Hospital, AP-HP and Université Paris Cité, Paris, France
e-mail: regis.peffaultdelatour@aphp.fr

FA is inherited mostly in an autosomal recessive manner; rarely, transmission is autosomal dominant (*RAD51*-related FA) or X-linked (*FANCB*-related FA) [2].

The carrier frequency of FA is 1:181 in the general population of North America and 1:93 in Israel. Specific populations have a founder effect with increased carrier frequencies (1 per 100 or less), e.g., Ashkenazi Jews (*FANCC* and *FANCD1*/BRCA2), Afrikaners (*FANCA*), sub-Saharan Africans (*FANCG*), Spanish gypsies (*FANCA*), and South Asians from India and Pakistan (*FANCL*).

Physical abnormalities, present in approximately 75% of affected individuals, include one or more of the following: short stature, abnormal skin pigmentation, skeletal malformations of the upper and/or lower limbs, microcephaly, and ophthalmic and genitourinary tract anomalies [2]. In the remaining 25% of cases, physical abnormalities can be either absent or very subtle.

In a cohort of 203 FA patients [3], the cumulative incidences of severe BMF, solid tumors, and leukemia as the first event were 70%, 20%, and 6.5%, respectively. Head and neck and gynecological cancers were the most common solid tumors, with a further increased risk after hematopoietic stem cell transplantation (HSCT). Overall, the median survival was 37 years; patients with leukemia or FANCD1/BRCA2 variants had the poorest survival.

To date, genotype/phenotype correlation is of a limited value in FA. To note, FA patients from the same kindred may have a very different phenotype and hematological outcome. The only exception is for patients mutated within downstream genes, typically *FANCD1/BRCA2,* for whom the risk of early and multiple cancers is very high [4].

Diagnosis

Diagnosis of FA should always be suspected in the presence of BMF with or without associated classical malformations and in young patients with de novo BMF, a positive family history for BMF, spontaneous chromosomal breaks, or unbalanced 1q, 3q, or 7q translocations found during the diagnostic workup for myelodysplasia (MDS) or AML. At best, FA diagnosis is suspected in patients without BMF but with evidence of classic FA extra-hematological phenotype; to note, isolated macrocytosis may be present very early. Furthermore, the presence of early-onset tumors in sites classical for FA and excessive toxicity after standard-dose chemotherapy should also trigger suspicion of an underlying FA diagnosis [1, 5].

The gold standard tests for FA diagnosis are based on the hypersensitivity of cells from FA patients to interstrand cross-linking (ICL) agents such as mitomycin C (MMC) and diepoxybutane (DEB). These tests should be performed in expert labs. False positives include tests done after chemotherapy and other syndromes like Nijmegen breakage syndrome, Warsaw breakage syndrome, Roberts breakage syndrome, and ERCC6 syndrome, which are all associated with chromosome breakages.

False negative tests are a classic feature in patients with somatic mosaicism, which can occur as a consequence of molecular events generating a correction of an

FA mutation in one allele in a hematopoietic stem cell or in a lymphocyte progenitor [6]. In this case, tests should be performed on "non-blood" chromosomes (skin fibroblasts or hair follicles). If positive, it leads to the identification of a mosaic FA.

Other tests for diagnosis are cell cycle study and the FANCD2 test. Lymphocytes from FA patients are unable to properly move through the cell cycle and, after exposure to an ICL agent, are arrested at the G2/M transition due to elevated levels of DNA damage. FANCD2 test (Western blot) allows us to distinguish native and monoubiquitinated FANCD2 isoforms; lack of monoubiquitination implies a defective FA pathway upstream of ubiquitination and, thus, mutation within the classical FA core genes (FANCA, FANCB, FANCC, FANCE, FANCF, FANCG, FANCL, and the FA-associated proteins (FAAP), FAAP20 and FAAP100) [7].

If the Chromosome Breakage Test (CBT) is positive (Fig. 16.1), a targeted FA gene panel should be performed. Next-generation sequencing (NGS) has proven to be efficient and accurate in the diagnosis of FA and other inherited marrow failures and is now part of the routine diagnostic workup. If the targeted panel is negative, whole exome sequencing (WES) or whole genome sequencing can be performed. However, it has to be outlined that, due to their wide availability, some centers adopt targeted NGS panels or WES upfront for the diagnosis of FA and CBT as the functional validation test in case of dubious/ambiguous genetic findings. Last, increased fetal hemoglobin (as in many inherited bone marrow failures (IBMFs)) and raised alpha-fetoprotein [8] can support the diagnosis of FA.

The recommended testing procedures are outlined in the flow chart in Fig. 16.1 (modified from FARF guidelines 2020).

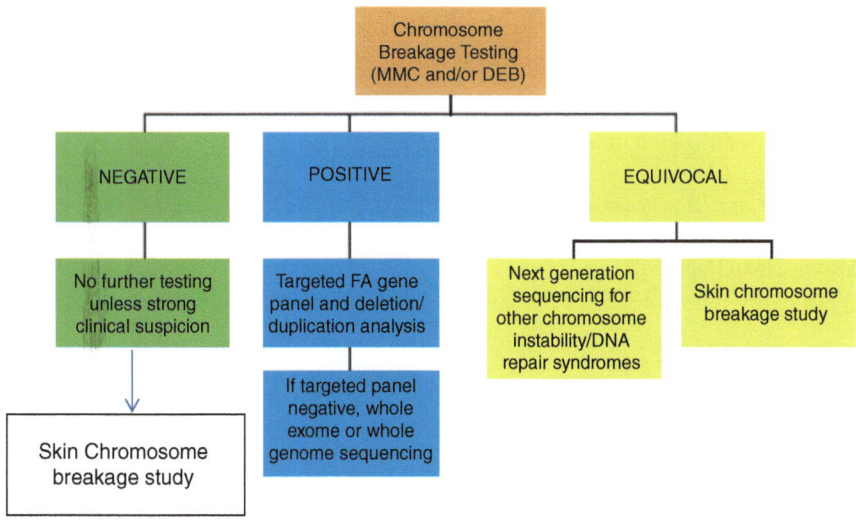

Fig. 16.1 Recommended testing procedures. (Modified from FARF guidelines 2020)

Follow-Up After Diagnosis

After diagnosis, patients with FA should undergo baseline extensive multiorgan assessment (Table 16.1) prior to entering a monitoring plan that is recommended to be performed in centers specialized in inherited bone marrow failure syndromes [1, 5, 9].

Post-diagnosis hematological monitoring plan is summarized in Fig. 16.2. The goal is to evaluate the degree of cytopenia, the presence of marrow dysplastic features or MDS or AML, and the presence and type of cytogenetic abnormalities in order to determine the best moment to perform hematopoietic stem cell transplantation (HSCT), the only curative option for FA hematological complications.

In Table 16.2, long-term follow-up of extra-hematological manifestations in non-transplanted FA patients is reported.

Table 16.1 Workup for patients with FA after diagnosis

Soon after diagnosis:
Hematological evaluation FBC with differential count Serum immunoglobulin levels, peripheral blood immunophenotyping, and response to vaccines Bone marrow aspiration for morphology, cytogenetics, and immunophenotyping Trephine bone marrow biopsy (definition of hematopoietic cellularity, abnormal localization of myeloid progenitors, and increased blasts on specific CD34 and CD117 staining)
Extensive extra-hematological evaluation Liver, kidney, heart, urinary tract, gastrointestinal tract, skeleton, and hearing and visual function evaluation Endocrinologic evaluation (thyroid, glucose tolerance, pituitary gland function, and gonads in postpubertal subjects) Psychological evaluation Brain magnetic resonance imaging with angiography for pituitary gland and moyamoya syndrome Assessment for cancers typically associated with FA, with special attention to the oral cavity
Chromosomal fragility tests in siblings and, possibly, in relatives
HLA typing of the patient, healthy sibling, and parents
Search for an HLA-matched unrelated donor (MUD) if no healthy HLA-matched sibling is found in the family
Modified from Dufour Abbreviations: *FBC* full blood count, *HLA* human leukocyte antigen

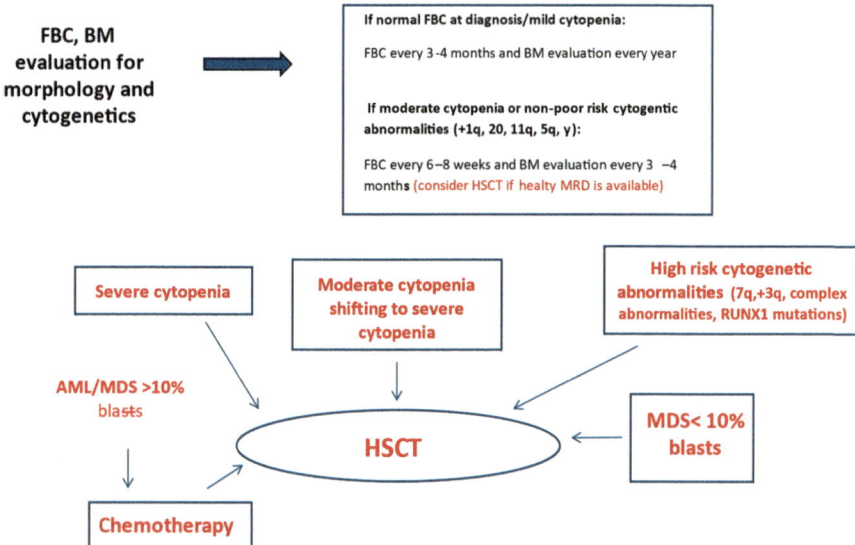

Fig. 16.2 Hematological monitoring plan and HSCT indications. (Modified from Dufour and Pierri [1])

Table 16.2 Follow-up recommendations for extra-hematological manifestations in non-transplanted FA patients

Organ or system affected	Recommended follow-up
General health status	Annual clinical evaluation
Iron overload in repeatedly Transfused patients	Ferritin and baseline MRI T2*; if iron overload, continue follow-up (ferritin and MRI T2*)
Immunology	Annual monitoring of lymphocyte subsets and Ig levels; vaccinations including HPV
Heart	If iron overload or congenital abnormalities
Liver	Liver function test every 3–6 months and ultrasound/elastography every 6–12 months if androgen therapy; ultrasound/elastography every 3–5 years in other cases. MRI is more sensitive than ultrasound in detecting hepatocellular adenomas
Kidney	If no malformations/abnormalities, monitor renal function (serum levels of electrolytes, BUN, and creatinine in the urine) once a year

(continued)

Table 16.2 (continued)

Organ or system affected	Recommended follow-up
Endocrine	Weight and height once a year
Measure the levels of IGF-1 and IGFBP-3 in patients younger than 18 years
Assess bone age in patients aged 5–18 years
Perform an oral glucose tolerance test (OGTT) if fasting glucose is abnormal
Measure the levels of TSH and FT4, 25-OH vitamin D, and calcium annually if previously normal
Measure the levels of FSH and LH in female patients older than 12 years, clinical evaluation, and AMH as a marker of ovarian failure
DXA scan every 5 years in patients older than 14 years, annually in females with hypogonadism or early menopause
Measure fasting lipid serum profile (total cholesterol, LDL, HDL, and triglycerides)
Cancer screening	Screen for head and neck cancers (performed by a head and neck specialist) every 6–12 months (every 6 months from 10 years)
Screen for anal cancer: proctologic evaluation (yearly) from 14 years
General gynecological evaluation and cancer screening in female
Patients older than 13 years (PAP test in patients older than 18 years or sexually active)
Evaluate nevi and check for skin cancers annually from the age of 18 years
Breast cancer screening *(ultrasound/MRI from age 25 years in FANCD1/BRCA2, FANCJ/BRIP1, FANCN/PALB2, FANCO/RAD51C, and FANCS/BRCA1) and then annual MRI until 30 years of age. From 30 years, twice a year (mammography alternating with MRI)*
In other genotypes, no consensus guidelines for breast cancer screening, indication to start earlier than the general population
Central nervous system	Angio-MRI annually to detect FA neuroinflammatory syndromes [10], vascular abnormalities (moyamoya), and other cerebral abnormalities
Gastrointestinal system	Endoscopy indicated if gastrointestinal symptoms
Dental evaluation	Every 6–12 months (every 6 months from 14 years)

Abbreviations: *AMH* anti-müllerian hormone, *BUN* Blood urea nitrogen, *DXA* Dual X-ray Absorptiometry, *FSH* follicle stimulating hormone, *FT4* Free thyroxine test, *HDL* high-density lipoprotein, *HPV* Human papilloma virus, *Ig* Immunoglobulin, *IGF-1* insulin-like growth factor 1, *IGFBP-3* Insulin-like growth factor-binding protein 3, *LDL* low-density lipoprotein, *LH* Luteinizing hormone, *PAP* Pulmonary alveolar proteinosis, *TSH* thyroid stimulating hormone

Clonal Evolution

Patients with FA have a 30%–40% cumulative risk of myeloid malignancies by the age of 40 years. They often arise from clonal karyotype abnormalities and unbalanced translocations, leading to gains or losses of chromosomes. Some cytogenetic changes, such as monosomy 7/del(7q), gain of chromosome 3q, and RUNX1 abnormalities, predict negative outcomes, and their identification is important to decide the timing of HSCT [11–14]. To note, HSCT prevents the risk of clonal evolution.

Gain of chromosome 1q is the most common abnormality in FA; it can occur without indication impending transformation and is not an indication for HSCT per se [11].

It has recently been shown that in FA patients who develop chromosome 1q gain, the molecular driver of hematopoiesis is Mouse Double Minute 4 (MDM4) copy number variation (CNV) (mainly trisomy) that down-modulates p53 signaling, which is followed by genomic alterations associated with secondary acute leukemia [15]. These findings point to new potential players in the clonal evolution monitoring plan and open horizons related to therapeutic applications, for instance, of polymerase (PARP) or MDM4 inhibitors, in combination with HSCT at the Myelodysplastic syndrome with excess blasts (MDS-EB)/AML stage or in post-transplant relapsing AML or complementary to gene therapy (GT).

Transplants performed with active MDS/AML have a significantly lower overall survival (OS) vs. those performed in complete remission [16]. This highlights the importance of accurate monitoring plans aimed at intercepting the "momentum" for the transplant. A cytoreductive approach, still withstanding the risks of undesired toxicity, should not be avoided because of the fear of negative toxic effects during the post-HSCT period.

The FLAG regimen (fludarabine 30 mg/m^2 daily, cytarabine 1 g/m^2 twice daily for 5 days, plus Granulocytes colony stimulating factor (G-CSF)), followed by HSCT in the aplastic phase, described in a French–Brazilian study [17], led to a 3-year progression-free survival and OS of 53% and 53%, respectively, although there was a high rate of fungal and viral infections.

Solid Tumors

FA is a cancer-prone disease.

Head and neck cancers at rates that were a hundredfold greater than those of the general population are diagnosed at a younger age (20–50 years) in patients with FA and often at an advanced stage, resulting in poor outcomes. FA patients also have an augmented risk for vulvar, anogenital, and esophageal squamous cell carcinomas (SCCs) and liver cancer [2]. In addition, patients with mutations within *FANCD1/BRCA2* have a very high and early risk of nephroblastoma, neuroblastoma, and medulloblastoma (potentially associated with early leukemia, including T cell leukemia) [4].

Clinically, three subsets of patients can be distinguished:

1. Transplanted FA patients for whom a systematic screening for SCC is warranted (Table 16.2). Causative well-defined risk factors in the general population, such as tobacco and alcohol use, should be avoided by patients with FA; immunization against papillomavirus should be done; and careful surveillance is recommended [18, 19]. Careful inspection of the oral cavity of individuals with FA, followed by brush biopsy–based cytology and DNA ploidy analysis, can help identify potentially malignant and premalignant lesions that warrant treatment, detecting approximately 63% of SCC and precursor lesions at a noninvasive or

early stage [20]. To note, the risk of solid tumors in patients who have undergone HSCT is significantly higher than in those who did not [18].
2. Patients with somatic mosaicism, in whom cancer may be the first clinical event. FA should be systematically suspected in a patient considered young for this cancer and without tobacco and alcohol use. FA should also be suspected in case of unexpected toxicity after the use of alkylating agents or radiotherapy.
3. Young children (age <5 years), *FANDC1/BRCA2*-mutated, with early and multiple cancers. The prognosis is very poor in this subgroup but may vary according to the variants [4].

Overall, the prognosis of secondary tumors (ST) in FA patients is very poor. Standard treatment (chemotherapy or radiotherapy) is very toxic in FA patients and not doable. The next challenge is to define the best therapeutic approaches, which may rely on innovative agents. For the time being, efforts must focus on screening for an early diagnosis. Chirurgical treatment of a precancerous lesion (leukoplakia) is most often effective.

Hematopoietic Stem Cell Transplantation

HSCT is the only cure for FA hematological manifestations. Indications for transplant should be carefully weighed, based on a thorough evaluation of risks and benefits, because this procedure has intrinsic morbidity and mortality and may increase the risk and accelerate the appearance of late malignancies [1].

Established indications for HSCT in FA include marrow failure, poor prognosis of cytogenetic aberrations, and overt MDS/AML [21].

Over the past 20 years, the outcome of HSCT in patients with FA has improved dramatically because of a reduction of the doses of alkylating agents and irradiation, the introduction of fludarabine, and the use of recipient T cell depletion (TCD) that improved engraftment and decreased graft-vs.-host disease (GvHD) rates [22]. In an European group for blood and marrow transplantation (EBMT) report published in July 2024, the 5-year OS of FA patients undergoing HSCT was 83%, with better results in matched related donor (MRD)- or MUD-HSCT vs. haplo or mismatched unrelated donor (MMUD) [23].

In patients lacking a matched sibling or unrelated donor, haploidentical HSCT is a promising strategy. The most frequent platforms used in this setting are ex vivo TCD with TCRαβ+/CD19+ depletion and T-repleted protocols with post transplantation cyclophosphamide (PTCy). Overall, T cell receptor (TCR)-αβ-depletion proved to have a positive effect compared to other platforms, being associated with a significantly lower incidence of graft failure (GF) ($p = 0.004$) and acute graft versus host disease (aGvHD) ($p = 0.046$) and, consequently, better OS ($p = 0.026$) and GRFS ($p = 0.007$) [24].

With the aim to ensure engraftment and improve immune reconstitution in FA patients undergoing transplantation from a haploidentical donor, an ongoing clinical trial (NCT04784052) is evaluating a radiation-free, reduced-intensity preparative

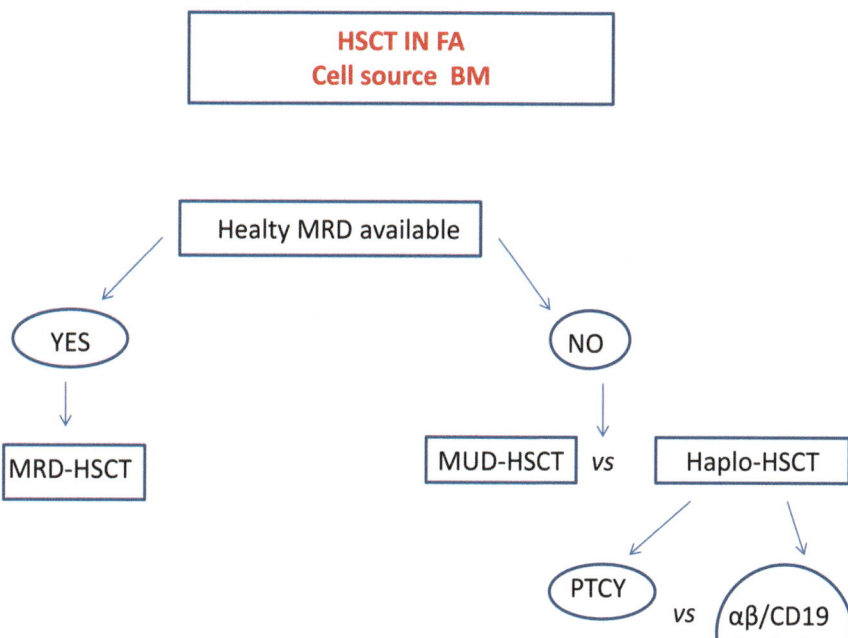

Fig. 16.3 From Dufour (2022)

regimen containing JSP191, a humanized monoclonal antibody that targets CD117 and causes stem cell death.

In Fig. 16.3, the HSCT decision-making process in FA patients is outlined.

A careful monitoring of the development of HNSCC and other malignancies, such as other FA manifestations, should be performed after HSCT [5].

Non-transplant Therapy

Drugs

Synthetic androgens produce a hematological response in FA patients, rendering this treatment a reasonable option in patients who cannot access HSCT at a given time, acting as a bridge treatment until the possibility of a transplant occurs [25, 26]. After the initial response, treatment should be reduced to the minimal active dose. The risk of liver tumor and clonal evolution is high.

Other drugs, such as metformin and quercetin, have been evaluated in clinical trials, without any evidence of clinical benefit at the moment [27, 28].

Eltrombopag is now under evaluation in a prospective phase 1/2 clinical trial (NCT03204188) in patients with FA, but its efficacy is currently not established, and its use should be restricted to clinical trials [29].

Gene Therapy

Hematopoietic gene therapy (GT) of autologous hematopoietic stem cells (HSCs) has become an important area of therapeutic development in FA patients.

At present, GT in FA is available only for the FA-A genotype and offers the best results if performed in the early stage of BMF and if a significant number of corrected CD34+ cells are infused [30].

Early results have shown that lentiviral-mediated GT can ameliorate BMF in nonconditioned FA patients because of the proliferative advantage of corrected FA hematopoietic stem and progenitor cells [31]. Furthermore, GT reverts the transcriptional signature of FA HSC, making it resemble that of a healthy donor HSC [32].

Trials using gene editing techniques in other FA genes, including *FANCB, FANCC, FANCD1,* and *FANCD2,* demonstrated that the non-homologous end joining (NHEJ)–editing approach restores MMC resistance in FA-deficient cells. Furthermore, the successful restoration of FA gene function by NHEJ-mediated gene editing approaches was also observed in FA-patient-derived CD34+ cells [33]. These studies clearly suggest the importance of NHEJ-mediated FA gene therapy in the development of effective and personalized FA patient treatment plans [34].

Conclusion

FA is a very heterogeneous disorder, with the main morbidities represented by BMF and increased cancer risk.

This condition leads to numerous bodily complications that require specific clinical care approaches and management by expert teams.

Currently, the main challenge is the early diagnosis and treatment of solid tumors.

Progress in the understanding of the biology of the disease will help develop new therapeutic strategies for FA-co-related complications.

References

1. Dufour C, Pierri F. Modern management of Fanconi anemia. Hematology Am Soc Hematol Educ Program. 2022;2022(1):649–57.
2. Peake JD, Noguchi E. Fanconi anemia: current insights regarding epidemiology, cancer, and DNA repair. Hum Genet. 2022;141(12):1811–36.

3. Altintas B, Giri N, McReynolds LJ, Best A, Alter BP. Genotype-phenotype and outcome associations in patients with Fanconi anemia: the National Cancer Institute cohort. Haematologica. 2023;108(1):69–82.
4. Alter BP, Rosenberg PS, Brody LC. Clinical and molecular features associated with biallelic mutations in FANCD1/BRCA2. J Med Genet. 2007;44(1):1–9.
5. Fanconi Anemia Research Fund, editor. Fanconi anemia clinical care guidelines. 5th ed. Eugene: Fanconi Anemia Research Fund; 2020.
6. Nicoletti E, Rao G, Bueren JA, Río P, Navarro S, Surrallés J, Choi G, Schwartz JD. Mosaicism in Fanconi anemia: concise review and evaluation of published cases with focus on clinical course of blood count normalization. Ann Hematol. 2020;99(5):913–24.
7. Soulier J, Leblanc T, Larghero J, et al. Detection of somatic mosaicism and classification of Fanconi anemia patients by analysis of the FA/BRCA pathway. Blood. 2005;105(3):1329–36.
8. Cassinat B, Guardiola P, Chevret S, et al. Constitutive elevation of serum alpha-fetoprotein in Fanconi anemia. Blood. 2000;96(3):859–63.
9. Olson TS. Management of Fanconi anemia beyond childhood. Hematology Am Soc Hematol Educ Program. 2023;2023(1):556–62.
10. Bartlett AL, Wagner JE, Jones BV, et al. Fanconi Anemia Neuroinflammatory Syndrome (FANS): brain lesions and neurologic injury in Fanconi anemia. Blood Adv. 2024;8(12):3027–37.
11. Choijilsuren HB, Park Y, Jung M. Mechanisms of somatic transformation in inherited bone marrow failure syndromes. Hematology Am Soc Hematol Educ Program. 2021;2021(1):390–8.
12. Tönnies H, Huber S, Kuhl J-S, Gerlach A, Ebell W, Neitzel H. Clonal chromosomal aberrations in bone marrow cells of Fanconi anemia patients: gains of the chromosomal segment 3q26q29 as an adverse risk factor. Blood. 2003;101(10):3872–4.
13. Marion W, Koppe T, Chen CC, et al. RUNX1 mutations mitigate quiescence to promote transformation of hematopoietic progenitors in Fanconi anemia. Leukemia. 2023;37(8):1698–708.
14. Quentin S, Cuccuini W, Ceccaldi R, et al. Myelodysplasia and leukemia of Fanconi anemia are associated with a specific pattern of genomic abnormalities that includes cryptic RUNX1/AML1 lesions. Blood. 2011;117(15):e161–70.
15. Sebert M, Gachet S, Leblanc T, et al. Clonal hematopoiesis driven by chromosome 1q/MDM4 trisomy defines a canonical route toward leukemia in Fanconi anemia. Cell Stem Cell. 2023;30(2):153–170.e9.
16. Giardino S, de Latour RP, Aljurf M, Severe Aplastic Anemia and Chronic Malignancies Working Parties of European Blood and Marrow Transplantation Group, et al. Outcome of patients with Fanconi anemia developing myelodysplasia and acute leukemia who received allogeneic hematopoietic stem cell transplantation: a retrospective analysis on behalf of EBMT group. Am J Hematol. 2020;95(7):809–16.
17. Debureaux PE, Sicre de Fontbrune F, Bonfim C, et al. FLAG-sequential regimen followed by bone marrow transplantation for myelodysplastic syndrome or acute leukemia in patients with Fanconi anemia: a Franco-Brazilian study. Bone Marrow Transplant. 2021;56(1):285–8.
18. Alter BP, Giri N, Savage SA, Rosenberg PS. Cancer in the National Cancer Institute inherited bone marrow failure syndrome cohort after fifteen years of follow-up. Haematologica. 2018;103(1):30–9.
19. Walsh MF, Chang VY, Kohlmann WK, et al. Recommendations for childhood cancer screening and surveillance in DNA repair disorders. Clin Cancer Res. 2017;23(11):e23–31.
20. Velleuer E, Dietrich R, Pomjanski N, et al. Diagnostic accuracy of brush biopsy-based cytology for the early detection of oral cancer and precursors in Fanconi anemia. Cancer Cytopathol. 2020;128(6):403–13.
21. Carreras E, et al., editors. The EBMT handbook: hematopoietic stem cell transplantation and cellular therapies. 7th ed. Cham: Springer; 2024. p. 718.
22. Ebens CL, MacMillan ML, Wagner JE. Hematopoietic cell transplantation in Fanconi anemia: current evidence, challenges and recommendations. Expert Rev Hematol. 2017;10(1):81–97.
23. Lum SH, Eikema DJ, Piepenbroek B, Wynn RF, Samarasinghe S, Dalissier A, Kalwak K, Ayas M, Hamladji RM, Yesilipek A, Dalle JH, Uckan-Cetinkaya D, Bierings M, Kupesiz

A, Halahleh K, Skorobogatova E, Öztürk G, Faraci M, Renard C, Evans P, Corbacioglu S, Locatelli F, Dufour C, Risitano A, Peffault de Latour R. Outcomes of hematopoietic stem cell transplantation in 813 pediatric patients with Fanconi anemia. Blood. 2024;144(12):1329–42. https://doi.org/10.1182/blood.2023022751. PMID: 38968140.
24. Giardino S, Eikema DJ, Piepenbroek B, et al. HLA-haploidentical stem cell transplantation in children with inherited bone marrow failure syndromes: a retrospective analysis on behalf of EBMT severe aplastic anemia and pediatric diseases working parties. Am J Hematol. 2024;99(6):1066–76.
25. Calado RT, Clé DV. Treatment of inherited bone marrow failure syndromes beyond transplantation. Hematology Am Soc Hematol Educ Program. 2017;2017(1):96–101.
26. Scheckenbach K, Morgan M, Filger-Brillinger J, et al. Treatment of the bone marrow failure in Fanconi anemia patients with danazol. Blood Cells Mol Dis. 2012;48(2):128–31.
27. Pollard JA, Furutani E, Liu S, et al. Metformin for treatment of cytopenias in children and young adults with Fanconi anemia. Blood Adv. 2022;6(12):3803–11.
28. Mehta PA, Fukuda T, Zhao J, et al. Quercetin: a novel targeted chemoprevention for patients with Fanconi anemia (FA). Blood. 2017;130(suppl 1):1178.
29. Barranta ME, Chinian F, Roskom K, et al. Prospective phase I/II study of eltrombopag for the treatment of bone marrow failure in Fanconi anemia. Poster session presented at: 508. Bone Marrow Failure: Poster II, 63th ASH Annual Meeting and Exposition, Atlanta, GA, 11–14 Dec 2021.
30. Sevilla J, Navarro S, Rio P, et al. Improved collection of hematopoietic stem cells and progenitors from Fanconi anemia patients for gene therapy purposes. Mol Ther Methods Clin Dev. 2021;22:66–75.
31. Lasaga M, Río P, Vilas-Zornoza A, et al. Gene therapy restores the transcriptional program of hematopoietic stem cells in Fanconi anemia. Haematologica. 2023;108(10):2652–63.
32. Diez B, Genovese P, Roman-Rodriguez FJ, et al. Therapeutic gene editing in CD34$^+$ hematopoietic progenitors from Fanconi anemia patients. EMBO Mol Med. 2017;9(11):1574–88.
33. Román-Rodríguez FJ, Ugalde L, Álvarez L, et al. NHEJ-mediated repair of CRISPR-Cas9-induced DNA breaks efficiently corrects mutations in HSPCs from patients with Fanconi anemia. Cell Stem Cell. 2019;25(5):607–621.e7.
34. Siegner SM, Ugalde L, Clemens A, et al. Adenine base editing efficiently restores the function of Fanconi anemia hematopoietic stem and progenitor cells. Nat Commun. 2022;13(1):6900.

Open Access This chapter is licensed under the terms of the Creative Commons Attribution 4.0 International License (http://creativecommons.org/licenses/by/4.0/), which permits use, sharing, adaptation, distribution and reproduction in any medium or format, as long as you give appropriate credit to the original author(s) and the source, provide a link to the Creative Commons license and indicate if changes were made.

The images or other third party material in this chapter are included in the chapter's Creative Commons license, unless indicated otherwise in a credit line to the material. If material is not included in the chapter's Creative Commons license and your intended use is not permitted by statutory regulation or exceeds the permitted use, you will need to obtain permission directly from the copyright holder.

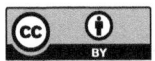

Chapter 17
Telomere Biology

Joshua Glass, Emma Groarke, and Neal S. Young

Introduction

Telomeres are located at the ends of linear chromosomes and protect them from damage (Fig. 17.1). Comprising tens to thousands of TTAGGG tandem repeats that do not code for a protein, telomeres are designed to function and protect human chromosomes over a normal lifespan [1]. Every time a cell undergoes mitosis, telomeres are shortened, ultimately promoting a signal for the arrest of cell proliferation and apoptosis [2].

Telomerase is an enzyme that drives the repair mechanism that helps minimize the loss of genetically encoded information with each cell division. The addition of new DNA to the ends of chromosomes is accomplished by the reverse transcription of an RNA molecule, TERC, and two copies of the telomerase reverse transcriptase (TERT). By copying a short region of TERC into the telomeric DNA, TERT is able to extend the 3′ end of the chromosome [3].

In addition to telomerase, other protective mechanisms have been identified. A capping protein structure, collectively referred to as shelterin, protects the telomere by preventing the DNA repair machinery from mistaking telomeres for double-stranded DNA breaks. The shelterin complex is composed of six proteins: TIN2, TRF1, TRF2, RAP1, POT1, and TPP1. The significance of this structure became evident upon discovery that mutations within *TINF2*, which encodes TIN2, are associated with the development of short telomeres and a clinical presentation consistent with dyskeratosis congenita (DC). This finding underscores the pivotal role of TIN2 in maintaining telomere integrity and highlights its relevance in understanding the molecular basis of dyskeratosis congenita. Other proteins, including

---

J. Glass (✉) · E. Groarke · N. S. Young
Hematology Branch, National Heart, Lung, and Blood Institute, National Institutes of Health, Bethesda, MD, USA
e-mail: joshua.glass@nih.gov

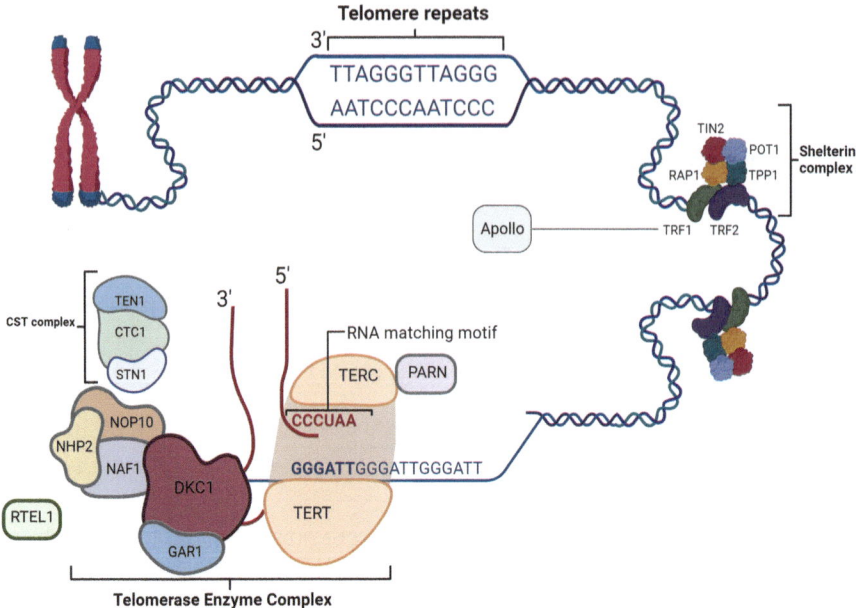

Fig. 17.1 The telomere, telomerase, and associated proteins. (Created with BioRender.com)

RTEL1, help maintain the structural integrity of the protein during cellular replication [4].

Telomere shortening contributes to aging and is affected by multiple factors. Exposure to toxic chemicals, treatment with chemotherapy, and bone marrow transplant conditioning regimens all cause tissue damage, which leads to an increased rate of telomere shortening. Viral infections have been implicated [5, 6]. Lifestyle factors, such as sedentary behavior, obesity, smoking, and stress, have also been linked to the presence of shorter telomeres [7–9].

The clinical ramifications associated with shortened telomeres have gained further clarity through the identification of genetic associations. Pathogenic variants in genes encoding the components of the telomerase complex (*DKC1*, *TERC*, *TERT*, or *PARN*), telomerase biogenesis (*NOP10*, *NHP2*, or *NAF1*), telomere trafficking (*WRAP53*), or telomerase recruitment (*ACD*) collectively lead to shortened telomere length. Similarly, defects in genes encoding proteins responsible for the various aspects of telomere protection and synthesis (*TINF2*, *CTC1*, *STN1*, *POT1*, and *RTEL1*) also contribute to telomere shortening [10, 11]. Collectively, these diseases are termed the telomere biology disorders (TBDs).

Telomere dysfunction, in the setting of normal telomere length, was identified in patients with a splice variant of *DCLRE1B*, the gene responsible for encoding the protein Apollo. The *DCLRE1B* mutation is associated with telomere maintenance and the DNA cross-link repair mechanism. Unlike the majority of individuals with TBD, who exhibit significantly shortened telomeres, cases involving the *DCLRE1B* splice variant are associated with chromosomal instability rather than a defect in telomere length [12–14].

The inheritance of TBDs and the level of penetrance are variable. Those presenting with autosomal dominant inheritance patterns, excluding *TINF2*, have been shown to have the best overall survival [15]. Individuals with very short telomeres (<1st percentile) in lymphocytes, even in the absence of an identified gene mutation, may have a TBD due to an undiscovered gene mutation, as occurs in ~25% of cases. The spectrum of genetic and etiological factors that lead to TBD is not complete [2].

Clinical Manifestations

The first described telomere biology disorder, dyskeratosis congenita, was initially characterized in the early 1900s in pediatric patients presenting with the mucocutaneous triad of reticulated skin pigmentation, nail dystrophy, and oral leukoplakia [16–18]. Dyskeratosis congenita and other more recently described TBDs comprise a wide phenotypic and genotypic spectrum (Fig. 17.2). Diagnosis is made through the quantitative analysis of telomere length and genetic testing. Currently, the only test that is validated for clinical purposes is fluorescent in situ hybridization (flow-FISH) [19, 20].

Dyskeratosis Congenita

Dyskeratosis congenita (DC) is at the severe end of the TBD spectrum. Common manifestations include bone marrow failure, increased susceptibility to cancer, systemic infections, pulmonary fibrosis, and liver fibrosis [10, 16–18]. Unfortunately, individuals affected by DC typically experience a shortened lifespan, with death occurring often before the age of 40 years [21].

The classic mucocutaneous triad associated with DC comprises nail dystrophy, reticulated hyperpigmentation of the skin, and mucous membrane leukoplakia [16–18]. Skin and nail alterations become apparent typically within the initial decade of life. Nail dystrophy manifests as atrophic and longitudinally ridged nails and even complete nail loss. Skin changes appear subsequent to nail changes and manifest with reticulated gray-brown skin pigmentation, atrophy, and telangiectasia that predominantly affects the neck, face, and chest. Additional characterized features include hyperhidrosis, hyperkeratosis of the palms and soles, sparse scalp hair, and heightened susceptibility to blistering on the hands and feet [17, 22, 23].

During the second and third decades of life, oral leukoplakia and excessive ocular tearing become notable. Lacrimal duct stenosis contributes to blepharitis, ectropion, and increased tearing. Oral leukokeratosis predisposes to squamous cell carcinoma. Other mucous membranes, including conjunctival, urethral, and genital, may be involved [22, 23].

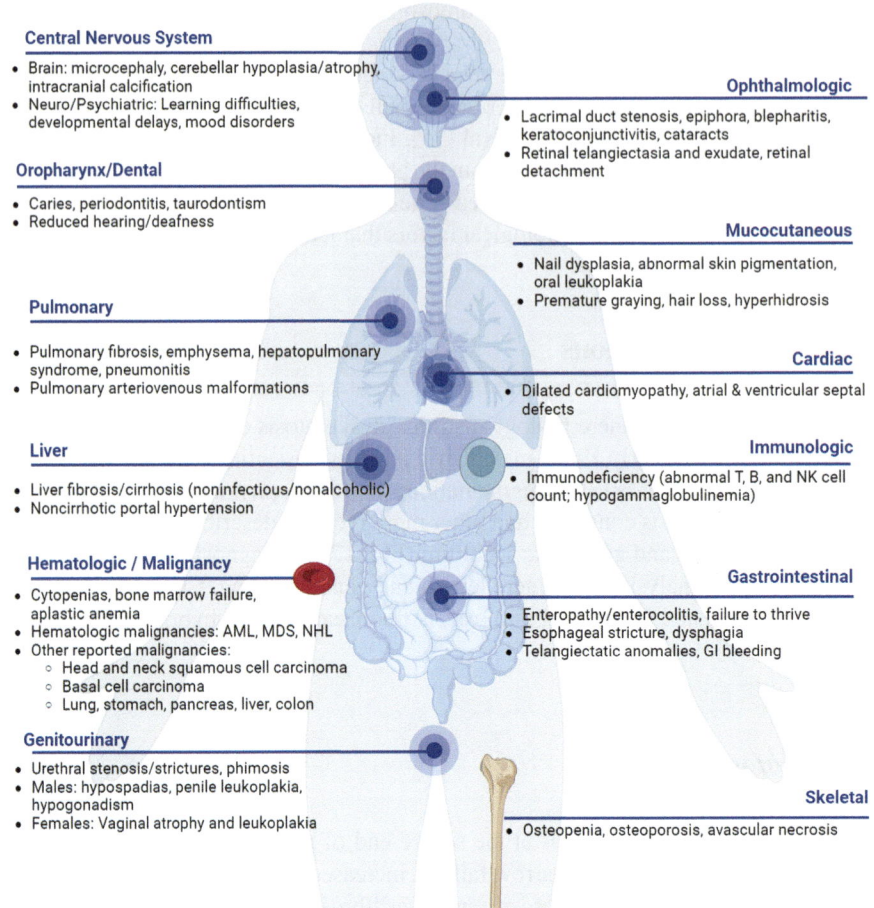

Fig. 17.2 Clinical manifestations of telomere biology disorders. (Created with BioRender.com)

Hematologic and immunologic anomalies are prominent components of the complex clinical profile of DC. The initial hematologic changes often involve thrombocytopenia and/or macrocytic anemia. Nearly 90% of patients will exhibit varying degrees of bone marrow failure, with severe aplastic anemia occurring in nearly half of the cases, typically manifesting in the second decade of life [20, 22–24]. Hematologic malignancy is also seen in older patients [25]. Immunologic abnormalities associated with DC include alterations in immunoglobulin levels (either reduced or elevated), diminished B- and/or T-lymphocyte counts, and a decrease or absence of the lymphocytic proliferative response [26].

Dyskeratosis congenita exhibits genetic heterogeneity, with different inheritance patterns associated with specific causative genes. The X-linked recessive inheritance pattern of *DKC1*, which encodes the nuclear protein dyskerin, accounts for the higher prevalence of male patients in many instances. Interestingly, despite the

X-linked nature, a considerable number of female patients present with features similar to their male counterparts [10, 23].

The autosomal dominant form of DC is attributed to mutations in *TINF2*, and less commonly in *TERC*, and *TERT*. Autosomal recessive DC is linked to mutations in *NOLA3*, *NOP10*, *NHP2*, *RTEL1*, *TCAB1*, and *CTC1* [3, 10, 23].

Hoyeraal–Hreidarsson Syndrome

A diagnosis of Hoyeraal–Hreidarsson syndrome (HHS) is considered in children meeting the diagnostic criteria of DC but with cerebellar hypoplasia [27, 28]. Enterocolitis is a prevalent defining feature and may be observed in the initial presentation [29]. Additional features include intrauterine growth restriction, developmental delay/intellectual disability, microcephaly, and immunodeficiency [13, 30–32].

Telomere maintenance defects represent the hallmark abnormality in HHS, highlighted by the identification of the heterozygous splice variant *DCLRE1B*, encoding the nuclease Apollo, identified in a child with HHS [12]. The syndrome is genetically diverse, with X-linked recessive cases involving *DKC1* mutations and autosomal recessive cases associated with homozygous mutations in *TERT*. *TINF2* mutations result in sporadic presentations of HHS [33–37].

Revesz Syndrome

Revesz syndrome is considered in children meeting the diagnostic criteria of dyskeratosis congenita and found with bilateral exudative retinopathy (bilateral Coats' disease). Additional features include intrauterine growth restriction, sparse hair, and intracranial calcification [38, 39]. Mutations in *TINF2* are also linked to Revesz syndrome, an autosomal dominant variant of dyskeratosis congenita [4, 40].

Coats Plus

Coats plus is a condition that is caused by biallelic mutations in *CTC1* and is characterized by retinal telangiectasia and exudates. This diagnosis presents with asymmetric intracranial calcifications involving the thalamus, basal ganglia, dentate, and deep cortex, accompanied by associated leukoencephalopathy and brain cysts. Other features of Coats plus include pre- and postnatal growth restriction, osteopenia that predisposes patients to fractures and impaired bone healing, and recurrent gastrointestinal (GI) hemorrhage due to vascular ectasias in the stomach, small intestines, and liver [41–45].

Bone Marrow Failure/Aplastic Anemia

Hematopoietic dysfunction resulting from compromised telomere structure and repair spans a diverse clinical spectrum. Marrow failure is the consequence of progressive attrition and depletion of hematopoietic stem cells due to premature senescence.

The initial cytopenia typically observed is thrombocytopenia, followed by the development of anemia and/or neutropenia [21]. The severity of bone marrow failure varies, encompassing a spectrum from no apparent abnormalities to pronounced pancytopenia consistent with severe aplastic anemia [2, 23, 46, 47].

Manifestations are observed across the lifespan, ranging in onset from birth to late adulthood. Infants or young children with severe forms of DC may present with progressive bone marrow failure early in life, sometimes preceding other clinical signs. In contrast, older individuals with TBD, particularly those with *TERC* or *TERT* variants, may develop blood cell abnormalities later in life [48, 49].

Cancer

Telomere shortening is generally (but not invariably) associated with increased cancer risk. Cancer manifests in nearly 15% of patients with DC, typically emerging in the third and fourth decades of life. DC patients are predisposed to the development of both myeloid neoplasms and solid tumors [23, 46, 47].

Patients with TBD are at an increased risk of developing hematologic malignancies, diagnosed two decades earlier when compared to the general population [50]. While TBDs are due to germline mutations in genes responsible for telomere maintenance and repair, clonal hematopoiesis driven by somatic mutations is associated with the development of myelodysplastic syndrome (MDS) and acute myeloid leukemia (AML). MDS and AML are the most common short telomere–associated malignancies [51–53]. Outcomes in patients diagnosed with malignancy are often inferior due to the poor tolerance of standard conditioning for allogeneic hematopoietic stem cell transplantation (HSCT) [52].

The clonal landscape in TBD is dominated by *PPM1D*, the *TERT* promoter (*TERTp*), *POT1*, and *U2AF1*. Somatic mutations in *TERTp*, *TP53*, and *U2AF1* correlate with worse overall survival. In TBD, *U2AF1* is associated with the development of myeloid malignancy. While *U2AF1* mutations occur in patients without cancer, they are considered premalignant, likely maladaptive, early events and secondary acquisition of subsequent mutations driving hematologic malignancy. In functional studies, *U2AF1^{S34}* mutations compensate for aberrant upregulation of TP53 and interferon pathways in telomere-dysfunctional hematopoietic stem cells [54, 55]. PPM1D mutations, typically associated with myeloid malignancy secondary to chemotherapy, in TBD are not associated with either cancer development or worse overall survival [56].

Solid tumors are more common in younger, male patients with *DKC1* mutations at a cumulative incidence of 20%–30% before age 50. Though the overall incidence in patients with TBD is much less compared to hematologic malignancies, solid tumors characterized include squamous cell carcinomas, primarily affecting the head and neck regions, including the tongue, mouth, and pharynx [25, 51]. Additionally, cancers of the skin and the gastrointestinal tract (involving the esophagus, stomach, colon, and anorectal areas) are commonly observed [23, 46, 47]. The risk of solid tumors in patients with DC following allogeneic hematopoietic stem cell transplantation is greater than in non-transplanted patients [47]. Short-term cancer outcomes with resectable solid tumors are generally favorable but poor in those with an invasive disease [51, 57].

Cancer predisposition with long telomeres has also been described, attributed to germline variants in the telomere maintenance genes *POT1* and *TINF2*. Long telomeres are associated with an increased cancer risk, including for melanoma, chronic lymphocytic leukemia, lymphoma, sarcoma, and thyroid cancer [58–60]. Of note, multiple solid tumors, including brain, kidney, lung, melanoma, and thyroid cancers, occur with relatively longer telomeres, within the normal range for the general population [58].

Liver Disease

There is a wide range of liver disease in TBD. Presentation may be limited to inflammation and transaminitis, though more extensive hepatic involvement is often identified via imaging or biopsy [61]. In patients with *TERT* or *TERC* mutations that do not present with any of the mucocutaneous symptoms seen in patients with DC, hepatic dysfunction may be the only symptom of a TBD. Liver disease can also be seen in the absence of bone marrow failure [2, 62].

Non-cirrhotic liver disease leads to the development of portosystemic varices and portal hypertension [22]. While patients with non-cirrhotic portal hypertension can develop edema, ascites, and varices, synthetic liver function is typically preserved [63]. Biopsy demonstrates hepatic nodular regenerative hyperplasia (NRH). A familial relationship between NRH and TBD-associated gene mutations has been characterized, even in the absence of bone marrow failure and/or pulmonary fibrosis [64, 65].

Severe hepatic disease is characterized by the development of late-stage cirrhosis and liver failure. Synthetic function of the liver is impaired, resulting in decreased albumin levels and prolonged prothrombin time. Patients may present with fatigue, jaundice, bleeding, ascites/peripheral edema, and hepatic encephalopathy in the most extreme cases [66].

Lung Disease and Pulmonary Fibrosis

Pulmonary disease is a lethal complication of TBD. Pulmonary function tests with diffusion capacity of the lung for carbon monoxide (DL_{CO}) are consistent with a restrictive pattern and can precede the development of fibrosis. Nearly 40% of patients with DC have lung disease, as the development of pulmonary fibrosis represents the most prevalent manifestation seen in patients with TBD [67, 68]. Pulmonary fibrosis may be symptomatic with cough, dyspnea, impaired gas exchange, and reduced lung volume. Approximately 25% of familial cases and up to 10% of sporadic cases of pulmonary fibrosis are linked to *TERT, TERC, DKC1, TINF2, RTEL1,* and/or *PARN* [68–80]. *NAF1* variants have been associated with pulmonary fibrosis–emphysema [81]. Pathologically, the condition is characterized by patchy fibrosis in the lungs, interstitial inflammation, and the alternation of normal lung tissue with areas of fibrosis, inflammation, and collagen deposition [68–81]. The spectrum of TBD includes patients with isolated pulmonary fibrosis; while they often have a telomere length <10th percentile, in some cases, telomere length may be normal [82, 83].

Patients with pulmonary fibrosis and shortened telomeres have been reported to present with cryptogenic hepatic cirrhosis, suggestive of the involvement of telomere loss in both fibrotic processes. This relationship between telomere dysfunction and various systemic manifestations highlights the broad impact of telomere biology disorders on multiple organ systems [62, 84, 85].

The hepatopulmonary syndrome occurs when intrapulmonary vascular dilations lead to an arterial oxygenation defect in the setting of liver disease [86–88]. Patients with TBD are at an increased risk of developing hepatopulmonary syndrome due to the presence of underlying liver disease. Concurrently, patients may develop pulmonary arteriovenous malformations (AVMs) that cause a deficit in arterial oxygenation as a result of the right-to-left shunting of blood [89]. The diagnosis of both hepatopulmonary syndrome and pulmonary AVM is challenging, as symptoms are similar to those of pulmonary fibrosis. Patients with hepatopulmonary syndrome and/or pulmonary AVM may present with significant clubbing and an exaggerated decrease in DL_{CO} [88, 89].

Vascular Anomalies

In addition to pulmonary arteriovenous malformations, the presence of gastrointestinal (GI) and retinal vascular telangiectasias has been characterized in patients with DC [42, 89, 90]. The mechanism of development is not well-understood, though it is hypothesized to be an effect of impaired wound healing causing vascular dysfunction [90]. As previously discussed, pulmonary AVM can lead to respiratory insufficiency.

Retinal telangiectasias is seen in patients diagnosed with Coats plus and is the reason that patients with DC/TBD should be regularly followed by ophthalmology [42–45].

GI telangiectasias can present with life-threatening GI bleeding and is more commonly seen in pediatric patients (median age 12.5 years). Diagnosis is made via endoscopy. While initially characterized in patients with Coats plus, individuals with DC, Revesz syndrome, and Hoyeraal–Hreidarsson syndrome have also been described to have GI telangiectasias. Most GI telangiectasias are identified in the stomach and small bowel, though some patients have AVM present in the colon [91].

In patients with TBD, AVM can occur throughout the body and may be identified in previously unreported locations.

Diagnosis

The gold standard for telomere length (TL) measurement is the flow-FISH assay. Results are reported as a percentile for age in both lymphocyte subsets and granulocytes. Telomere length less than the 1st percentile is sensitive and specific for a TBD; however, some patients may have TL in the 1st–10th percentile, and in these cases, the clinical phenotype is of key importance. Short TL in granulocytes is less specific for TBD and can occur in states of marrow stress, including immune marrow failure and MDS [19, 20, 23].

Genetic testing for telomere-related gene mutations should be performed, as normal telomere length does not exclude a TBD diagnosis [82, 83]. Additionally, approximately 25% of cases of TBD are due to unknown germline defects, and thus, even a negative genetic test is not definitive and may confuse the evaluation of an otherwise typical patient and pedigree [92].

Somatic reversion occurs in patients with TBD, described in patients with autosomal dominant DC with a germline *TERC* mutation found in skin fibroblasts [93, 94]. As a result of reversion, a TBD-associated gene variant may not be detectable in the peripheral blood; telomere length normalizes, and there is effective hematopoiesis. Because revertant somatic mosaicism obscures the genetic diagnosis, a skin biopsy is essential to determine the germline genotype [10, 93–97].

Treatment

Unfortunately, treatment options remain limited for patients with TBD, with no targeted therapies available. Depending on the disease severity and affected organ(s), patients may be observed or given medical therapy, or they can undergo either hematopoietic or solid organ transplantation.

Surveillance

Hematologic monitoring includes regular complete blood counts, performed every 3–6 months, depending on clinical status. Due to increased risk of myeloid malignancy, some guidelines recommend yearly bone marrow examination, though in practice, this is not always performed when patients exhibit stable blood counts. A drop in blood counts or the presence of a new cytogenetic abnormality should prompt a reevaluation.

While there are no prospective studies on cancer surveillance in TBD patients, guidelines recommend regular screening for early identification. In particular, patients should undergo regular oral and ENT exams due to the increased risk of head and neck squamous cell carcinoma, as well as regular gynecologic and skin exams.

Full screening recommendations can be found in the Diagnosis and Management Guidelines for patients with TBD (https://teamtelomere.org/telomere-biology-disorders-diagnosis-and-management-guidelines-downloads/) [98].

Androgens

Androgens are often prescribed to improve blood counts in TBD patients. Clinical studies have demonstrated efficacy in patients. In a prospective analysis of 16 patients on androgen therapy (oxymetholone, fluoxymesterone, and nandrolone), which included mostly children with DC, 11 achieved clinically significant hematologic responses [99]. In a prospective trial, Townsley et al. demonstrated hematologic responses in 79% of patients after only 3 months of treatment [100].

In vitro studies of peripheral blood and bone marrow samples have also suggested that telomere length can be modulated by sex hormones. Exposure of normal peripheral blood lymphocytes and human bone marrow–derived CD34+ stem cells to androgens increased telomerase activity in vitro [101]. In cells collected from individuals carrying a loss-of-function *TERT* mutation, in vitro androgen exposure resulted in increased telomerase activity. In a prospective protocol of high doses of danazol, based on in vitro experiments, Townsley et al. demonstrated that increases in telomere length, assessed by polymerase chain reaction (PCR) assays, were observed in all evaluable patients after 6 months of therapy [100, 101]. A subsequent prospective study from Cle et al. also demonstrated telomere elongation in TBD patients using nandrolone [102].

Retrospective studies have reported the role of androgens in telomere elongation, both positive and negative. One study compared the rate of telomere attrition in younger patients with clinical DC who did or did not receive androgens and demonstrated no significant difference in lymphocyte telomere attrition between groups [103]. The second study of seven patients with TBD treated with androgen therapy showed an improvement in cytopenias and an increase in lymphocyte telomere length in all patients [104]. There was a significant difference in age (median 7 years in the first study and 40 years in the second) and genotype (*DKC1* and *TINF2* predominating in the first and *TERT/TERC* in the second). Given the heterogeneity of TBD, androgen therapy may be more beneficial in certain subgroups. The use of androgens to treat lung and liver fibrosis remains investigational.

Hematopoietic Stem Cell Transplantation

Hematopoietic stem cell transplantation (HSCT) is reserved for patients with severe marrow failure or those who develop MDS or AML. Outcomes had traditionally been poor, with less than one-third overall survival. This was due to post-transplant organ toxicity related to conditioning regimens, most commonly lung or endovascular [105, 106]. More recently, outcomes have improved, with an overall survival of 60%–70% due to the reduction or elimination of alkylating agents and radiation in preparative regimens in patients without neoplasia and an increasing use of fludarabine and antibody-based immunosuppressive conditioning [107, 108]. It is important to note that HSCT only treats the marrow manifestations of TBD and is not a therapeutic approach for other organ manifestations.

Solid Organ Transplantation

Solid organ transplantation may be the only therapy available for patients with end-stage lung or liver disease. There are limited specific data on the use of lung and liver transplants in the TBD setting. There is evidence that in patients undergoing lung transplant, short telomeres can predispose them to an increased risk of immunosuppression-induced cytopenias and lung allograft dysfunction [109, 110]. TBD patients referred for solid organ transplantation should undergo testing to assess for other significant organ involvement, which may impact management. Importantly, the diagnosis of TBD is not a contraindication for transplant, and suitable patients should be referred for assessment at a transplant center [111, 112].

Future Directions

Currently, there are a few ongoing clinical trials using novel agents in TBD, and further research is needed to develop therapeutics. One active study (NCT04211714) is an autologous cellular therapy in which ex vivo telomere elongation occurs; results are pending. Another promising compound is the PAPD5 inhibitor, a compound that reverses TERC oligoadenylation and increased TERC levels, which has shown promise in TBD cell lines and mouse models [113]. For now, options remain limited, and the development of treatments is a key priority for the telomere community.

References

1. Moyzis RK, Buckingham JM, Cram LS, et al. A highly conserved repetitive DNA sequence, (TTAGGG)n, present at the telomeres of human chromosomes. Proc Natl Acad Sci USA. 1988;85(18):6622–6. https://doi.org/10.1073/pnas.85.18.6622.
2. Calado RT, Young NS. Telomere diseases. N Engl J Med. 2009;361(24):2353–65. https://doi.org/10.1056/NEJMra0903373.
3. Young NS. Telomere biology and telomere diseases: implications for practice and research. Hematology Am Soc Hematol Educ Program. 2010;2010:30–5. https://doi.org/10.1182/asheducation-2010.1.30.
4. Savage SA, Giri N, Baerlocher GM, Orr N, Lansdorp PM, Alter BP. TINF2, a component of the shelterin telomere protection complex, is mutated in dyskeratosis congenita. Am J Hum Genet. 2008;82(2):501–9. https://doi.org/10.1016/j.ajhg.2007.10.004.
5. Bellon M, Nicot C. Telomere dynamics in immune senescence and exhaustion triggered by chronic viral infection. Viruses. 2017;9(10):289. https://doi.org/10.3390/v9100289. Published 5 Oct 2017.
6. Sanchez-Vazquez R, Guío-Carrión A, Zapatero-Gaviria A, Martínez P, Blasco MA. Shorter telomere lengths in patients with severe COVID-19 disease. Aging (Albany NY). 2021;13(1):1–15. https://doi.org/10.18632/aging.202463.
7. Mirabello L, Huang WY, Wong JY, et al. The association between leukocyte telomere length and cigarette smoking, dietary and physical variables, and risk of prostate cancer. Aging Cell. 2009;8(4):405–13. https://doi.org/10.1111/j.1474-9726.2009.00485.x.
8. Bekaert S, De Meyer T, Rietzschel ER, et al. Telomere length and cardiovascular risk factors in a middle-aged population free of overt cardiovascular disease. Aging Cell. 2007;6(5):639–47. https://doi.org/10.1111/j.1474-9726.2007.00321.x.
9. Nordfjäll K, Eliasson M, Stegmayr B, Lundin S, Roos G, Nilsson PM. Increased abdominal obesity, adverse psychosocial factors and shorter telomere length in subjects reporting early ageing; the MONICA Northern Sweden Study. Scand J Public Health. 2008;36(7):744–52. https://doi.org/10.1177/1403494808090634.
10. Savage SA. Dyskeratosis congenita and telomere biology disorders. Hematology Am Soc Hematol Educ Program. 2022;2022(1):637–48. https://doi.org/10.1182/hematology.2022000394.
11. Savage S, Vulliamy T. The genetics of dyskeratosis congenita and telomere biology disorders. In: Agarwal S, Savage SA, Stevens K, Raj H, Carson HK, editors. Telomere biology disorders: diagnosis and management guidelines. Team Telomere Inc; 2022. p. 69–82.
12. Touzot F, Callebaut I, Soulier J, et al. Function of Apollo (SNM1B) at telomere highlighted by a splice variant identified in a patient with Hoyeraal-Hreidarsson syndrome. Proc Natl Acad Sci USA. 2010;107(22):10097–102. https://doi.org/10.1073/pnas.0914918107.
13. Touzot F, Gaillard L, Vasquez N, et al. Heterogeneous telomere defects in patients with severe forms of dyskeratosis congenita. J Allergy Clin Immunol. 2012;129(2):473–482.e4823. https://doi.org/10.1016/j.jaci.2011.09.043.
14. Kermasson L, Churikov D, Awad A, et al. Inherited human Apollo deficiency causes severe bone marrow failure and developmental defects. Blood. 2022;139(16):2427–40. https://doi.org/10.1182/blood.2021010791.

15. Niewisch MR, Giri N, McReynolds LJ, et al. Disease progression and clinical outcomes in telomere biology disorders. Blood. 2022;139(12):1807–19. https://doi.org/10.1182/blood.2021013523.
16. Drachtman RA, Alter BP. Dyskeratosis congenita: clinical and genetic heterogeneity. Report of a new case and review of the literature. Am J Pediatr Hematol Oncol. 1992;14(4):297–304.
17. Ward SC, Savage SA, Giri N, et al. Beyond the triad: inheritance, mucocutaneous phenotype, and mortality in a cohort of patients with dyskeratosis congenita. J Am Acad Dermatol. 2018;78(4):804–6. https://doi.org/10.1016/j.jaad.2017.10.017.
18. Dokal I. Dyskeratosis congenita: an inherited bone marrow failure syndrome. Br J Haematol. 1996;92(4):775–9. https://doi.org/10.1046/j.1365-2141.1996.355881.x.
19. Baerlocher GM, Vulto I, de Jong G, Lansdorp PM. Flow cytometry and FISH to measure the average length of telomeres (flow FISH). Nat Protoc. 2006;1(5):2365–76. https://doi.org/10.1038/nprot.2006.263.
20. Baerlocher GM, Mak J, Tien T, Lansdorp PM. Telomere length measurement by fluorescence in situ hybridization and flow cytometry: tips and pitfalls. Cytometry. 2002;47(2):89–99. https://doi.org/10.1002/cyto.10053.
21. Savage SA, Alter BP. Dyskeratosis congenita. Hematol Oncol Clin North Am. 2009;23(2):215–31. https://doi.org/10.1016/j.hoc.2009.01.003.
22. Niewisch MR, Savage SA. An update on the biology and management of dyskeratosis congenita and related telomere biology disorders. Expert Rev Hematol. 2019;12(12):1037–52. https://doi.org/10.1080/17474086.2019.1662720.
23. Savage SA, Bertuch AA. The genetics and clinical manifestations of telomere biology disorders. Genet Med. 2010;12(12):753–64. https://doi.org/10.1097/GIM.0b013e3181f415b5.
24. Kirwan M, Dokal I. Dyskeratosis congenita: a genetic disorder of many faces. Clin Genet. 2008;73(2):103–12. https://doi.org/10.1111/j.1399-0004.2007.00923.x.
25. Alter BP, Giri N, Savage SA, et al. Malignancies and survival patterns in the National Cancer Institute inherited bone marrow failure syndromes cohort study. Br J Haematol. 2010;150(2):179–88. https://doi.org/10.1111/j.1365-2141.2010.08212.x.
26. Hodes RJ, Hathcock KS, Weng NP. Telomeres in T and B cells. Nat Rev Immunol. 2002;2(9):699–706. https://doi.org/10.1038/nri890.
27. Hoyeraal HM, Lamvik J, Moe PJ. Congenital hypoplastic thrombocytopenia and cerebral malformations in two brothers. Acta Paediatr Scand. 1970;59(2):185–91. https://doi.org/10.1111/j.1651-2227.1970.tb08986.x.
28. Sznajer Y, Baumann C, David A, et al. Further delineation of the congenital form of X-linked dyskeratosis congenita (Hoyeraal-Hreidarsson syndrome). Eur J Pediatr. 2003;162(12):863–7. https://doi.org/10.1007/s00431-003-1317-5.
29. Jonassaint NL, Guo N, Califano JA, Montgomery EA, Armanios M. The gastrointestinal manifestations of telomere-mediated disease. Aging Cell. 2013;12(2):319–23. https://doi.org/10.1111/acel.12041.
30. Zhang MJ, Cao YX, Wu HY, Li HH. Brain imaging features of children with Hoyeraal-Hreidarsson syndrome. Brain Behav. 2021;11(5):e02079. https://doi.org/10.1002/brb3.2079.
31. Ballew BJ, Joseph V, De S, et al. A recessive founder mutation in regulator of telomere elongation helicase 1, RTEL1, underlies severe immunodeficiency and features of Hoyeraal Hreidarsson syndrome. PLoS Genet. 2013;9(8):e1003695. https://doi.org/10.1371/journal.pgen.1003695.
32. Lamm N, Ordan E, Shponkin R, Richler C, Aker M, Tzfati Y. Diminished telomeric 3′ overhangs are associated with telomere dysfunction in Hoyeraal-Hreidarsson syndrome. PLoS One. 2009;4(5):e5666. https://doi.org/10.1371/journal.pone.0005666. Published 22 May 2009.
33. Knight SW, Heiss NS, Vulliamy TJ, et al. Unexplained aplastic anaemia, immunodeficiency, and cerebellar hypoplasia (Hoyeraal-Hreidarsson syndrome) due to mutations in the dyskeratosis congenita gene, DKC1. Br J Haematol. 1999;107(2):335–9. https://doi.org/10.1046/j.1365-2141.1999.01690.x.

34. Cossu F, Vulliamy TJ, Marrone A, Badiali M, Cao A, Dokal I. A novel DKC1 mutation, severe combined immunodeficiency (T+B-NK-SCID) and bone marrow transplantation in an infant with Hoyeraal-Hreidarsson syndrome. Br J Haematol. 2002;119(3):765–8. https://doi.org/10.1046/j.1365-2141.2002.03822.x.
35. Marrone A, Walne A, Tamary H, et al. Telomerase reverse-transcriptase homozygous mutations in autosomal recessive dyskeratosis congenita and Hoyeraal-Hreidarsson syndrome. Blood. 2007;110(13):4198–205. https://doi.org/10.1182/blood-2006-12-062851.
36. Walne AJ, Vulliamy T, Beswick R, Kirwan M, Dokal I. TINF2 mutations result in very short telomeres: analysis of a large cohort of patients with dyskeratosis congenita and related bone marrow failure syndromes. Blood. 2008;112(9):3594–600. https://doi.org/10.1182/blood-2008-05-153445.
37. Vulliamy T, Beswick R, Kirwan MJ, Hossain U, Walne AJ, Dokal I. Telomere length measurement can distinguish pathogenic from non-pathogenic variants in the shelterin component, TIN2. Clin Genet. 2012;81(1):76–81. https://doi.org/10.1111/j.1399-0004.2010.01605.x.
38. Revesz T, Fletcher S, al-Gazali LI, DeBuse P. Bilateral retinopathy, aplastic anaemia, and central nervous system abnormalities: a new syndrome? J Med Genet. 1992;29(9):673–5. https://doi.org/10.1136/jmg.29.9.673.
39. Karremann M, Neumaier-Probst E, Schlichtenbrede F, et al. Revesz syndrome revisited. Orphanet J Rare Dis. 2020;15(1):299. https://doi.org/10.1186/s13023-020-01553-y. Published 23 Oct 2020.
40. Sasa GS, Ribes-Zamora A, Nelson ND, Bertuch AA. Three novel truncating TINF2 mutations causing severe dyskeratosis congenita in early childhood. Clin Genet. 2012;81(5):470–8. https://doi.org/10.1111/j.1399-0004.2011.01658.x.
41. Crow YJ, McMenamin J, Haenggeli CA, et al. Coats' plus: a progressive familial syndrome of bilateral Coats' disease, characteristic cerebral calcification, leukoencephalopathy, slow pre- and post-natal linear growth and defects of bone marrow and integument. Neuropediatrics. 2004;35(1):10–9. https://doi.org/10.1055/s-2003-43552.
42. Anderson BH, Kasher PR, Mayer J, et al. Mutations in CTC1, encoding conserved telomere maintenance component 1, cause Coats plus. Nat Genet. 2012;44(3):338–42. https://doi.org/10.1038/ng.1084. Published 22 Jan 2012.
43. Polvi A, Linnankivi T, Kivelä T, et al. Mutations in CTC1, encoding the CTS telomere maintenance complex component 1, cause cerebroretinal microangiopathy with calcifications and cysts. Am J Hum Genet. 2012;90(3):540–9. https://doi.org/10.1016/j.ajhg.2012.02.002.
44. Savage SA. Connecting complex disorders through biology. Nat Genet. 2012;44(3):238–40. https://doi.org/10.1038/ng.2206. Published 27 Feb 2012.
45. Keller RB, Gagne KE, Usmani GN, et al. CTC1 mutations in a patient with dyskeratosis congenita. Pediatr Blood Cancer. 2012;59(2):311–4. https://doi.org/10.1002/pbc.24193.
46. Alter BP, Giri N, Savage SA, Rosenberg PS. Cancer in dyskeratosis congenita. Blood. 2009;113(26):6549–57. https://doi.org/10.1182/blood-2008-12-192880.
47. Alter BP, Giri N, Savage SA, Rosenberg PS. Cancer in the National Cancer Institute inherited bone marrow failure syndrome cohort after fifteen years of follow-up. Haematologica. 2018;103(1):30–9. https://doi.org/10.3324/haematol.2017.178111.
48. Dokal I. Dyskeratosis congenita in all its forms. Br J Haematol. 2000;110(4):768–79. https://doi.org/10.1046/j.1365-2141.2000.02109.x.
49. Dokal I. Dyskeratosis congenita. Hematology Am Soc Hematol Educ Program. 2011;2011:480–6. https://doi.org/10.1182/asheducation-2011.1.480.
50. Ma X, Does M, Raza A, Mayne ST. Myelodysplastic syndromes: incidence and survival in the United States. Cancer. 2007;109(8):1536–42. https://doi.org/10.1002/cncr.22570.
51. Schratz KE, Haley L, Danoff SK, et al. Cancer spectrum and outcomes in the Mendelian short telomere syndromes. Blood. 2020;135(22):1946–56. https://doi.org/10.1182/blood.2019003264.
52. Mangaonkar AA, Patnaik MM. Short telomere syndromes in clinical practice: bridging bench and bedside. Mayo Clin Proc. 2018;93(7):904–16. https://doi.org/10.1016/j.mayocp.2018.03.020.

53. Fabre MA, de Almeida JG, Fiorillo E, et al. The longitudinal dynamics and natural history of clonal haematopoiesis. Nature. 2022;606(7913):335–42. https://doi.org/10.1038/s41586-022-04785-z.
54. Ferrer A, Lasho T, Fernandez JA, et al. Patients with telomere biology disorders show context specific somatic mosaic states with high frequency of U2AF1 variants. Am J Hematol. 2023;98(12):E357–9. https://doi.org/10.1002/ajh.27086.
55. Groarke EM, Gutierrez-Rodrigues F, Ma X, et al. U2AF1 and other splicing factor gene mutations in telomere biology disorders are associated with hematologic neoplasia and worse overall survival. Blood. 2021;138(Supplement 1):862. https://doi.org/10.1182/blood-2021-146946.
56. Gutierrez-Rodrigues F, Groarke EM, Clé D, et al. Clonal hematopoiesis in telomere biology disorders associates with the underlying germline defect and somatic mutations in POT1, PPM1D, and TERT promoter. Blood. 2021;138(Supplement 1):1111. https://doi.org/10.1182/blood-2021-151199.
57. Savage S, Vasta L, Niewisch M. Solid tumors. In: Telomere biology disorders diagnosis and management guidelines. 2nd ed; 2022. p. 149–58. https://teamtelomere.org.
58. Savage SA. Telomere length and cancer risk: finding Goldilocks. Biogerontology. 2024;25(2):265–78. https://doi.org/10.1007/s10522-023-10080-9.
59. Nakao T, Natarajan P. Familial clonal hematopoiesis in a long telomere syndrome. N Engl J Med. 2023;389(16):1535. https://doi.org/10.1056/NEJMc2309139.
60. Codd V, Wang Q, Allara E, et al. Polygenic basis and biomedical consequences of telomere length variation. Nat Genet. 2021;53(10):1425–33. https://doi.org/10.1038/s41588-021-00944-6.
61. Kapuria D, Ben-Yakov G, Ortolano R, et al. The spectrum of hepatic involvement in patients with telomere disease. Hepatology. 2019;69(6):2579–85. https://doi.org/10.1002/hep.30578.
62. Calado RT, Regal JA, Kleiner DE, et al. A spectrum of severe familial liver disorders associate with telomerase mutations. PLoS One. 2009;4(11):e7926. https://doi.org/10.1371/journal.pone.0007926. Published 20 Nov 2009.
63. Schouten JN, Garcia-Pagan JC, Valla DC, Janssen HL. Idiopathic noncirrhotic portal hypertension. Hepatology. 2011;54(3):1071–81. https://doi.org/10.1002/hep.24422.
64. Talbot-Smith A, Syn WK, MacQuillan G, Neil D, Elias E, Ryan P. Familial idiopathic pulmonary fibrosis in association with bone marrow hypoplasia and hepatic nodular regenerative hyperplasia: a new "trimorphic" syndrome. Thorax. 2009;64(5):440–3. https://doi.org/10.1136/thx.2008.099796.
65. González-Huezo MS, Villela LM, Zepeda-Florencio Mdel C, Carrillo-Ponce CS, Mondragón-Sánchez RJ. Nodular regenerative hyperplasia associated to aplastic anemia: a case report and literature review. Ann Hepatol. 2006;5(3):166–9.
66. Runyon BA. A primer on detecting cirrhosis and caring for these patients without causing harm. Int J Hepatol. 2011;2011:801983. https://doi.org/10.4061/2011/801983.
67. Giri N, Ravichandran S, Wang Y, et al. Prognostic significance of pulmonary function tests in dyskeratosis congenita, a telomere biology disorder. ERJ Open Res. 2019;5(4):00209–2019. https://doi.org/10.1183/23120541.00209-2019. Published 15 Nov 2019.
68. Armanios M. Telomerase and idiopathic pulmonary fibrosis. Mutat Res. 2012;730(1–2):52–8. https://doi.org/10.1016/j.mrfmmm.2011.10.013.
69. Armanios MY, Chen JJ, Cogan JD, et al. Telomerase mutations in families with idiopathic pulmonary fibrosis. N Engl J Med. 2007;356(13):1317–26. https://doi.org/10.1056/NEJMoa066157.
70. Cronkhite JT, Xing C, Raghu G, et al. Telomere shortening in familial and sporadic pulmonary fibrosis. Am J Respir Crit Care Med. 2008;178(7):729–37. https://doi.org/10.1164/rccm.200804-550OC.
71. Diaz de Leon A, Cronkhite JT, Katzenstein AL, et al. Telomere lengths, pulmonary fibrosis and telomerase (TERT) mutations. PLoS One. 2010;5(5):e10680. https://doi.org/10.1371/journal.pone.0010680. Published 19 May 2010.

72. Newton CA, Batra K, Torrealba J, et al. Telomere-related lung fibrosis is diagnostically heterogeneous but uniformly progressive. Eur Respir J. 2016;48(6):1710–20. https://doi.org/10.1183/13993003.00308-2016.
73. Borie R, Bouvry D, Cottin V, et al. Regulator of telomere length 1 (*RTEL1*) mutations are associated with heterogeneous pulmonary and extra-pulmonary phenotypes. Eur Respir J. 2019;53(2):1800508. https://doi.org/10.1183/13993003.00508-2018. Published 7 Feb 2019.
74. Stuart BD, Choi J, Zaidi S, et al. Exome sequencing links mutations in PARN and RTEL1 with familial pulmonary fibrosis and telomere shortening. Nat Genet. 2015;47(5):512–7. https://doi.org/10.1038/ng.3278.
75. Kannengiesser C, Borie R, Ménard C, et al. Heterozygous RTEL1 mutations are associated with familial pulmonary fibrosis. Eur Respir J. 2015;46(2):474–85. https://doi.org/10.1183/09031936.00040115.
76. Cogan JD, Kropski JA, Zhao M, et al. Rare variants in RTEL1 are associated with familial interstitial pneumonia. Am J Respir Crit Care Med. 2015;191(6):646–55. https://doi.org/10.1164/rccm.201408-1510OC.
77. Kropski JA, Mitchell DB, Markin C, et al. A novel dyskerin (DKC1) mutation is associated with familial interstitial pneumonia. Chest. 2014;146(1):e1–7. https://doi.org/10.1378/chest.13-2224.
78. Kropski JA, Reiss S, Markin C, et al. Rare genetic variants in PARN are associated with pulmonary fibrosis in families. Am J Respir Crit Care Med. 2017;196(11):1481–4. https://doi.org/10.1164/rccm.201703-0635LE.
79. Alder JK, Stanley SE, Wagner CL, Hamilton M, Hanumanthu VS, Armanios M. Exome sequencing identifies mutant TINF2 in a family with pulmonary fibrosis. Chest. 2015;147(5):1361–8. https://doi.org/10.1378/chest.14-1947.
80. Borie R, Tabeze L, Thabut G, et al. Prevalence and characteristics of TERT and TERC mutations in suspected genetic pulmonary fibrosis. Eur Respir J. 2016;48(6):1721–31. https://doi.org/10.1183/13993003.02115-2015.
81. Stanley SE, Gable DL, Wagner CL, et al. Loss-of-function mutations in the RNA biogenesis factor NAF1 predispose to pulmonary fibrosis-emphysema. Sci Transl Med. 2016;8(351):351ra107. https://doi.org/10.1126/scitranslmed.aaf7837.
82. Alder JK, Hanumanthu VS, Strong MA, et al. Diagnostic utility of telomere length testing in a hospital-based setting [published correction appears in Proc Natl Acad Sci U S A. 2018 May 1;115(18):E4312. doi: 10.1073/pnas.1805407115]. Proc Natl Acad Sci USA. 2018;115(10):E2358–65. https://doi.org/10.1073/pnas.1720427115.
83. Diaz de Leon A, Cronkhite JT, Yilmaz C, et al. Subclinical lung disease, macrocytosis, and premature graying in kindreds with telomerase (TERT) mutations. Chest. 2011;140(3):753–63. https://doi.org/10.1378/chest.10-2865.
84. Calado RT, Brudno J, Mehta P, et al. Constitutional telomerase mutations are genetic risk factors for cirrhosis. Hepatology. 2011;53(5):1600–7. https://doi.org/10.1002/hep.24173.
85. Hartmann D, Srivastava U, Thaler M, et al. Telomerase gene mutations are associated with cirrhosis formation. Hepatology. 2011;53(5):1608–17. https://doi.org/10.1002/hep.24217.
86. Rodríguez-Roisin R, Krowka MJ, Hervé P, Fallon MB, ERS Task Force Pulmonary-Hepatic Vascular Disorders (PHD) Scientific Committee. Pulmonary-hepatic vascular disorders (PHD). Eur Respir J. 2004;24(5):861–80. https://doi.org/10.1183/09031936.04.00010904.
87. Rodríguez-Roisin R, Krowka MJ. Hepatopulmonary syndrome—a liver-induced lung vascular disorder. N Engl J Med. 2008;358(22):2378–87. https://doi.org/10.1056/NEJMra0707185.
88. Gorgy AI, Jonassaint NL, Stanley SE, et al. Hepatopulmonary syndrome is a frequent cause of dyspnea in the short telomere disorders. Chest. 2015;148(4):1019–26. https://doi.org/10.1378/chest.15-0825.
89. Khincha PP, Bertuch AA, Agarwal S, et al. Pulmonary arteriovenous malformations: an uncharacterised phenotype of dyskeratosis congenita and related telomere biology disorders.

Eur Respir J. 2017;49(1):1601640. https://doi.org/10.1183/13993003.01640-2016. Published 25 Jan 2017.
90. Higgs C, Crow YJ, Adams DM, et al. Understanding the evolving phenotype of vascular complications in telomere biology disorders. Angiogenesis. 2019;22(1):95–102. https://doi.org/10.1007/s10456-018-9640-7.
91. Himes RW, Chiou EH, Queliza K, et al. Gastrointestinal hemorrhage: a manifestation of the telomere biology disorders. J Pediatr. 2021;230:55–61.e4. https://doi.org/10.1016/j.jpeds.2020.09.038.
92. Savage SA, Niewisch MR. Dyskeratosis congenita and related telomere biology disorders. In: GeneReviews® – NCBI bookshelf. Published 19 Jan 2023. https://www.ncbi.nlm.nih.gov/books/NBK22301/.
93. Jongmans MC, Verwiel ET, Heijdra Y, et al. Revertant somatic mosaicism by mitotic recombination in dyskeratosis congenita. Am J Hum Genet. 2012;90(3):426–33.
94. Simon AJ, Lev A, Zhang Y, et al. Mutations in STN1 cause Coats plus syndrome and are associated with genomic and telomere defects. J Exp Med. 2016;213(8):1429–40.
95. Bertuch A. Diagnosing telomere biology disorders. In: Telomere biology disorders diagnosis and management guidelines. 2nd ed; 2022. p. 31–68. https://teamtelomere.org.
96. Sharma R, Sahoo SS, Honda M, et al. Gain-of-function mutations in RPA1 cause a syndrome with short telomeres and somatic genetic rescue. Blood. 2022;139(7):1039–51. https://doi.org/10.1182/blood.2021011980.
97. Revy P, Kannengiesser C, Fischer A. Somatic genetic rescue in Mendelian haematopoietic diseases. Nat Rev Genet. 2019;20(10):582–98. https://doi.org/10.1038/s41576-019-0139-x.
98. Savage S, Agarwal S, Stevens K, editors. Telomere biology disorders diagnosis and management guidelines. 2nd ed; 2022. https://teamtelomere.org.
99. Khincha PP, Wentzensen IM, Giri N, Alter BP, Savage SA. Response to androgen therapy in patients with dyskeratosis congenita. Br J Haematol. 2014;165(3):349 57. https://doi.org/10.1111/bjh.12748.
100. Townsley DM, Dumitriu B, Liu D, et al. Danazol treatment for telomere diseases. N Engl J Med. 2016;374(20):1922–31. https://doi.org/10.1056/NEJMoa1515319.
101. Calado RT, Yewdell WT, Wilkerson KL, et al. Sex hormones, acting on the TERT gene, increase telomerase activity in human primary hematopoietic cells. Blood. 2009;114(11):2236–43. https://doi.org/10.1182/blood-2008-09-178871.
102. Clé DV, Catto LFB, Gutierrez-Rodrigues F, et al. Effects of nandrolone decanoate on telomere length and clinical outcome in patients with telomeropathies: a prospective trial. Haematologica. 2023;108(5):1300–12. https://doi.org/10.3324/haematol.2022.281808. Published 1 May 2023.
103. Khincha PP, Bertuch AA, Gadalla SM, Giri N, Alter BP, Savage SA. Similar telomere attrition rates in androgen-treated and untreated patients with dyskeratosis congenita. Blood Adv. 2018;2(11):1243–9. https://doi.org/10.1182/bloodadvances.2018016964.
104. Kirschner M, Vieri M, Kricheldorf K, et al. Androgen derivatives improve blood counts and elongate telomere length in adult cryptic dyskeratosis congenita. Br J Haematol. 2021;193(3):669–73. https://doi.org/10.1111/bjh.16997.
105. Gadalla SM, Sales-Bonfim C, Carreras J, et al. Outcomes of allogeneic hematopoietic cell transplantation in patients with dyskeratosis congenita. Biol Blood Marrow Transplant. 2013;19(8):1238–43. https://doi.org/10.1016/j.bbmt.2013.05.021.
106. Barbaro P, Vedi A. Survival after hematopoietic stem cell transplant in patients with dyskeratosis congenita: systematic review of the literature. Biol Blood Marrow Transplant. 2016;22(7):1152–8. https://doi.org/10.1016/j.bbmt.2016.03.001.
107. Ayas M, Nassar A, Hamidieh AA, et al. Reduced intensity conditioning is effective for hematopoietic SCT in dyskeratosis congenita-related BM failure. Bone Marrow Transplant. 2013;48(9):1168–72. https://doi.org/10.1038/bmt.2013.35.

108. Nelson AS, Marsh RA, Myers KC, et al. A reduced-intensity conditioning regimen for patients with dyskeratosis congenita undergoing hematopoietic stem cell transplantation. Biol Blood Marrow Transplant. 2016;22(5):884–8. https://doi.org/10.1016/j.bbmt.2016.01.026.
109. Swaminathan AC, Neely ML, Frankel CW, et al. Lung transplant outcomes in patients with pulmonary fibrosis with telomere-related gene variants. Chest. 2019;156(3):477–85. https://doi.org/10.1016/j.chest.2019.03.030.
110. Borie R, Kannengiesser C, Hirschi S, et al. Severe hematologic complications after lung transplantation in patients with telomerase complex mutations. J Heart Lung Transplant. 2015;34(4):538–46. https://doi.org/10.1016/j.healun.2014.11.010.
111. Courtwright A, Hayes D Jr, El-Chemaly S. Lung transplantation. In: Telomere biology disorders diagnosis and management guidelines. 2nd ed; 2022. p. 255–63. https://teamtelomere.org.
112. Nastasio S, Lee C. Liver transplantation. In: Telomere biology disorders diagnosis and management guidelines. 2nd ed; 2022. p. 289–308. https://teamtelomere.org.
113. Nagpal N, Wang J, Zeng J, et al. Small-molecule PAPD5 inhibitors restore telomerase activity in patient stem cells. Cell Stem Cell. 2020;26(6):896–909.e8. https://doi.org/10.1016/j.stem.2020.03.016.

Open Access This chapter is licensed under the terms of the Creative Commons Attribution 4.0 International License (http://creativecommons.org/licenses/by/4.0/), which permits use, sharing, adaptation, distribution and reproduction in any medium or format, as long as you give appropriate credit to the original author(s) and the source, provide a link to the Creative Commons license and indicate if changes were made.

The images or other third party material in this chapter are included in the chapter's Creative Commons license, unless indicated otherwise in a credit line to the material. If material is not included in the chapter's Creative Commons license and your intended use is not permitted by statutory regulation or exceeds the permitted use, you will need to obtain permission directly from the copyright holder.

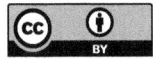

Chapter 18
Dyskeratosis Congenita

Mouhab Ayas and Syed Osman Ahmed

Background

Dyskeratosis congenita (DC), also known eponymously as Zinsser–Cole–Engman syndrome after the three physicians who separately described the clinical features in the early 1900s, is a rare inherited multisystem disorder characterized by mucocutaneous features of reticulated skin pigmentation, oral leukoplakia, and nail dystrophy and progressive bone marrow (BM) failure, which is often the main cause of death. The disorder can affect other organs, including, but not limited to, the lungs, liver, and genitourinary and skeletal systems, and is associated with a predisposition to the development of cancers.

Pathobiology

The process of understanding and diagnosing DC has undergone a paradigmatic shift over the past decade, with a recognition that abnormalities of telomere maintenance, resulting from one of a number of mutations, underlie the syndrome. Telomeres are repetitive nucleotide sequences that cap the ends of chromosomes and that shorten with successive cell division; these sequences are replenished by functioning telomerase, which is a ribonucleoprotein (RNA) complex. Heiss et al.

M. Ayas (✉)
Department of Pediatric Hematology/Oncology, King Faisal Specialist Hospital and Research Center, Riyadh, Saudi Arabia
e-mail: mouhab@kfshrc.edu.sa

S. O. Ahmed
Department of Hematology, Stem Cell Transplant & Cellular Therapy, Cancer Center of Excellence, King Faisal Specialist Hospital and Research Center, Riyadh, Saudi Arabia
e-mail: syedahmed@kfshrc.edu.sa

© The Author(s) 2026
M. Aljurf et al. (eds.), *Textbook of Bone Marrow Failure*,
https://doi.org/10.1007/978-3-032-02386-5_18

identified a gene coding for dyskerin, *DKC1*, as being mutated in X-linked DC in 1998 [1]; dyskerin is a nucleolar protein and is also a component of the telomerase complex. That DC was caused by mutations affecting the telomerase function was further uncovered in a number of families with autosomal dominant (AD) inheritance of DC, with mutations in the telomerase RNA component, TERC [2]. Mutations affecting the protein component of the telomerase enzyme, TERT, were subsequently described in patients with acquired and inherited bone marrow failure syndromes [3, 4]. In 2008, mutations in *TINF2* affecting shelterin—a protein complex that protects the telomeres by controlling the synthesis of telomeric DNA—were implicated in autosomal dominant DC by more than one group [5, 6]. Mutations affecting NOP10—a small nucleolar ribonucleoprotein component of the telomerase complex—were described in a large consanguineous Saudi Arabian family, leading to autosomal recessive (AR) DC; homozygous individuals had shortened telomeres and reduced TERC levels. Currently, around ten genes have been implicated with either X-linked, autosomal dominant (AD), or autosomal recessive (AR) inheritance patterns, with a tendency for X-linked forms to have the mildest and the AR forms to have the most severe phenotype (Table 18.1) [7, 8]. Mutations affecting telomerase—and the accelerated telomere loss that ensues—lead to the clinical manifestations seen in DC: The depletion of the stem cell compartment leads to bone marrow failure, often the main cause of mortality; accelerated cell senescence leads to mucocutaneous abnormalities, and the chromosomal instability predisposes to other malignancies.

Short telomeres in hematopoietic cells are dysfunctional in general. They mediate chromosomal instability and, hence, the predisposition to malignant transformation [9]. Cancer susceptibility in patients with DC is, therefore, part of the spectrum of the disease. In fact, it has been shown that DC closely resembles Fanconi anemia (FA) in both the rates and types of neoplastic events [10]. The crude rate of malignancy in DC has been reported to be approximately 10% [11]. In one study, the actuarial risk of cancer was 40% by age 50 years and more than 60% by age 68 years [12]. The most frequent solid tumors are head and neck squamous cell carcinomas,

Table 18.1 List of genes that have been identified in patients and families with DC [7]

Gene	Chromosomal location	Inheritance
DKC1	Xq28	X-linked recessive
TINF2	17p13.1	Autosomal dominant
TERC	3q26.2	Autosomal dominant
TERT	5p15.33	Autosomal dominant/recessive
NOP10	15q14	Autosomal recessive
NHP2	5q35.3	Autosomal recessive
USB1	16q21	Autosomal recessive
TCAB1	17p13.1	Autosomal recessive
CTC1	17p13.1	Autosomal recessive
RTEL1	20q13.3	Autosomal recessive

and the incidence of acute myeloid leukemia is reported to be 10% between the ages of 30 and 40. The general cancer predisposition may well also vary according to the underlying mutation.

Clinical Features

The clinical presentation of DC can be highly variable. While manifestations of DC often appear and are diagnosed in childhood, some cases may only be diagnosed when they present with a severe bone marrow failure syndrome, a malignancy such as acute leukemia, or pulmonary abnormalities. Diagnosis requires the presence of two out of four major features (BM failure, nail dystrophy, abnormal skin pigmentation, and leukoplakia) and at least two other systemic features (Table 18.2). Bone

Table 18.2 Clinical features of dyskeratosis congenita syndromes

Hematological	**Bone marrow failure** Isolated cytopenias Macrocytosis Elevated fetal hemoglobin
Dermatologic (90%)	**Nail dystrophy** **Abnormal skin pigmentation** Thinning/early graying of hair Hyperhidrosis and hyperkeratosis of soles and palms Adermatoglyphia Acrocyanosis
Oral	Leukoplakia Erythematous patches Brown/black patches Short tooth roots Enlarged dental pulp chambers Increased rate of dental decay
Ophthalmic	**Epiphora** Conjunctivitis Blepharitis Strabismus Cataracts Ectropion Entropion Sparse eyelashes Optic nerve atrophy Retinal vessel fragility and hemorrhages, exudative retinopathy
Neurological	**Learning disability** Ataxia Cerebellar hypoplasia Microcephaly Deafness

(continued)

Table 18.2 (continued)

Pulmonary disease	**Pulmonary fibrosis**
	Pulmonary vasculopathy
Musculoskeletal	**Short stature**
	Osteoporosis
	Long bone fractures
	Avascular necrosis
	Scoliosis
	Mandibular hypoplasia
Gastrointestinal (GI)	Esophageal strictures
	Hepatomegaly
	Cirrhosis
	Peptic ulceration
	Enteropathy
Genitourinary	Hypogonadism
	Undescended testes
	Hypospadias
	Phimosis
	Urethral stenosis
	Horseshoe kidney
Cancer predisposition	Myelodysplastic syndrome
	Acute myeloid leukemia
	Solid cancers (oropharynx, GI)
Other	Intrauterine growth retardation

Features in bold occur at a frequency of ≥20% [13, 14]

marrow failure occurs in over 90% of patients by the age of 40 and is the main cause of mortality [13, 14].

DKC1 mutations are associated with X-linked childhood DC, and the affected males usually demonstrate the classical mucocutaneous features [1]. A less common but more severe variant of DC, the Hoyeraal–Hreidarsson syndrome (severe DC, growth retardation, immune deficiency, and cerebellar hypoplasia) has also been associated with other mutations of the DKC1 gene [15]. Another severe manifestation, Revesz syndrome, in which classic DC features occur, along with exudative retinopathy, is caused by mutations in TINF2 and is also transmitted in an autosomal dominant fashion [5, 16]. Autosomal dominant DC is heterogeneous, and mutations in *TERC, TERT, and TINF1* can cause telomeropathies in both children and adults [17–19].

The lungs have been well-documented as target organs for telomeropathies. Idiopathic pulmonary fibrosis is the classical lung disease and accounts for 65% of telomere-mediated lung pathology. *TERT, TERC, PANR,* and *RTEL1* have been closely associated with the development of idiopathic pulmonary fibrosis [17, 20]. Pulmonary fibrosis is also well-described in patients with the classical DC. It is usually age related in both types (idiopathic and in patients with DC) and is considered a frequent cause of mortality in adults with DC. Smoking has been blamed as a likely cofactor that accelerates the development of lung fibrosis, at least in patients with the idiopathic form.

Diagnosis

In making the diagnosis, the importance of a careful investigation of personal and family history and detailed clinical examination cannot be overstated. Investigations may reveal a pancytopenia that usually develops within the first two decades of life; less frequently, patients may have an isolated cytopenia. There is often a macrocytosis, and fetal hemoglobin may be elevated. Imaging may reveal cerebellar hypoplasia, pulmonary fibrosis, renal abnormalities, and osteopenia.

Telomere length can be determined by the measurement of telomere length in leukocyte subsets by flow cytometry and fluorescence in situ hybridization (flow-FISH) and compared to a population control [21]. Telomere length in patients with DC appears to be a fundamental measure of clinical severity [22]. Interestingly, unlike patients with DC, patients with non-DC inherited bone marrow failure syndromes usually tend to have the telomere lengths within the normal range, albeit shorter than in unaffected individuals [23]. With the advent and greater accessibility of next-generation sequencing (NGS) technologies, the underlying mutation can now be more rapidly identified in patients and families. Many labs can now offer an NGS-based bone marrow failure gene panel that can be customized to test for a variable number of gene mutations implicated in inherited bone marrow failure syndromes; such panels have been shown to be efficient and accurate in detecting mutations in IBMFS [24, 25].

Management

Given the multisystem nature of the disease, patients are best managed in conjunction with or with consultation of pediatricians, hematologists, dermatologists, dentists, and oncologists. Patients and their families will need to be seen by a medical geneticist for confirmation of the diagnosis, identification of mutations, and appropriate counseling to identify potential affected members in the family, as it has been clearly demonstrated that some telomere biology disorders (TBDs) can be present late, in what is referred to as late-onset TBDs or adult-onset TBDs [26–28]. Such identification is pivotal for future stem cell transplant decisions.

Management recommendations should include general measures such as dental hygiene, skin care, and avoidance of smoking and alcohol, given the propensity for the lungs and liver to be affected by the disease and the risk of cancer. Because the manifestations in DC are more of a spectrum, therapy should be tailored according to the manifestations and the underlying genetic abnormality. Special attention should be paid to pulmonary fibrosis and liver cirrhosis as potential cryptic presentations that may precedes the hematological manifestations.

Bone marrow failure is reported to be the leading cause of death in patients with DC and is estimated to occur in over 80% of patients in DC [11, 12]. Hematopoietic stem cell transplantation (HSCT) is eventually required in the majority of patients to restore normal hematopoiesis; it should be considered when there is evidence of failing hematopoiesis. In addition to bone marrow failure, DC patients are at risk of clonal/leukemic evolution, and periodic monitoring should be performed if HSCT is not done. Until that time, some therapeutic modalities have been shown, at least transiently, to ameliorate hematopoiesis in these patients.

1. *Androgens*

    Androgens have been used to treat inherited bone marrow failure syndromes, even in the current era of HSCT, particularly when a suitable donor is not readily available or when the patient is not an HSCT candidate. There are data to suggest that these patients are particularly sensitive to androgen therapy, even with lower doses; one observational study evaluated the hematological response and side effects of androgen therapy in 16 patients with DC, with a cohort of untreated patients serving as controls; 70% of treated DC patients had a hematological response with red blood cell and/or platelet transfusion independence, suggesting that androgen therapy for the pancytopenia in DC patients may be a viable option while awaiting HSCT; of note is that in this study, the expected age-related decline in telomere length was noted in androgen-treated patients [17, 29–32]. Another prospective trial using danazol over 24 months in adults with TBDs reported a hematological response in about 80% [32]. Of note is that the use of androgens is associated with a multitude of side effects, such as elevated liver enzymes and virilization, and many patients end up discontinuing the medication due to side effects. The mechanism of action of androgens has been attributed to many etiologies; it has been suggested that androgens increase erythropoietin production, which, in turn, stimulates erythropoietic stem cells and, to a lesser extent, myeloid progenitor cells in the bone marrow [33]. More recent studies suggest that androgens, such as testosterone, do not increase erythropoietin levels but rather work at the level of the erythropoietin receptor to elicit a hematological response [34]. It has also been shown that, in view of the telomerase defect observed in DC patients, androgens and their derivatives may upregulate and increase the telomerase activity by slowing the rate of telomere attrition and enhancing cell regeneration [26, 29, 30]. Interestingly, this hypothesis may suggest that androgens could improve not only hematopoiesis but also other organ dysfunction [35].

2. *Immune Suppressive Therapy*

    Immune suppressive therapy is probably not an appropriate option for patients with DC, but there have been some reported observations in adult patients with *TERT* and *TERC* mutations that have shown blood count improvement after immune suppressive therapy, suggesting that such genetic mutations may act as risk factors in stem cell susceptibility to immune attacks [17, 36].

3. *Growth Factors*

    Although the clinical availability of recombinant hematopoietic growth factors was initially thought to be a breakthrough in the treatment of bone marrow failure syndromes, severe congenital neutropenia is probably the only marrow failure syndrome where long-term administration of granulocyte colony-

stimulating factor (G-CSF) was associated with a maintained increase in the absolute neutrophil count (ANC) and a reduction of severe bacterial infections. In other bone marrow failure syndromes, however, only transient benefits were noted, and overall, the results have been disappointing [30]. In patients with DC, one report described excellent neutrophil and hemoglobin responses with granulocyte-macrophage colony-stimulating factor and erythropoietin [37]. If the decision is made to treat with growth factors, it is strongly recommended to monitor patients for clonal aberrations prior to and during long-term treatment with growth factors.
4. *Allogeneic Hematopoietic Stem Cell Transplantation*

Allogeneic hematopoietic stem cell transplantation (HSCT) has been shown to restore hematopoiesis in hereditary bone marrow failure syndromes with favorable results. HSCT is currently considered the only widely used modality to treat bone failure in DC. The long-term results of HSCT in DC, however, are less satisfactory compared to other syndromes. Given the complicated nature of the telomeropathy disorders, the decision to perform HSCT should be studied very carefully, looking at the best and least toxic conditioning regimens and ensuring the use of a suitable donor.

Choice of a Suitable Conditioning Regimen

Despite many similarities, the heterogeneity of the bone marrow failure syndromes precludes the implementation of general rules and guidelines when deciding about the process of HSCT; hence, what is now considered the standard conditioning for patients with Fanconi anemia (FA), which is a more prevalent hereditary bone marrow failure syndrome, may not necessarily be the best for DC patients. In FA patients who suffer from abnormal DNA damage repair mechanisms, the sensitivity of FA cells to alkylating agents and radiation has been clearly established, and thus, the use of lower doses of alkylating agents and radiation conditioning in FA patients has been pivotal in avoiding undue transplant toxicity [18]. In patients with DC, on the other hand, such evidence supporting the use of reduced-intensity conditioning (RIC) transplants is lacking, and whether the use of RIC would lead to a lower incidence of pulmonary fibrosis or liver cirrhosis in the long term is still not clear. Pulmonary fibrosis is reported to be the second leading cause of death in DC. Many series reported increased pulmonary and hepatic toxicities when conventional intensity regimens were used for conditioning, and it has been speculated that the use of RIC may result in milder toxicity and, consequently, better survival, presumably by reducing the need for the extensive cellular repair associated with higher doses of chemotherapy and limiting the role of the already defective telomeres and telomerases in tissues of the DC patients undergoing HSCT. Given the rarity of the disease, the results of RIC in the literature are rather sketchy [38–43]. Nishio et al. reported a favorable outcome in three DC patients who had HSCT from mismatched related bone marrow ($n = 2$) and unrelated BM ($n = 1$) donors, all using RIC; patients were engrafted successfully and were alive at 10, 66, and 72 months after transplantation [39]. Dietz et al. reported that in six DC patients who underwent allogeneic HSCT using a non-myeloablative conditioning regimen, with graft sources including related PBSCs ($n = 1$), unrelated BM ($n = 2$), and unrelated double umbilical cord blood ($n = 3$) and with a median follow-up of 26.5 months, four patients are alive, three of whom were recipients of unrelated grafts [41]. A report from the Eastern Mediterranean Blood and Marrow Transplantation Registry described nine patients with a homogeneous donor source (all underwent matched related HSCT); out of the eight who received RIC, seven were reported to be alive and hematologically stable at a median follow-up of 61 months (0.8–212 months); one patient was reported to have developed liver cirrhosis [19]. Of note, although some survival advantages and a lower incidence of complications have been reported with reduced-intensity conditioning (RIC), most available data derive from small series and are confounded by multiple factors, including heterogeneous donor sources and varying pre-transplant comorbidity profiles. This precludes the ability to make solid recommendations regarding the use of RIC in DC patients [35]. Furthermore, a systematic review of the literature by Barbaro et al. concluded that RIC was not associated with improved survival [43]. Thus, concerns over graft failure remain realistic. A recent study compared the outcome of RIC in DC patients to a similar cohort but with total body irradiation and concluded that RIC patients were less likely to achieve full donor chimerism and had delayed immune reconstitution [44]. Additionally, it was shown that in patients with DC, the skeletal stem cells within the bone marrow stromal population (known as bone marrow–derived mesenchymal stem cells), which are responsible for the creation of the hematopoietic environment, may contribute (along with the defect in hematopoietic stem cells) to the DC phenotype, which may further emphasize the role of adequate marrow ablation in creating the necessary environment for the donor cells and may account for the primary and secondary graft failures noted in several reports [20]. Interestingly, in one study from Center for International Blood and Marrow Transplant Research (CIBMTR) on 34 patients with DC, cyclophosphamide, an alkylating agent that remains the backbone of conditioning regimens in patients with Fanconi anemia, was used alone at 200 mg/kg in ten patients (eight matched related and two matched unrelated) and was found to be associated with the longest survival [45]. A more recent study by Nichele et al. reported a large series of 29 patients, 28 of whom had RIC; only 14 patients were reported to be alive at the last follow-up (median follow-up of 6 years); most patients died due to non-hematological disease progression or complications of chronic graft-versus-host disease (GVHD) [42].

Choice of a Suitable Donor

1. *Matched Related Donors*

    In general, matched related donor stem cell transplants for bone marrow failure syndromes are associated with a superior outcome when compared with alternative donor HSCT. In telomere biology disorders, however, the reported outcomes of matched related donor HSCT remain suboptimal. In the cohort of patients reported by the CIBMTR, 18 received grafts from related donors, and only eight of them were reported to be alive at the time of publication [45]. Others had marginally better survival; seven of the nine patients in the study by Ayas et al. were reported to be alive (median follow-up of 61 months) [19]. Advancements in supportive care and early recognition of potential complications peculiar to DC patients obviously play a pivotal role in improving the outcome; in the CIBMTR study, the 5-year probability of overall survival was significantly better in those who underwent HSCT after the year 2000 [45]. In the study by Nichele et al., the 5-year overall survival was better in matched sibling donor 88.9% vs. 47.7% in non-matched related donor recipients. Additionally, most of the existing reports on matched related HSCT in patients with DC do not address the carrier status of the donor, and thus, its impact on the eventual outcome is not well-delineated. Should the carrier status be determined in related donors for DC patients undergoing related HSCT? It has now been established that the first manifestations of telomere disease may not be till adolescence or early adulthood; furthermore, TDB manifestations are highly variable and may be subtle and, hence, may go undiagnosed for some time. Improved understanding of the so-called late-onset TBDs, also referred to as cryptic TBDs or adult-onset TBDs [26–28, 46], has led to better decision when it comes to donor selection and it is now largely accepted that related donors in families with TBD must be evaluated by genetic and/or telomere length testing because of the phenotypic variability in the telomere disorders and poor outcomes associated with using affected donors [47]. Silent carriers should thus be avoided as donors [48]. Furthermore, in addition to concerns about the hematological stem cells, the study by Balakumaran et al., cited above, suggests that the issue may not only be in the hematopoietic cells, as it may also be indirectly evoked that carriers are not suitable donors as their shorter telomeres of the stromal stem cells (SSCs)/bone marrow stromal cells (BMSCs) may fail to produce the necessary healthy hematopoietic environment after transplant and, hence, contribute to graft failure [20].

2. *Alternative Donors*

Thus far, the results of unrelated donor HSCT in patients with DC have been equally disappointing. The largest review of the outcomes of unrelated donor HSCT in DC patients is probably the CIBMTR report cited above; out of the 34 DC patients, 16 had unrelated donors, and only six were alive at the time of publication. Of note, graft failure was the most common cause of early death; all but one of those who developed graft failure (four primary and six secondary) were recipients of mismatched related or unrelated donor transplants [45]. More recent reports offer more optimistic results, but the follow-up time is too short to allow us to draw solid recommendations. Lu et al. reported a series of seven patients with DC who underwent allo-HSCT from an alternative donor (matched unrelated/haplo) using RIC; all patients were reported alive with full engraftment at the last follow-up [49] (longest follow-up was 4 years). Other stem cell sources also appear to be associated with dismal outcomes for patients with DC. In a study by the European Society for Blood and Marrow Transplantation (EBMT) group about outcomes after cord blood transplantation in non-FA hereditary bone marrow failures, eight patients had DC (two related and six unrelated), and all patients died except one who is alive at 126 months after an HLA-matched sibling UCBT. In the group given unrelated grafts, three had been conditioned with conventional intensity conditioning with cyclophosphamide (120 mg/kg), busulfan (16 mg/kg), and antithymocyte globulin; three had RIC with fludarabine and reduced doses of busulfan or cyclophosphamide. All six died of transplant-related toxicity [50].

HSCT from haplo-identical donors is gaining momentum in hereditary bone marrow failure syndromes, and encouraging data are reported in FA [51–53]. Data are, however, scarcer in DC patients; one patient was recently reported to be alive and transfusion-independent 26 months after T-cell-depleted haplo-identical HSCT from a family donor [54]. In a recent report from EBMT on the outcome of hereditary bone marrow failure syndrome after haplo-HSCT, nine of the 150 patients in the cohort had DC, but no solid conclusions could be drawn on the outcome of this subset due to the small number [51]. It is noteworthy here that even in unrelated donor HSCT, the telomere length in the donor leukocyte might play a crucial role in transplant outcome. In the analysis of 330 patients who received HSCT for severe aplastic anemia (235 acquired and 95 hereditary), it was demonstrated that longer leukocyte telomere length was associated with significantly increased five-year survival. None of the patients in the study had DC, but these findings may be particularly pertinent in DC, where telomeropathy is the underlying pathology of the disease [25, 55]. Interestingly, in the same study, patient leukocyte telomere length was not associated with survival after HSCT.

Does Transplantation Accelerate Pulmonary Complications?

Mortality due to pulmonary complications has been reported to be a major cause of late death in the literature of DC patients after HSCT, even for those who underwent reduced-intensity conditioning; the impact of donor source on the incidence of such complications is not clear either; in one study, none of the patients who died of pulmonary complications were reported to have lung disease at transplantation. Hence, it is strongly recommended that preparative regimens should be carefully selected to minimize the risk of pulmonary toxicity. Thorough and regular pre- and post-transplant pulmonary function assessment should be done on these patients for the early detection of pulmonary insufficiency.

Conditioning and Cancer Risk

As outlined above, patients with DC have a significantly higher risk of developing solid and hematological malignancies. Whereas in FA patients, it has been suggested that better prevention and treatment of GVHD and avoiding the use of radiation-containing regimens might reduce the risk of late tumor development, such data are lacking, however, in patients with DC. It might be safer, however, to recommend that radiation be avoided in the conditioning of DC patients.

Conclusions

Long strides have been made in understanding the biology of DC and in the diagnosis of DC. The classically described clinical features, combined with the current state of the art of genomic technologies, should allow specialists to accurately diagnose the disease and the underlying mutations. Our knowledge reservoir as it relates to definitive management, however, remains deficient, especially with respect to HSCT, as many of the available studies on the role of HSCT in DC are limited by the lack of power to evaluate the impact of different key factors on outcomes due to small sample size. More work is clearly needed; larger collaborative studies with well-defined clinical and laboratory characterization of the subtype of DC and a more uniform approach to the choice of conditioning regimens and donors are warranted to be able to make solid recommendations. Meanwhile, however, stem cell transplantation remains the ultimate and only curative modality for marrow failure/clonal evolution in this disorder; conditioning regimens, preferably of lesser intensity, should be selected carefully. Matched related or unrelated donors are both viable options, but telomere length measurements should be included in the assessment of any potential donor.

References

1. Heiss NS, Knight SW, Vulliamy TJ, et al. X-linked dyskeratosis congenita is caused by mutations in a highly conserved gene with putative nucleolar functions. Nat Genet. 1998;19(1):32–8.
2. Vulliamy T, Marrone A, Goldman F, et al. The RNA component of telomerase is mutated in autosomal dominant dyskeratosis congenita. Nature. 2001;413(6854):432–5.
3. Vulliamy TJ, Walne A, Baskaradas A, Mason PJ, Marrone A, Dokal I. Mutations in the reverse transcriptase component of telomerase (TERT) in patients with bone marrow failure. Blood Cells Mol Dis. 2005;34(3):257–63.
4. Yamaguchi H, Calado RT, Ly H, et al. Mutations in TERT, the gene for telomerase reverse transcriptase, in aplastic anemia. N Engl J Med. 2005;352(14):1413–24.
5. Savage SA, Giri N, Baerlocher GM, Orr N, Lansdorp PM, Alter BP. TINF2, a component of the shelterin telomere protection complex, is mutated in dyskeratosis congenita. Am J Hum Genet. 2008;82(2):501–9.

6. Walne AJ, Vulliamy T, Beswick R, Kirwan M, Dokal I. TINF2 mutations result in very short telomeres: analysis of a large cohort of patients with dyskeratosis congenita and related bone marrow failure syndromes. Blood. 2008;112(9):3594–600.
7. Dokal I, Vulliamy T, Mason P, Bessler M. Clinical utility gene card for: dyskeratosis congenita – update 2015. Eur J Hum Genet. 2015;23(4). https://doi.org/10.1038/ejhg.2014.170.
8. Walne AJ, Vulliamy T, Marrone A, et al. Genetic heterogeneity in autosomal recessive dyskeratosis congenita with one subtype due to mutations in the telomerase-associated protein NOP10. Hum Mol Genet. 2007;16(13):1619–29.
9. Calado RT, Cooper JN, Padilla-Nash HM, et al. Short telomeres result in chromosomal instability in hematopoietic cells and precede malignant evolution in human aplastic anemia. Leukemia. 2012;26(4):700–7.
10. Alter BP, Giri N, Savage SA, et al. Malignancies and survival patterns in the National Cancer Institute inherited bone marrow failure syndromes cohort study. Br J Haematol. 2010;150(2):179–88.
11. Vulliamy T, Dokal I. Dyskeratosis congenita. Semin Hematol. 2006;43(3):157–66.
12. Alter BP, Giri N, Savage SA, Rosenberg PS. Cancer in dyskeratosis congenita. Blood. 2009;113(26):6549–57.
13. Dokal I. Dyskeratosis congenita in all its forms. Br J Haematol. 2000;110(4):768–79.
14. Dokal I. Dyskeratosis congenita. Hematology Am Soc Hematol Educ Program. 2011;2011:480–6.
15. Hoyeraal HM, Lamvik J, Moe PJ. Congenital hypoplastic thrombocytopenia and cerebral malformations in two brothers. Acta Paediatr Scand. 1970;59(2):185–91.
16. Revesz T, Fletcher S, al-Gazali LI, DeBuse P. Bilateral retinopathy, aplastic anaemia, and central nervous system abnormalities: a new syndrome? J Med Genet. 1992;29(9):673–5.
17. Townsley DM, Dumitriu B, Young NS. Bone marrow failure and the telomeropathies. Blood. 2014;124(18):2775–83.
18. Gluckman E. Radiosensitivity in Fanconi anemia: application to the conditioning for bone marrow transplantation. Radiother Oncol. 1990;18(Suppl 1):88–93.
19. Ayas M, Nassar A, Hamidieh AA, et al. Reduced intensity conditioning is effective for hematopoietic SCT in dyskeratosis congenita-related BM failure. Bone Marrow Transplant. 2013;48(9):1168–72.
20. Balakumaran A, Mishra PJ, Pawelczyk E, et al. Bone marrow skeletal stem/progenitor cell defects in dyskeratosis congenita and telomere biology disorders. Blood. 2015;125(5):793–802.
21. Alter BP, Baerlocher GM, Savage SA, et al. Very short telomere length by flow fluorescence in situ hybridization identifies patients with dyskeratosis congenita. Blood. 2007;110(5):1439–47.
22. Alter BP, Rosenberg PS, Giri N, Baerlocher GM, Lansdorp PM, Savage SA. Telomere length is associated with disease severity and declines with age in dyskeratosis congenita. Haematologica. 2012;97(3):353–9.
23. Alter BP, Giri N, Savage SA, Rosenberg PS. Telomere length in inherited bone marrow failure syndromes. Haematologica. 2015;100(1):49–54.
24. Ghemlas I, Li H, Zlateska B, et al. Improving diagnostic precision, care and syndrome definitions using comprehensive next-generation sequencing for the inherited bone marrow failure syndromes. J Med Genet. 2015;52(9):575–84.
25. Ayas M. Unrelated hematopoietic cell transplantation in aplastic anemia: there is more to a successful outcome than meets the eye. JAMA Oncol. 2015;1(8):1164–5.
26. Rolles B, Tometten M, Meyer R, Kirschner M, Beier F, Brummendorf TH. Inherited telomere biology disorders: pathophysiology, clinical presentation, diagnostics, and treatment. Transfus Med Hemother. 2024;51(5):292–309.
27. Tometten M, Kirschner M, Meyer R, et al. Identification of adult patients with classical dyskeratosis congenita or cryptic telomere biology disorder by telomere length screening using age-modified criteria. Hemasphere. 2023;7(5):e874.
28. Niewisch MR, Beier F, Savage SA. Clinical manifestations of telomere biology disorders in adults. Hematology Am Soc Hematol Educ Program. 2023;2023(1):563–72.

29. Khincha PP, Wentzensen IM, Giri N, Alter BP, Savage SA. Response to androgen therapy in patients with dyskeratosis congenita. Br J Haematol. 2014;165(3):349–57.
30. Calado RT, Yewdell WT, Wilkerson KL, et al. Sex hormones, acting on the TERT gene, increase telomerase activity in human primary hematopoietic cells. Blood. 2009;114(11):2236–43.
31. Vieri M, Kirschner M, Tometten M, et al. Comparable effects of the androgen derivatives danazol, oxymetholone and nandrolone on telomerase activity in human primary hematopoietic cells from patients with dyskeratosis congenita. Int J Mol Sci. 2020;21(19):7196.
32. Townsley DM, Dumitriu B, Liu D, et al. Danazol treatment for telomere diseases. N Engl J Med. 2016;374(20):1922–31.
33. Shahidi NT. A review of the chemistry, biological action, and clinical applications of anabolic-androgenic steroids. Clin Ther. 2001;23(9):1355–90.
34. Maggio M, Snyder PJ, Ceda GP, et al. Is the haematopoietic effect of testosterone mediated by erythropoietin? The results of a clinical trial in older men. Andrology. 2013;1(1):24–8.
35. de la Fuente J, Dokal I. Dyskeratosis congenita: advances in the understanding of the telomerase defect and the role of stem cell transplantation. Pediatr Transplant. 2007;11(6):584–94.
36. Comoli P, Basso S, Huanga GC. Intensive immunosuppression therapy for aplastic anemia associated with dyskeratosis congenita: report of a case. Int J Hematol. 2005;82(1):35–7.
37. Erduran E, Hacisalihoglu S, Ozoran Y. Treatment of dyskeratosis congenita with granulocyte-macrophage colony-stimulating factor and erythropoietin. J Pediatr Hematol Oncol. 2003;25(4):333–5.
38. Kharfan-Dabaja MA, Otrock ZK, Bacigalupo A, Mahfouz RA, Geara F, Bazarbachi A. A reduced intensity conditioning regimen of fludarabine, cyclophosphamide, antithymocyte globulin, plus 2 Gy TBI facilitates successful hematopoietic cell engraftment in an adult with dyskeratosis congenita. Bone Marrow Transplant. 2012;47(9):1254–5.
39. Nishio N, Takahashi Y, Ohashi H, et al. Reduced-intensity conditioning for alternative donor hematopoietic stem cell transplantation in patients with dyskeratosis congenita. Pediatr Transplant. 2011;15(2):161–6.
40. Dror Y, Freedman MH, Leaker M, et al. Low-intensity hematopoietic stem-cell transplantation across human leucocyte antigen barriers in dyskeratosis congenita. Bone Marrow Transplant. 2003;31(10):847–50.
41. Dietz AC, Orchard PJ, Baker KS, et al. Disease-specific hematopoietic cell transplantation: nonmyeloablative conditioning regimen for dyskeratosis congenita. Bone Marrow Transplant. 2011;46(1):98–104.
42. Nichele S, Bonfim C, Junior LGD, et al. Hematopoietic cell transplantation for telomere biology diseases: a retrospective single-center cohort study. Eur J Haematol. 2023;111(3):423–31.
43. Barbaro P, Vedi A. Survival after hematopoietic stem cell transplant in patients with dyskeratosis congenita: systematic review of the literature. Biol Blood Marrow Transplant. 2016;22(7):1152–8.
44. Dimitrov M, Merkle S, Cao Q, et al. Allogeneic hematopoietic cell transplant for bone marrow failure or myelodysplastic syndrome in dyskeratosis congenita/telomere biology disorders: single-center, single-arm, open-label trial of reduced-intensity conditioning without radiation. Transplant Cell Ther. 2024;30(10):1005.e1–e17.
45. Gadalla SM, Sales-Bonfim C, Carreras J, et al. Outcomes of allogeneic hematopoietic cell transplantation in patients with dyskeratosis congenita. Biol Blood Marrow Transplant. 2013;19(8):1238–43.
46. Kapuria D, Ben-Yakov G, Ortolano R, et al. The spectrum of hepatic involvement in patients with telomere disease. Hepatology. 2019;69(6):2579–85.
47. Fogarty PF, Yamaguchi H, Wiestner A, et al. Late presentation of dyskeratosis congenita as apparently acquired aplastic anaemia due to mutations in telomerase RNA. Lancet. 2003;362(9396):1628–30.
48. Bessler M, Du HY, Gu B, Mason PJ. Dysfunctional telomeres and dyskeratosis congenita. Haematologica. 2007;92(8):1009–12.

49. Lu Y, Xiong M, Sun RJ, et al. Hematopoietic stem cell transplantation for inherited bone marrow failure syndromes: alternative donor and disease-specific conditioning regimen with unmanipulated grafts. Hematology. 2021;26(1):134–43.
50. Bizzetto R, Bonfim C, Rocha V, et al. Outcomes after related and unrelated umbilical cord blood transplantation for hereditary bone marrow failure syndromes other than Fanconi anemia. Haematologica. 2011;96(1):134–41.
51. Giardino S, Eikema DJ, Piepenbroek B, et al. HLA-haploidentical stem cell transplantation in children with inherited bone marrow failure syndromes: a retrospective analysis on behalf of EBMT severe aplastic anemia and pediatric diseases working parties. Am J Hematol. 2024;99(6):1066–76.
52. Zubicaray J, Pagliara D, Sevilla J, et al. Haplo-identical or mismatched unrelated donor hematopoietic cell transplantation for Fanconi anemia: results from the Severe Aplastic Anemia Working Party of the EBMT. Am J Hematol. 2021;96(5):571–9.
53. Ayas M, Siddiqui K, Al-Jefri A, et al. Successful outcome in patients with Fanconi anemia undergoing T cell-replete mismatched related donor hematopoietic cell transplantation using reduced-dose cyclophosphamide post-transplantation. Biol Blood Marrow Transplant. 2019;25(11):2217–21.
54. Algeri M, Comoli P, Strocchio L, et al. Successful T-cell-depleted haploidentical hematopoietic stem cell transplantation in a child with dyskeratosis congenita after a fludarabine-based conditioning regimen. J Pediatr Hematol Oncol. 2015;37(4):322–6.
55. Gadalla SM, Wang T, Haagenson M, et al. Association between donor leukocyte telomere length and survival after unrelated allogeneic hematopoietic cell transplantation for severe aplastic anemia. JAMA. 2015;313(6):594–602.

Open Access   This chapter is licensed under the terms of the Creative Commons Attribution 4.0 International License (http://creativecommons.org/licenses/by/4.0/), which permits use, sharing, adaptation, distribution and reproduction in any medium or format, as long as you give appropriate credit to the original author(s) and the source, provide a link to the Creative Commons license and indicate if changes were made.

The images or other third party material in this chapter are included in the chapter's Creative Commons license, unless indicated otherwise in a credit line to the material. If material is not included in the chapter's Creative Commons license and your intended use is not permitted by statutory regulation or exceeds the permitted use, you will need to obtain permission directly from the copyright holder.

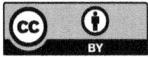

Chapter 19
Pathophysiology of Ribosomal Disorders

Lydie Da Costa and Alan J. Warren

Introduction: Eukaryotic Ribosomes

Ribosomes are essential for protein synthesis in all cells. The mature 80S ribosome is composed of the small (40S) and large (60S) ribosomal subunits, containing 78 ribosomal proteins (RPs) and four ribosomal RNAs (rRNA) that carry more than 200 known chemical modifications (Fig. 19.1). The small ribosomal subunit contains 32 RPs and only one rRNA (18S), while the large ribosomal subunit contains 46 RPs and three rRNAs (5S, 5.8S, and 28S) (Tables 19.1 and 19.2). Ribosomes are, therefore, ribonucleoprotein (RNP) complexes in which the catalytic activity of peptide bond formation is carried out by the rRNA. Each ribosome carries one binding site for the mRNA and three for the transfer RNA (tRNA), oriented from 5′ to 3′ on the mRNA, called the exit (E), peptidyl (P), and aminoacyl (A) sites [1]. The small subunit is responsible for decoding the mRNA through the recognition of codon pairing. The large subunit harbors the peptidyl transferase center (PTC), which catalyzes polypeptide bond formation and peptide release.

L. Da Costa (✉)
Laboratory of Hematology, Bicêtre University Hospital, Le Kremlin-Bicêtre, France
e-mail: lydie.dacosta@aphp.fr

A. J. Warren
Department of Hematology, Cambridge Institute for Medical Research, University of Cambridge, Cambridge, UK

Department of Hematology, Cambridge Stem Cell Institute, University of Cambridge, Cambridge, UK

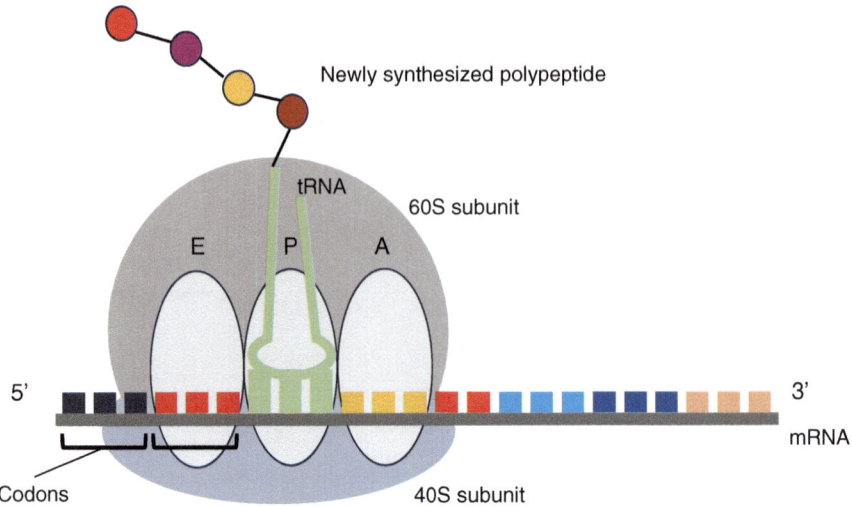

Fig. 19.1 Ribosomes catalyze new protein synthesis. Schematic showing the roles of the 40S and 60S subunits in mRNA decoding and peptide bond formation, respectively. A (aminoacyl), P (peptidyl), and E (exit) tRNA binding sites are indicated

Table 19.1 New nomenclature of ribosomal proteins

New name	Old yeast name	Old human name
Small ribosomal subunit		
eS1	S1	S3A
uS2	S0	SA
uS3	S3	S3
uS4	S9	S9
eS4	S4	S4
uS5	S2	S2
eS6	S6	S6
uS7	S5	S5
eS7	S7	S7
uS8	S22	S15A
eS8	S8	S8
uS9	S16	S16
uS10	S20	S20
eS10	S10	S10
uS11	S14	S14
uS12	S23	S23
eS12	S12	S12
uS13	S18	S18
uS14	S29	S29
uS15	S13	S13
uS17	S11	S11

(continued)

Table 19.1 (continued)

New name	Old yeast name	Old human name
uS19	S15	S15
eS21	S21	S21
eS24	S24	S24
eS25	S25	S25
eS26	S26	S26
eS27	S27	S27
eS28	S28	S28
eS30	S30	S30
eS31	S31	S27A
eS32 (see [3])	L41	L41
RACK1	Asc1	RACK1
Large ribosomal subunit		
uL1	L1	L10A
uL2	L2	L8
uL3	L3	L3
uL4	L4	L4
uL5	L11	L11
uL6	L9	L9
eL6	L6	L6
eL8	L8	L7A
uL10	P0	P0
uL11	L12	L12
uL13	L16	L13A
eL13	L13	L13
uL14	L23	L23
eL14	L14	L14
uL15	L28	L27A
eL15	L15	L15
uL16	L10	L10
uL18	L5	L5
eL18	L18	L18
eL19	L19	L19
eL20	L20	L18A
eL21	L21	L21
uL22	L17	L17
eL22	L22	L22
uL23	L25	L23A
uL24	L26	L26
eL24	L24	L24
eL27	L27	L27
eL28	–	L28

(continued)

Table 19.1 (continued)

uL29	L35	L35
eL29	L29	L29
uL30	L7	L7
eL30	L30	L30
eL31	L31	L31
eL32	L32	L32
eL33	L33	L35A
eL34	L34	L34
eL36	L36	L36
eL37	L37	L37
eL38	L38	L38
eL39	L39	L39
eL40	L40	L40
eL41	L41	eS32 (see [3])
eL42	L42	L36A
eL43	L43	L37A
P1/P2	P1/P2 (AB)	P1/P2 ($\alpha\beta$)

Table 19.2 Composition of the eukaryotic ribosome

	Eukaryotic ribosome content
Large ribosomal subunit	
Svedberg	60S
Number of ribosomal proteins	46
rRNAs	5S, 5.8S, 28S
Small ribosomal subunit	
Svedberg	40S
Number of ribosomal proteins	32
rRNAs	18S

Ribosome biogenesis is a highly coordinated process in time and space [2]. RPs from the small and large subunits are assembled in a defined order [3]. In the nucleolus, an rRNA precursor is transcribed and co-transcriptionally joined by RPs and ribosomal binding factors (RBFs), giving rise to the 90S pre-ribosomal particle [4, 5]. Ribosome maturation continues in a hierarchical, ordered pathway through the nucleolus and nucleoplasm, with the completion of the final steps of this complex process in the cytoplasm [6–8].

RNA polymerase I (RNA Pol I) synthesizes the 47S pre-rRNA, which triggers the self-assembly of the nucleolus in the nucleolar organizer regions. This pre-rRNA carries the 18S, 5.8S, and 28S rRNAs, flanked on each side by the 5′ and 3′ external transcribed spacers (ETSs) and two internal transcribed spacers (ITS1 and ITS2) [9, 10]. The transcribed spacers contain cleavage sites that are cut by endonucleases to release the 18S, 5.8S, and 28S rRNAs in an ordered sequence. These steps take place within three sub-nucleolar compartments: the fibrillar center, which is surrounded by the dense fibrillar component and the granular component. The 47S pre-rRNA is further processed in the dense fibrillar component by specific cleavages and posttranscriptional modifications carried out by snoRNPs, while the assembly of the rRNA with ribosomal proteins occurs in the granular component. The 5S rRNA, which joins the pre-60S particles in the nucleolus, is separately transcribed by the RNA polymerase III (RNA Pol III). The 5S ribonucleoprotein complex comprises the 5S rRNA and ribosomal proteins uL18 (RPL5) and uL5 (RPL11). The complex is incorporated relatively early into nucleolar pre-60S particles but, during later nucleoplasmic stages of 60S subunit processing, undergoes a 180° rotation in conjunction with the ITS2 processing by the multi-protein rixosome complex [11, 12].

RNA polymerase II (RNA Pol II) has two distinct roles: the transcription of protein and snoRNA (small nucleolar RNA) genes. SnoRNAs can be classified into three categories: H/ACA box snoRNAs, C/D box snoRNAs, and small Cajal RNAs (scaRNAs). H/ACA box snoRNAs and C/D box snoRNAs guide the methyltransferase fibrillarin and the pseudouridine synthase dyskerin (encoded by the *DKC1* gene, mutated in X-linked dyskeratosis congenita (DC)) to mediate rRNA 2'-O-methylation and pseudouridylation, respectively [13]. ScaRNAs are in Cajal bodies and function in the modification and maturation of small nuclear RNAs. In human cells, H/ACA box snoRNAs bind to proteins such as NHP2, DKC1, GAR1, and NOP10, while C/D box snoRNAs bind to SNU13, fibrillarin, NOP56, and NOP58 to generate functional snoRNPs [14]. RNA Pol II transcribes mRNAs from all the RP genes and RBF genes. RP and RBF mRNAs are translated by the 80S ribosome in the cytoplasm and then imported into the nucleus to participate in the ribosome assembly process.

In human cells, after ETS1 cleavage (sites A' and A_0), the endonuclease RNase mitochondrial RNA processing (RMRP) (mutated in cartilage–hair hypoplasia (CHH)) cuts the 47S pre-rRNA at site 2 of ITS1 to release the early 40S pre-ribosome particle containing the 18S rRNA and recruits small subunit RPs in the nucleolus [2] (Fig. 19.2). The remaining pre-rRNA combines with the large subunit RPs to form the 60S pre-ribosome. After cleavage of the 47S pre-rRNA, the pre-40S and pre-60S particles mature independently in the nucleolus and the nucleoplasm. In the nucleus, the installation of NOP53 into the nuclear pre-60S ribosome is critical to recruit the RNA exosome to cut ITS2 at site 4 and disassemble the "foot" structure (Fig. 19.2). After export through the nuclear pore complex [15, 16], final maturation occurs in the cytoplasm.

In the cytoplasm, pre-40S particles are very similar to their mature equivalents. This means that a pre-40S particle could structurally interact with the translation apparatus before it is properly primed. To prevent this, several RBFs occupy the binding sites for other translation factors (bystin/ENP1, LTV1, RIO2, TSR1, DIM2/PNO1, and NOB1) [17]. The domains harboring the binding sites undergo several remodeling stages to release the RBFs. The final step in forming a mature and functional small ribosomal subunit is the cleavage of the 18S rRNA at the 3' end and the release of the last two RBFs, DIM2 and NOB1, an important checkpoint [17, 18]. Processing of the 3'end of the 18S rRNA is achieved by the endonuclease NOB1.

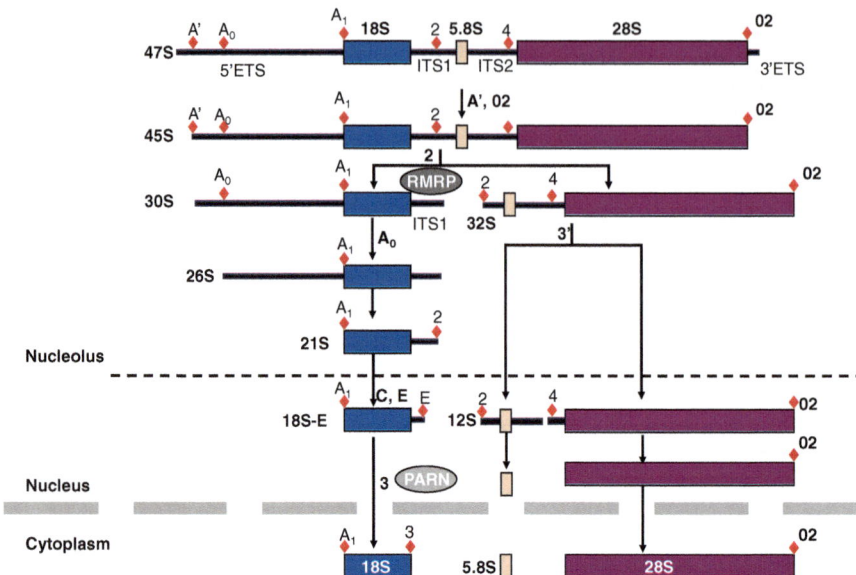

Fig. 19.2 Schematic of human rRNA maturation. Schematic of the major steps in human pre-rRNA processing. Assembly of both ribosomal subunits starts with the transcription of the mutual 47S rRNA precursor. RNA cleavage at site A2 by the endonuclease RMRP separates the two branches into the 40S (green) and 60S pre-ribosomes. Cleavage sites are indicated by red diamonds

However, NOB1 is restricted from cleaving the rRNA (site D) by the assembly factor DIM2, which contacts NOB1 in the particle and masks the rRNA cleavage site. ATP-bound RIO1 cooperates with ribosomal protein eS26 to displace DIM2 from the 3′ end of the 18S rRNA, triggering cleavage of the rRNA by NOB1. The final step of 40S subunit maturation is thereby controlled by a dual key lock mechanism [18]. In addition, NOB1 also occupies the mRNA binding site, thereby preventing the association of mRNAs with the pre-40S particle.

Following their initial assembly in the nucleolus, the large ribosomal subunit precursor is exported through the nuclear pore by recruiting the exportin Crm1/Xpo1 via the assembly factor Nmd3 to complete final cytoplasmic maturation [7, 8, 16, 19–23]. These steps include the recruitment of the final ribosomal proteins (eL40 and uL16) to complete the catalytic PTC [7, 8, 24–26]. In addition, a range of inhibitory assembly factors, including Nmd3, must be removed from the intersubunit face of the particle to allow the nascent 60S and 40S subunits to join to form actively translating 80S ribosomes [7, 8, 21, 23]. In the final step of 60S subunit maturation, SBDS cooperates with the GTPase EFL1 to release eIF6, a critical quality control checkpoint that licenses the entry of structurally and functionally competent 60S ribosomal subunits into the actively translating pool of ribosomes [27–32] (Fig. 19.3).

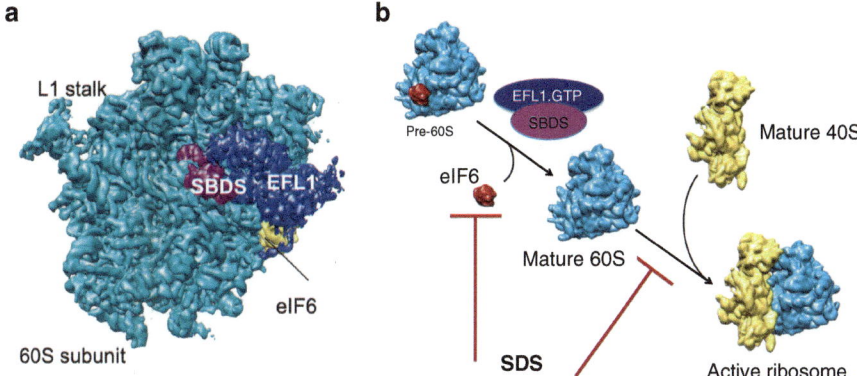

Fig. 19.3 SDS pathophysiology. (**a**). SBDS and EFL1 cooperate to release the anti-association factor eIF6 from the nascent 60S ribosomal subunit. (**b**). Release of eIF6 is required to allow the joining of the 40S and 60S subunits to form actively translating ribosomes. In SDS, the deficiency of the SBDS protein (or more rarely EFL1) impairs the release of eIF6, physically preventing the joining of the 40S and 60S subunits to form actively translating 80S ribosomes

Pathophysiology of Ribosomopathies

Overview

Ribosomopathies are a growing class of rare human diseases caused by impaired ribosome biogenesis and/or function (Table 19.3) [33, 34]. Ribosomal dysfunctions can be either congenital or acquired (somatic ribosomopathies) [35]. In this article, we will focus on congenital ribosomopathies. Congenital ribosomopathies are usually considered precancer states [36–39]; however, the mechanisms underlying malignant transformation are poorly understood [40]. Ribosomopathies are caused by mutations in genes encoding components of the ribosome assembly machinery, including RPs, RBFs, or rDNA transcription factors. While these diseases are clinically heterogeneous and affect a range of organs and developmental processes, ribosomopathies include several of the inherited bone marrow failure syndromes (IBMFSs), a group of rare genetic disorders affecting one or more hematopoietic lineages that are also characterized by short stature and a range of congenital malformations, including craniofacial, thumb, heart, and kidney abnormalities, with increased susceptibility to malignancies (hematological and solid tumors). These rare diseases highlight a still incompletely understood link between ribosome dysfunction and bone marrow failure. In Diamond–Blackfan anemia (DBA) syndrome and Shwachman–Diamond syndrome (SDS), impaired ribosome biogenesis appears

Table 19.3 Summary of known ribosomopathies: clinical characteristics, cancer risk, and associated mutations. (Adapted from [177])

Ribosomopathy	Gene defect	Clinical feature	Cancer risk	Congenital or acquired
Diamond–Blackfan anemia (DBA) syndrome	RPS19, RPS10, RPS17, RPS24, RPS26, RPL5, RPL11, RPL35A (≈ 70%–75% of the patients, including large deletions (20%) in these genes) Less frequent genes involved < 1% for each: RPS7, RPS15, RPS27, RPS27A, RPS28, RPS29, RPL4, RPL9, RPL13, RPL15, RPL17, RPL26, RPL27, RPL31, RPL36, TSR2, HEATR3 GATA1, EPO, TP53	Macrocytic anemia, short stature, craniofacial defects, thumb abnormalities	Colon, osteosarcoma, MDS	Congenital
5q- syndrome	RPS14	Macrocytic anemia, hypolobulated micromegakaryocytes	10% progression to AML	Acquired
Shwachman–Diamond Syndrome (SDS)	SBDS, EFL1, DNAJC21, SRP54	Neutropenia, pancreatic insufficiency, short stature, infections	MDS and AML	Congenital
X-linked dyskeratosis congenita	DKC1	Cytopenia, skin hyperpigmentation, nail dystrophy, oral leukoplakia, pulmonary fibrosis	MDS, AML, and head and neck tumors	Congenital
Cartilage–hair hypoplasia	RMRP	Hypoplastic anemia, short-limbed dwarfism, hypoplastic hair	Non-Hodgkin lymphoma, basal cell carcinoma	Congenital
Treacher Collins syndrome	TCOF1, POLR1D, POLR1C, POLR1B	Craniofacial abnormalities	None reported	Congenital

to be the primary pathophysiological mechanism [28, 29, 32, 41, 42]. Although the primary disease etiology in DC is defective telomere maintenance, a subset of genes mutated in this disorder are also involved in ribosome biogenesis or RNA metabolism (e.g., *DKC1, PARN, NPM1, DUT, TYMS-ENOSF1,* and *USB1*) [43–51]. The difference between the clinical phenotypes among ribosomopathies highlights how the disruption of different points during the ribosome assembly process or the overlapping roles for the mutated genes in distinct processes such as telomere maintenance or nucleotide metabolism may result in very different impacts on cellular physiology and the ultimate clinical phenotype.

Tissue Specificity of Ribosomopathies

Given the ubiquitous nature of ribosomes, the tissue specificity and proclivity in the range of affected tissues toward the hematopoietic, skeletal, and neurological systems in the ribosomopathies remain puzzling.

Some studies have sought to provide clues regarding the issue of tissue specificity. In normal physiology, mRNA translation levels vary throughout differentiation, with lower rates of protein synthesis in embryonic and hematopoietic stem cells compared to mature cells [52, 53]. Several studies have highlighted the role of ribosome biogenesis in the maintenance of stem cell homeostasis in *Drosophila* germ stem cells [54–57], *Drosophila* neuroblasts [58], endoplasmic reticulum (ES) cells [59, 60], and hematopoietic cells [61]. Lower translation rates in undifferentiated cells could reflect the reduced need for a diverse proteome in stem cells compared to mature cells (differentiation switch) [62, 63]. Control and regulation of protein synthesis and, therefore, of the ribosome and its associated factors are essential for stem cells, both to maintain their self-renewal and for their ability to differentiate. Indeed, in the context of *Drosophila* germline stem cells, ribosome biogenesis and translation are uncoupled to create the conditions required for terminal differentiation [54]. This combination of low protein synthesis but high ribosome biogenesis activity likely maintains stem cells in a state of readiness, primed to efficiently differentiate by enabling rapid reassembly of the proteome. The cell is held in a critical state where any defect (such as reduced ribosome numbers or dysregulated translation) that tips this delicate balance may inhibit differentiation. Once the cell receives the appropriate signal, ribosome biogenesis may be temporarily downregulated to outsource resources to differentiation. Once differentiation is completed, cells enter a stable state in which protein synthesis is increased compared to stem cells to fulfill specific cellular functions. In ribosomopathies, diminished quantity or quality of ribosomes might affect both stem cell self-renewal and differentiation, depending on the specific tissue.

Ribosome heterogeneity posits that ribosome composition varies temporally or under different conditions in individual cells or tissues and is proposed as a hypothesis to explain the tissue proclivity in ribosomopathies [64–66]. Ribosome heterogeneity can be seen on several levels:

- rRNA modifications: rRNAs are post-translationally modified, most commonly 2′-O-methylation of the ribose and the isomerization of uridine to pseudouridine (Ψ) [67–70]. These modifications may significantly influence the ribosome structure and function, conferring additional layers of regulation to the translation process by modulating the speed or fidelity of translation of specific subsets of mRNA with the potential to influence cell fate [71]. Modifications of rRNA are guided by snoRNAs. Nucleophosmin (*NPM1*) is an essential regulator of 2'-O-methylation of rRNA that directly binds C/D box snoRNAs to regulate translation. Germline *NPM1* mutations in DC lead to altered rRNA 2'-O-methylation. Importantly, mice harboring a DC-related germline *NPM1* mutation recapitulate both the hematological and non-hematological features of DC [45]. These findings implicate impaired 2'-O-methylation of rRNA in the pathogenesis of IBMFSs. Furthermore, in X-linked DC, mutations in the *DKC1* gene alter the translational efficiency and fidelity of transcripts carrying internal ribosome entry site (IRES) elements [72]. Taken together, these data support the hypothesis that altered rRNA modifications contribute to the pathogenesis of ribosomopathies by modulating the translation of specific mRNAs.

- Ribosomal proteins may vary in their stoichiometry, composition, posttranslational modifications, or expression of paralogs [73]. About a quarter of RPs have tissue-specific expression, with unanticipated plasticity across normal and malignant cells [74]. In cancer, the expression pattern of RPs is dysregulated compared to healthy tissues. Heterogenous ribosomes may preferentially translate a certain class of transcripts [67, 75]. Post-translational modifications on RPs can include phosphorylation, methylation, ubiquitination, acetylation, and hydroxylation. In hematopoietic tissue, specifically during erythroid differentiation, expression of the hybrid E2–E3 ubiquitin ligase UBE2O is upregulated in reticulocytes and allows the transition from reticulocytes to erythrocytes by ubiquitinating certain RPs to target them for degradation, thereby decreasing ribosome biogenesis and, consequently, remodeling the proteome [76]. Moreover, several RPs are ubiquitinated in response to stress, including RPS2/uS5, RPS3/uS3, and RSP20/uS10, whose ubiquitylation occurs on assembled cytoplasmic ribosomes and is positively regulated by the unfolded protein response [77, 78]. Defective ubiquitylation of these RPs increases cellular sensitivity to ER stress and leads to apoptosis [64]. Structural and biochemical analyses suggest a role for the E3 ubiquitin ligase UFM1 in post-termination release and recycling of the large ribosomal subunit from the ER membrane through UFMylation of ribosomal protein uL24 on the cytoplasmic face of the ER membrane [79].
- Specialized ribosomes refer to the concept that functional translation of specific mRNAs is modulated by structural variations of the ribosome. A recent striking example supporting the concept of specialized ribosomes is the ability of cytokines linked to tumor immunity to reshape the ribosome by regulating P-stalk incorporation to rewire the cellular proteome through translational regulation [80].
- Adding to the core RPs, several other proteins may associate with the ribosome (ribosome-associated protein (RAP)) or bind to the rRNA (RNA-binding protein (RBP)), a group commonly referred to as the "ribo-interactome." The ribo-interactome is composed of over 400 diverse proteins that can impact both the structure and the function of the ribosome [64, 66]. RAPs may also have tissue-specific expression patterns.

All these elements may contribute to the tissue specificity of ribosomopathies and are not mutually exclusive.

Pathophysiological Mechanisms of Ribosomopathies

Several hypotheses may explain the pathophysiological mechanisms through which germline mutations drive the clinical phenotypes associated with ribosomopathies. Ribosomal RNAs mature from a common precursor, and defects in pre-rRNA cleavage are a hallmark of ribosomopathies, including DBA, SDS, and CHH [29, 41, 42, 81] (Fig. 19.4). The defect in rRNA maturation may be identified by northern blotting using specific probes. Alterations of ribosome biogenesis perturb one of the most energy-demanding and complex biosynthetic pathways in the cell. Approximately $5-10 \times 10^6$ ribosomes are produced per cell cycle in mammals, and mRNAs encoding ribosomal proteins may constitute up to 50% of cellular mRNAs [82]. If you consider that for the erythroid lineage, 2×10^6 red blood cells are produced each second (2×10^{11} cells/day), we may easily imagine how a defect in such a major cellular component as the ribosome may negatively impact erythropoiesis. In DBA, while the number of available ribosomes is reduced, ribosome composition remains constant [83]. Somatic ribosomopathies may result in altered translation efficiency of a subset of mRNAs involved in hematopoiesis or cancer evolution [35, 40, 84]. Suboptimal numbers of ribosomes may preferentially affect the translation of mRNAs with low initiation rates [34]. An important example is the reduced translation of the major erythroid transcription factor *GATA1* to confer the erythroid

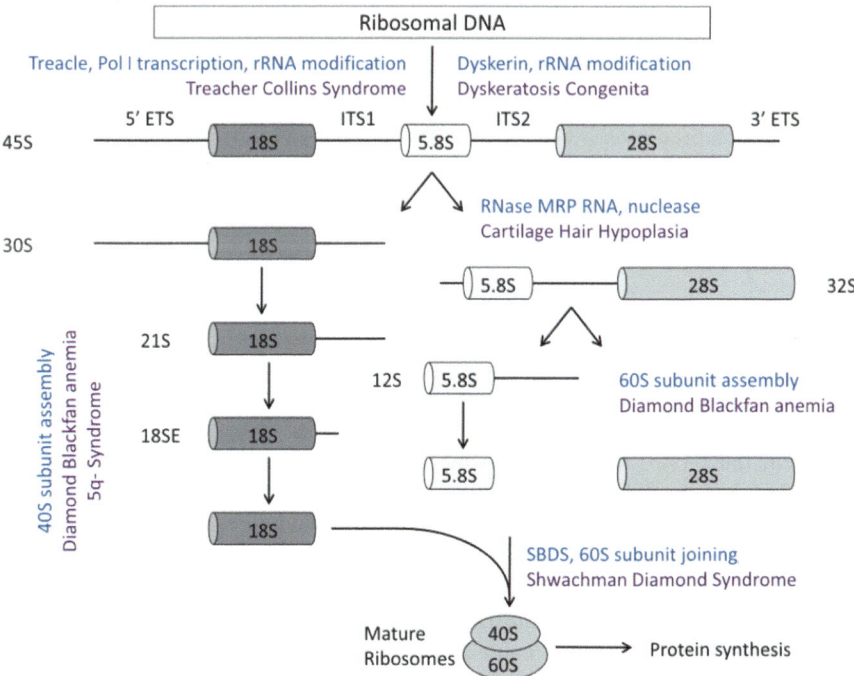

Fig. 19.4 Ribosomopathies mapped to multiple steps in the ribosome assembly pathwaySpecific ribosomopathies are mapped to the human rRNA processing pathway. (From [177])

tissue specificity in DBA [83, 85–87]. It is also important to consider the role of general translation factors, including ABCE1 and the ribosome rescue factors PELOTA and HBS1L, in calibrating the sensitivity of terminally differentiating erythroid cells in response to defects in ribosome supply and, more generally, in the maintenance of mammalian tissue homeostasis [34, 88, 89].

Impaired pre-rRNA processing and ribosome biogenesis may cause nucleolar stress and apoptotic death of hematopoietic progenitor cells, triggering cytostatic and proapoptotic responses [90, 91]. The p53 tumor suppressor protein is stabilized by the nucleolar stress generated by ribosome assembly defects induced by germline ribosomal protein gene variants that increase free 5S ribonucleoprotein particles (5S rRNA, RPL5/uL11, and RPL11/uL18) in the nucleus, which, in turn, sequester HDM2, preventing it from binding to p53 [92–94]. HDM2 is an E3 ubiquitin ligase that ubiquitinates p53 and promotes its degradation by the proteasome. During ribosomal stress, there is reduced binding of HDM2 to p53, thereby stabilizing the levels of p53 in the cell [90, 91, 95, 96]. The recently discovered HDM2 antagonist SURF2, which is overexpressed in many cancers, buffers free 5S RNP particles and can modulate their activity [97].

Pathophysiological p53-dependent anemia was initially recognized in mouse mutants with dominantly inherited dark skin–carrying germline *Rps19* or *Rps20* missense mutations and in morpholino-induced RPS19- or RPL11-deficient zebrafish and has been confirmed in human DBA-derived cells [98–101]. Indeed, the stabilization of p53 is detected in the majority of ribosomopathies [102–105]. In summary, the pathophysiology of the ribosomopathies is multifaceted due to the many outcomes of defective protein synthesis and altered rates of translation initiation in ribosome-deficient cells, with downstream impacts on multiple signaling pathways, DNA damage, metabolism, regulation of survival, proliferation, and cell differentiation processes.

Pathophysiology of the Most Frequent Ribosomopathies

Diamond–Blackfan Anemia Syndrome

DBA is an IBMFS characterized by erythroid tropism, which is caused by a defect in rRNA maturation as a consequence of mutations in *RP* genes (24 genes so far involved, Table 19.3) or genes encoding ribosome biogenesis factors, such as *TSR2* or *HEATR3* [106–109]. DBA-like disorders may also be caused by mutations in genes without any direct role in rRNA maturation, such as *GATA1* [110], erythropoietin (*EPO*) [111], and *TP53* [112] (for review [113–125]). Erythroblastopenia in DBA is the result of a developmental blockade that occurs during the BFU-e to CFU-e erythroid progenitor transition stage [126]. As previously discussed, the defect in ribosome biogenesis caused by a heterozygous mutation in an *RP* gene induces a defect in rRNA maturation, generating nucleolar stress, leading to p53 stabilization. Stabilization of p53, the guardian of the genome, provokes cell cycle arrest and increased apoptosis, at least in part, causing the characteristic erythroid defect in the proliferation and differentiation in DBA [90, 91]. However, as p53-independent pathways have also been implicated [109, 127–129] and given that p53 is activated in all ribosomopathies, p53 stabilization alone is not considered the major actor responsible for the erythroid tropism in DBA.

The HSP70/*GATA1* complex has been shown by several groups to be central to DBA pathophysiology [85, 87, 130, 131]. Splice site mutations in the *GATA1* gene impair the production of the full-length form of the protein by promoting translation initiation from an internal start site to generate the short protein isoform *GATA1s* [87]. RP gene mutations also reduce the efficiency of translation of the long *GATA1* isoform [110]. In addition, the *GATA1* chaperone HSP70, which protects *GATA1* from caspase-3 cleavage during terminal erythroid differentiation upon erythropoietin stimulation, is also involved [130]. Any factor that reduces *GATA1* or HSP70 expression is likely to induce a DBA phenotype. In addition, the inhibition of the p53 pathway by *GATA1* may be essential for erythroid cell development and survival [131]. By restoring *GATA1* expression, the overexpression of wild-type HSP70 or *GATA1* decreases p53 activation in RPL5/uL18- and RPL11/uL5-depleted erythroid cells [87, 130, 131]. Decreased expression of *GATA1* could thus also contribute to p53 activation in DBA.

Cell metabolism and free heme overload also play an important role in DBA pathophysiology. Our group and others found that in DBA, unbalanced globin/heme synthesis leads to excess free heme and increased production of reactive oxygen species (ROS), which result in cell death and apoptosis [131, 132]. The deleterious effect of the free heme excess in DBA was further strengthened by findings showing (1) an increased production of ROS in primary cells from DBA patients, with the extent of the increase dependent on the RP mutation; (2) the importance of the *GATA1*/HSP70 complex in DBA primary erythroid cells in controlling globin synthesis and limiting heme synthesis by decreasing ALAS2 and ferrochelatase expression to adapt the level of heme for decreased globin synthesis; and (3) the attempt of erythroid DBA cells to increase globin synthesis by repressing eIF2α phosphorylation and limit free heme toxicity by increasing the expression of the cell membrane heme exporter, FLVCR1 [131].

In addition, an autoregulated heme–*GATA1* feedback loop regulates normal erythroid differentiation. In early erythroid cells, heme upregulates RP and globin transcripts, while in later erythroid cells, heme decreases *GATA1* and *GATA1* target gene expression [133]. Thus, free heme excess and the globin/heme disequilibrium may indeed be the major modulators of the DBA phenotype. Autophagy and cell metabolism may also play important roles in modulating DBA phenotypes [134, 135], particularly arginine-dependent regulation of erythroid differentiation through hypusination of eIF5A [136]. DBA pathophysiology, therefore, involves multiple processes, with the erythroid-specific transcription factor *GATA1* at the center (summarized in Fig. 19.5, adapted from [113]).

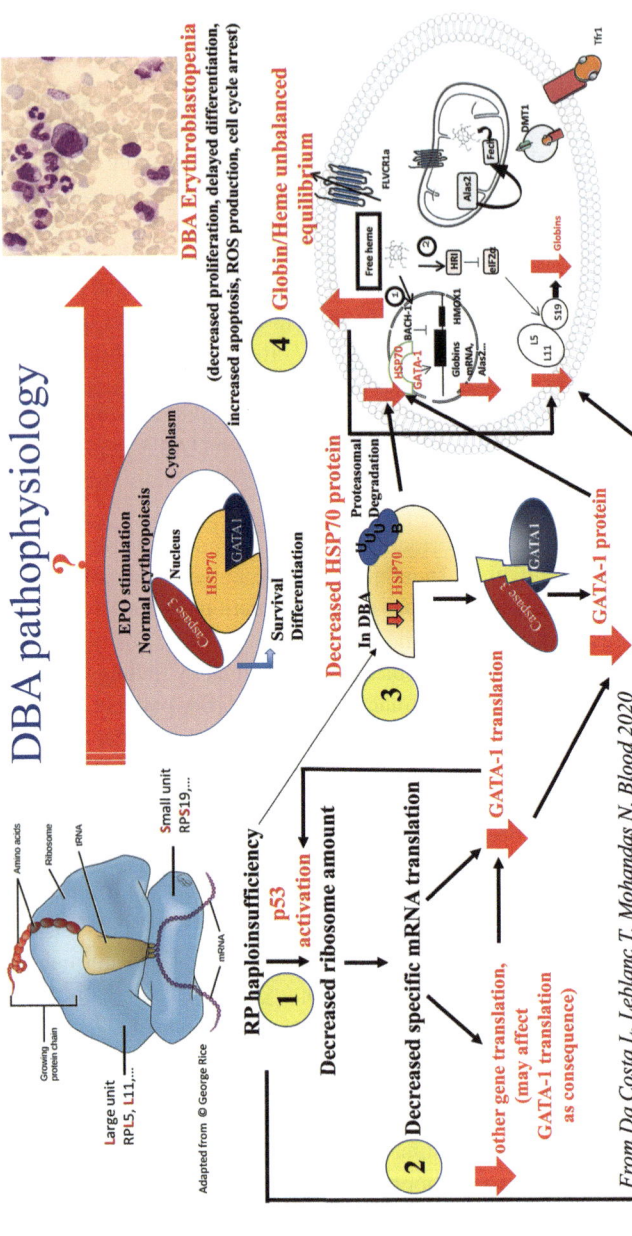

Fig. 19.5 DBA pathophysiology. Erythroid defect in DBA (DBA-like or other <1% of DBA syndrome cases not included) is the result of a mutated gene in an RP gene or a gene involved in ribosome biogenesis, which will generate a nucleolar stress, responsible for p53 activation. p53 activation is responsible for the erythroblastopenia, at least in part, by cell cycle arrest in G_0/G_1 and apoptosis induction. Ribosome biogenesis defect is also responsible for the translational alteration of specific transcripts, in particular, the *GATA1* mRNA. In addition, in RP- (except RPS19) depleted erythroid cells, HSP70, the chaperone of *GATA1*, is addressed for proteasomal degradation. *GATA1* is, therefore, no longer protected and cleaved by caspase-3 during terminal erythroid differentiation and EPO stimulation. Both mechanisms lead to decreased *GATA1* protein expression. A defect in *GATA1* is responsible for decreased hemoglobin levels and free heme overload due to the unbalanced globin/heme equilibrium. (From [113])

Shwachman–Diamond Syndrome

SDS is a rare autosomal recessive IBMFS caused by compound heterozygous germline mutations in the *SBDS* gene in over 90% of patients [137–139]. SDS-like phenotypes are also more rarely associated with mutations in *DNAJC21* [140, 141], *EFL1* [142, 143], and *SRP54* [144, 145]. The SBDS protein is a ribosome assembly factor that binds to late cytoplasmic pre-60S ribosomes to cooperate with the GTPase EFL1 in catalyzing the release of the anti-association factor eIF6 from the inter-subunit face of the large ribosomal subunit, a key quality control step that not only licenses the entry of nascent 60S subunits into active translation but also promotes ribosome recycling [27–29, 31, 32, 146]. The ribosome assembly defect and reduced protein synthesis in SDS results in bone marrow failure, with over one-third of individuals subsequently developing myelodysplastic syndrome (MDS) and acute myeloid leukemia (AML) by the fourth decade of life [147].

A few SDS patients (less than 3%) carry mutations in the elongation factor–like 1 (*EFL1*) or *DNAJC21* gene encoding the 60S assembly factor DNAJ heat shock protein family (HSP40) member 21, reinforcing the signature of SDS as a disorder of impaired late 60S ribosomal subunit maturation [141–143]. Mutations in the signal recognition particle 54 gene (*SRP54*) may also be associated with an SDS-like phenotype, highlighting defective proteostasis more broadly in SDS pathophysiology [144, 145].

How and why a defect in a process as ubiquitous as ribosome biogenesis more severely affects the pancreas and granulocytic differentiation in SDS remain incompletely understood. Differences in mRNA-specific rates of initiation and changes in ribosome concentration likely explain tissue-specific changes in gene expression [34]. As proposed for the defect in *GATA1* mRNA translation in DBA [85, 87], reduced cellular ribosome concentration may disproportionately impact inefficiently translated mRNAs with upstream reading frames or complex 5′ or 3′ untranslated regions [148]. In addition, the ablation of the *Sbds* gene in mice superimposes tissue-specific p53-dependent cell death and arrest pathways upon the underlying translational insufficiency to induce apoptosis in the fetal brain and senescence in the mature exocrine pancreas [149].

Strikingly, the phenomenon of somatic genetic rescue (SGR) provides multiple routes to help improve hematopoietic clonal fitness in SDS [150–155]. Adaptive somatic mutations try to restore ribosome homeostasis either by increasing the gene dosage of *SBDS* (i (7)(q10) structural variant) or *EFL1* or by reducing the eIF6 function through the selection of *EIF6* somatic mutations, *EIF6* gene deletion (del(20q)), or chromosomal translocation [151–153]. Although convergent somatic mutation of the p53-dependent nucleolar surveillance pathway may restore ribosome homeostasis, such maladaptive mutations increase the opportunity for *TP53*-mutated cancer evolution [151, 152, 156]. By providing important insights into genetic rescue mechanisms and their relative risk in driving leukemic evolution, emerging single-cell technologies are helping to inform the development of personalized medicine approaches in SDS and other IBMFSs [157]. Figure 19.6 summarizes the pathophysiology of MDS/AML evolution in SDS.

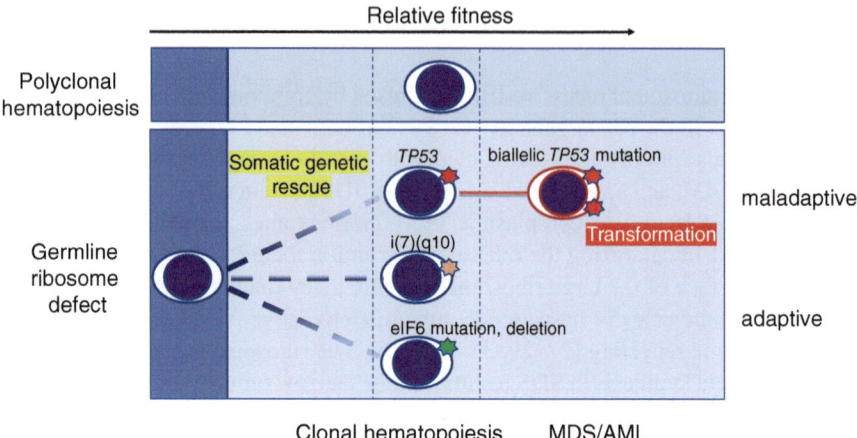

Fig. 19.6 Mechanism of evolution to blood cancer in SDS. Germline ribosome deficiency in SDS impairs hematopoietic stem cell fitness. Adaptive mutations that increase the dose of SBDS or reduce the amount of eIF6 restore ribosome homeostasis to improve cell fitness. Maladaptive *TP53* mutations offset the deleterious effects of germline ribosomopathy but provide an opportunity for biallelic *TP53* mutation acquisition and cancer evolution

Telomeropathy/Ribosomopathy: X-Linked Dyskeratosis Congenita

Mutations of the *DKC1, NHP2, NOP10,* or *PARN* genes have been associated with DC and the related Hoyeraal–Hreidarsson syndrome [43, 158–163]. Both syndromes are linked to deficient telomere maintenance [164].

The *DKC1* gene encodes dyskerin, which is a component of the telomerase holoenzyme complex that binds to the telomerase RNA component (TERC) H/ACA domain, thus increasing its stability in vivo. Dyskerin is a pseudouridine synthase that catalyzes the isomerization of uridine to pseudouridine in noncoding RNAs. Dyskerin forms a heterotrimer with NOP10 and NHP2 that binds snoRNAs or scaRNAs to form H/ACA snoRNPs or scaRNPs. By hybridizing with the RNA target sequences, sno- and sca-RNAs guide dyskerin-catalyzed pseudouridylation on preribosomal RNAs in the nucleolus and on spliceosomal snRNA in Cajal bodies, respectively. It has been proposed that *DKC1* mutations in X-linked DC were linked to the perturbation of the rRNA pseudouridylation pattern, as the depletion of dyskerin by RNA interference leads to a loss of translational fidelity [49]. However, in *DKC1* mutant models corrected for telomere maintenance defects, the levels of pseudouridine modification and the maturation kinetics of newly transcribed rRNA were normal [165], with no apparent defects in rRNA processing. In addition, ribosomal protein content was maintained, suggesting that ribosome biogenesis was not affected by the *DKC1* mutation [165]. These results obtained in fibroblast cell lines from patients with X-linked DC have been validated in immortalized pluripotent cells carrying three different *DKC1* mutations (*DKC1*[A353V], *DKC1*[Q31E], and *DKC1*[ΔL37]) [166]. Hence, the primary pathogenic defect in DC is telomere dysfunction [51, 166]. Indeed, telomerase is a ribonucleoparticle structured like an H/ACA snoRNP and requires functional DKC1, NOP10, and NHP2 for assembly. Similarly, the PARN exoribonuclease is involved in the maturation of both ribosomal RNAs and the telomerase RNA. It seems plausible that defective ribosome biogenesis in *DKC1*- (or indeed *PARN*-) mutated forms of DC exacerbates the clinical phenotype caused by telomere dysfunction.

Cartilage–Hair Hypoplasia: Anauxetic Dysplasia Spectrum

CHH is a rare autosomal recessive IBMFS described by McKusick in 1965 [167], which is characterized primarily by short-limbed dwarfism, sparse hypoplastic hair, defective T cell immunity, hypoplastic anemia, and as with other IBMFSs, an increased risk of developing malignancies. The molecular defect was identified in 2001 as mutations in the *RMRP* gene that encodes the RNA component of RNase mitochondrial RNA processing (RMRP) [168]. RMRP is a long noncoding RNA (lncRNA) that associates with the RNase MRP ribonucleoprotein complex, with around ten proteins, most of which are shared with the RNase P complex that functions in pre-tRNA processing. The role of human RMRP in pre-rRNA cleavage was demonstrated by using complementary strategies, including the analysis of pre-rRNA processing in CHH-patient-derived cells or by using CRISPR/Cas9 either to disrupt *RMRP* in HeLa cells or T cells or to introduce the most common CHH-associated mutation (70^{AG}) into K562 cells [81, 169]. These studies revealed that human RMRP is an endonuclease that cleaves the precursor rRNA at site 2 of ITS1 (see Fig. 19.2), leading to the generation of increased levels of ITS1-containing rRNA precursors, reduced levels of rRNA per cell, and reduced intact cytosolic ribosomes relative to the mitochondrial pool [170]. CHH may thus be considered as a ribosomopathy. Interestingly, children with CHH caused by *RMRP* mutations have short telomeres, suggesting a potential link between *RMRP* and telomerase function [171].

Treacher Collins Syndrome

Treacher Collins syndrome (TCS) is a rare craniofacial disorder that is classified as a ribosomopathy but is not associated with anemia or other cytopenias [172, 173]. This autosomal dominant disorder is linked to the mutation in the *TCOF1* gene that encodes the treacle protein, which is involved in recruiting RNA Pol I to the nucleolus to transcribe the pre-rRNA [172, 173]. TCOF1 co-localizes with the upstream binding factor and RNA Pol I and is involved in the transcription of active ribosomal DNA genes. In addition, mutations in the *POLR1D*, *POLR1C*, and *POLR1B* genes, which are also involved in rDNA transcription and thus ribosome biogenesis, have been identified in patients with TCS [174, 175]. The clinical phenotype in TCS arises from the intersection between p53 activation, apoptosis, ROS production, and the activation of the DNA damage response pathway [102, 176].

In conclusion, the pathophysiology of the heterogeneous clinical phenotypes of the ribosomopathies likely reflects the complex interplay between the impact of specific germline mutations in different components of the ribosome assembly pathway on cellular ribosome concentration and mRNA-specific rates of translation initiation with added tissue- or cell-specific stress responses, including p53-dependent pathways. However, there remains much more to learn about the etiology of these fascinating disorders. Harnessing these insights to improve patient risk stratification and develop new and effective disease-modifying therapeutics remains an urgent goal.

Acknowledgments Our special thanks go to the affected individuals, their families, to the DBA French patient association (AFMBD), and to SDS UK. We thank Prof. T. Leblanc (Pediatric Hematology, R. Debré hospital); I. Marie, L. David-Nguyen, and D. David-Ponn (hematology diagnostic laboratory, Bicêtre hospital, Le Kremlin-Bicêtre, France) for our fruitful collaboration in DBA care since 1999; and Prof. PE Gleizes and MF O'Donohue for our fruitful scientific discussions. I deeply thank my two mentors and dear friends, Prof. G. Tchernia and Mohandas Narla (NYBC, NY, USA). We deeply thank all our collaborators and colleagues in DBA and SDS research.

LDC is supported by #ANR-23-CE14-0011-02, the Laboratory of Excellence for Red Cells [(LABEX GR-Ex)-ANR Avenir-11-LABX-0005-02], and the French National PHRC OFABD (DBA registry).

A.J.W thanks all members of the lab for discussions. A.J.W is supported by Cancer Research UK (DRCNPG-Jun24/100002), the UK Medical Research Council (MR/T012412/1), the Rosetrees Trust, the European Cooperation in Science and Technology (COST) Action Translacore CA21154, SDS Foundation, SDS UK, Butterfly Guild, and the Shwachman–Diamond Project. A.J.W is a consultant for SDS Therapeutics.

Conflict of Interest The authors have no disclosure to make and no conflict of interest.

Author Contributions L.D.C and A.J.W wrote the manuscript. Both authors had fruitful discussions to improve the manuscript.

References

1. Holvec S, et al. The structure of the human 80S ribosome at 1.9 A resolution reveals the molecular role of chemical modifications and ions in RNA. Nat Struct Mol Biol. 2024;31:1251–64. https://doi.org/10.1038/s41594-024-01274-x.
2. Vanden Broeck A, Klinge S. Eukaryotic ribosome assembly. Annu Rev Biochem. 2024;93:189–210. https://doi.org/10.1146/annurev-biochem-030222-113611.
3. Ayers TN, Woolford JL. Putting it all together: the roles of ribosomal proteins in nucleolar stages of 60S ribosomal assembly in the yeast Saccharomyces cerevisiae. Biomolecules. 2024;14 https://doi.org/10.3390/biom14080975.

4. Dragon F, et al. A large nucleolar U3 ribonucleoprotein required for 18S ribosomal RNA biogenesis. Nature. 2002;417:967–70. https://doi.org/10.1038/nature00769.
5. Kornprobst M, et al. Architecture of the 90S pre-ribosome: a structural view on the birth of the eukaryotic ribosome. Cell. 2016;166:380–93. https://doi.org/10.1016/j.cell.2016.06.014.
6. Vanden Broeck A, Klinge S. Principles of human pre-60S biogenesis. Science. 2023;381:eadh3892. https://doi.org/10.1126/science.adh3892.
7. Kargas V, et al. Mechanism of completion of peptidyltransferase centre assembly in eukaryotes. elife. 2019;8:e44904. https://doi.org/10.7554/eLife.44904.
8. Zhou Y, Musalgaonkar S, Johnson AW, Taylor DW. Tightly-orchestrated rearrangements govern catalytic center assembly of the ribosome. Nat Commun. 2019;10:958. https://doi.org/10.1038/s41467-019-08880-0.
9. Fernandez-Pevida A, Kressler D, de la Cruz J. Processing of preribosomal RNA in Saccharomyces cerevisiae. Wiley Interdiscip Rev RNA. 2015;6:191–209. https://doi.org/10.1002/wrna.1267.
10. Moss T, Langlois F, Gagnon-Kugler T, Stefanovsky V. A housekeeper with power of attorney: the rRNA genes in ribosome biogenesis. Cell Mol Life Sci. 2007;64:29–49. https://doi.org/10.1007/s00018-006-6278-1.
11. Thoms M, et al. Structural insights into coordinating 5S RNP rotation with ITS2 pre-RNA processing during ribosome formation. EMBO Rep. 2023;24:e57984. https://doi.org/10.15252/embr.202357984.
12. Gordon J, et al. Cryo-EM reveals the architecture of the PELP1-WDR18 molecular scaffold. Nat Commun. 2022;13:6783. https://doi.org/10.1038/s41467-022-34610-0.
13. Kufel J, Grzechnik P. Small nucleolar RNAs tell a different tale. Trends Genet. 2019;35:104–17. https://doi.org/10.1016/j.tig.2018.11.005.
14. Massenet S, Bertrand E, Verheggen C. Assembly and trafficking of box C/D and H/ACA snoRNPs. RNA Biol. 2017;14:680–92. https://doi.org/10.1080/15476286.2016.1243646.
15. Delavoie F, Soldan V, Rinaldi D, Dauxois JY, Gleizes PE. The path of pre-ribosomes through the nuclear pore complex revealed by electron tomography. Nat Commun. 2019;10:497. https://doi.org/10.1038/s41467-019-08342-7.
16. Li Z, et al. Nuclear export of pre-60S particles through the nuclear pore complex. Nature. 2023;618:411–8. https://doi.org/10.1038/s41586-023-06128-y.
17. Ameismeier M, Cheng J, Berninghausen O, Beckmann R. Visualizing late states of human 40S ribosomal subunit maturation. Nature. 2018;558:249–53. https://doi.org/10.1038/s41586-018-0193-0.
18. Plassart L, et al. The final step of 40S ribosomal subunit maturation is controlled by a dual key lock. elife. 2021;10:e61254. https://doi.org/10.7554/eLife.61254.
19. Lo KY, et al. Defining the pathway of cytoplasmic maturation of the 60S ribosomal subunit. Mol Cell. 2010;39:196–208. https://doi.org/10.1016/j.molcel.2010.06.018.
20. Liang X, et al. Structural snapshots of human pre-60S ribosomal particles before and after nuclear export. Nat Commun. 2020;11:3542. https://doi.org/10.1038/s41467-020-17237-x.
21. Prattes M, et al. Visualizing maturation factor extraction from the nascent ribosome by the AAA-ATPase Drg1. Nat Struct Mol Biol. 2022;29:942–53. https://doi.org/10.1038/s41594-022-00832-5.
22. Klingauf-Nerurkar P, et al. The GTPase Nog1 co-ordinates the assembly, maturation and quality control of distant ribosomal functional centers. elife. 2020;9:e52474. https://doi.org/10.7554/eLife.52474.
23. Ma C, et al. Structural snapshot of cytoplasmic pre-60S ribosomal particles bound by Nmd3, Lsg1, Tif6 and Reh1. Nat Struct Mol Biol. 2017;24:214–20. https://doi.org/10.1038/nsmb.3364.
24. Lo KY, Li Z, Wang F, Marcotte EM, Johnson AW. Ribosome stalk assembly requires the dual-specificity phosphatase Yvh1 for the exchange of Mrt4 with P0. J Cell Biol. 2009;186:849–62. https://doi.org/10.1083/jcb.200904110.

25. Fernandez-Pevida A, Rodriguez-Galan O, Diaz-Quintana A, Kressler D, de la Cruz J. Yeast ribosomal protein L40 assembles late into precursor 60 S ribosomes and is required for their cytoplasmic maturation. J Biol Chem. 2012;287:38390–407. https://doi.org/10.1074/jbc.M112.400564.
26. Kemmler S, Occhipinti L, Veisu M, Panse VG. Yvh1 is required for a late maturation step in the 60S biogenesis pathway. J Cell Biol. 2009;186:863–80. https://doi.org/10.1083/jcb.200904111.
27. Ceci M, et al. Release of eIF6 (p27BBP) from the 60S subunit allows 80S ribosome assembly. Nature. 2003;426:579–84. https://doi.org/10.1038/nature02160.
28. Finch AJ, et al. Uncoupling of GTP hydrolysis from eIF6 release on the ribosome causes Shwachman-Diamond syndrome. Genes Dev. 2011;25:917–29. https://doi.org/10.1101/gad.623011.
29. Menne TF, et al. The Shwachman-Bodian-Diamond syndrome protein mediates translational activation of ribosomes in yeast. Nat Genet. 2007;39:486–95. https://doi.org/10.1038/ng1994.
30. Senger B, et al. The nucle(ol)ar Tif6p and Efl1p are required for a late cytoplasmic step of ribosome synthesis. Mol Cell. 2001;8:1363–73. https://doi.org/10.1016/s1097-2765(01)00403-8.
31. Weis F, et al. Mechanism of eIF6 release from the nascent 60S ribosomal subunit. Nat Struct Mol Biol. 2015;22:914–9. https://doi.org/10.1038/nsmb.3112.
32. Wong CC, Traynor D, Basse N, Kay RR, Warren AJ. Defective ribosome assembly in Shwachman-Diamond syndrome. Blood. 2011;118:4305–12. https://doi.org/10.1182/blood-2011-06-353938.
33. Freed EF, Bleichert F, Dutca LM, Baserga SJ. When ribosomes go bad: diseases of ribosome biogenesis. Mol BioSyst. 2010;6:481–93. https://doi.org/10.1039/b919670f.
34. Mills EW, Green R. Ribosomopathies: there's strength in numbers. Science. 2017;358:eaan2755. https://doi.org/10.1126/science.aan2755.
35. Kampen KR, Sulima SO, Vereecke S, De Keersmaecker K. Hallmarks of ribosomopathies. Nucleic Acids Res. 2020;48:1013–28. https://doi.org/10.1093/nar/gkz637.
36. Alter BP, Giri N, Savage SA, Rosenberg PS. Cancer in the National Cancer Institute inherited bone marrow failure syndrome cohort after fifteen years of follow-up. Haematologica. 2018;103:30–9. https://doi.org/10.3324/haematol.2017.178111.
37. Lipton JM, et al. Colorectal cancer screening and surveillance strategy for patients with Diamond Blackfan anemia: preliminary recommendations from the Diamond Blackfan anemia registry. Pediatr Blood Cancer. 2021;68:e28984. https://doi.org/10.1002/pbc.28984.
38. Vlachos A, Rosenberg PS, Atsidaftos E, Alter BP, Lipton JM. Incidence of neoplasia in Diamond Blackfan anemia: a report from the Diamond Blackfan anemia registry. Blood. 2012;119:3815–9. https://doi.org/10.1182/blood-2011-08-375972.
39. Martin ES, et al. Spectrum of hematological malignancies, clonal evolution and outcomes in 144 Mayo Clinic patients with germline predisposition syndromes. Am J Hematol. 2021;96:1450–60. https://doi.org/10.1002/ajh.26321.
40. De Keersmaecker K, Sulima SO, Dinman JD. Ribosomopathies and the paradox of cellular hypo- to hyperproliferation. Blood. 2015;125:1377–82. https://doi.org/10.1182/blood-2014-10-569616.
41. Choesmel V, et al. Impaired ribosome biogenesis in Diamond-Blackfan anemia. Blood. 2007;109:1275–83. https://doi.org/10.1182/blood-2006-07-038372.
42. Leger-Silvestre I, et al. Specific role for yeast homologs of the Diamond Blackfan anemia-associated Rps19 protein in ribosome synthesis. J Biol Chem. 2005;280:38177–85. https://doi.org/10.1074/jbc.M506916200.
43. Heiss NS, et al. X-linked dyskeratosis congenita is caused by mutations in a highly conserved gene with putative nucleolar functions. Nat Genet. 1998;19:32–8. https://doi.org/10.1038/ng0598-32.
44. Montellese C, et al. Poly(A)-specific ribonuclease is a nuclear ribosome biogenesis factor involved in human 18S rRNA maturation. Nucleic Acids Res. 2017;45:6822–36. https://doi.org/10.1093/nar/gkx253.

45. Nachmani D, et al. Germline NPM1 mutations lead to altered rRNA 2'-O-methylation and cause dyskeratosis congenita. Nat Genet. 2019;51:1518–29. https://doi.org/10.1038/s41588-019-0502-z.
46. Hilcenko C, et al. Aberrant 3′ oligoadenylation of spliceosomal U6 small nuclear RNA in poikiloderma with neutropenia. Blood. 2012;121:1028–38. https://doi.org/10.1182/blood-2012-10-461491.
47. Tummala H, et al. Germline thymidylate synthase deficiency impacts nucleotide metabolism and causes dyskeratosis congenita. Am J Hum Genet. 2022;109:1472–83. https://doi.org/10.1016/j.ajhg.2022.06.014.
48. Dos Santos RS, et al. dUTPase (DUT) is mutated in a novel monogenic syndrome with diabetes and bone marrow failure. Diabetes. 2017;66:1086–96. https://doi.org/10.2337/db16-0839.
49. Jack K, et al. rRNA pseudouridylation defects affect ribosomal ligand binding and translational fidelity from yeast to human cells. Mol Cell. 2011;44:660–6. https://doi.org/10.1016/j.molcel.2011.09.017.
50. Ruggero D, et al. Dyskeratosis congenita and cancer in mice deficient in ribosomal RNA modification. Science. 2003;299:259–62. https://doi.org/10.1126/science.1079447.
51. Thumati NR, et al. Severity of X-linked dyskeratosis congenita (DKCX) cellular defects is not directly related to dyskerin (DKC1) activity in ribosomal RNA biogenesis or mRNA translation. Hum Mutat. 2013;34:1698–707. https://doi.org/10.1002/humu.22447.
52. Signer RA, Magee JA, Salic A, Morrison SJ. Haematopoietic stem cells require a highly regulated protein synthesis rate. Nature. 2014;509:49–54. https://doi.org/10.1038/nature13035.
53. Corsini NS, et al. Coordinated control of mRNA and rRNA processing controls embryonic stem cell pluripotency and differentiation. Cell Stem Cell. 2018;22:543–558 e512. https://doi.org/10.1016/j.stem.2018.03.002.
54. Sanchez CG, et al. Regulation of ribosome biogenesis and protein synthesis controls germline stem cell differentiation. Cell Stem Cell. 2016;18:276–90. https://doi.org/10.1016/j.stem.2015.11.004.
55. Fichelson P, et al. Live-imaging of single stem cells within their niche reveals that a U3snoRNP component segregates asymmetrically and is required for self-renewal in Drosophila. Nat Cell Biol. 2009;11:685–93. https://doi.org/10.1038/ncb1874.
56. Zhang Q, Shalaby NA, Buszczak M. Changes in rRNA transcription influence proliferation and cell fate within a stem cell lineage. Science. 2014;343:298–301. https://doi.org/10.1126/science.1246384.
57. Yu J, et al. Protein synthesis and degradation are essential to regulate germline stem cell homeostasis in Drosophila testes. Development. 2016;143:2930–45. https://doi.org/10.1242/dev.134247.
58. Neumuller RA, et al. Genome-wide analysis of self-renewal in Drosophila neural stem cells by transgenic RNAi. Cell Stem Cell. 2011;8:580–93. https://doi.org/10.1016/j.stem.2011.02.022.
59. Fortier S, MacRae T, Bilodeau M, Sargeant T, Sauvageau G. Haploinsufficiency screen highlights two distinct groups of ribosomal protein genes essential for embryonic stem cell fate. Proc Natl Acad Sci USA. 2015;112:2127–32. https://doi.org/10.1073/pnas.1418845112.
60. You KT, Park J, Kim VN. Role of the small subunit processome in the maintenance of pluripotent stem cells. Genes Dev. 2015;29:2004–9. https://doi.org/10.1101/gad.267112.115.
61. Le Bouteiller M, et al. Notchless-dependent ribosome synthesis is required for the maintenance of adult hematopoietic stem cells. J Exp Med. 2013;210:2351–69. https://doi.org/10.1084/jem.20122019.
62. Gay DM, Lund AH, Jansson MD. Translational control through ribosome heterogeneity and functional specialization. Trends Biochem Sci. 2022;47:66–81. https://doi.org/10.1016/j.tibs.2021.07.001.
63. Saba JA, Liakath-Ali K, Green R, Watt FM. Translational control of stem cell function. Nat Rev Mol Cell Biol. 2021;22:671–90. https://doi.org/10.1038/s41580-021-00386-2.

64. Genuth NR, Barna M. The discovery of ribosome heterogeneity and its implications for gene regulation and organismal life. Mol Cell. 2018;71:364–74. https://doi.org/10.1016/j.molcel.2018.07.018.
65. Shi Z, et al. Heterogeneous ribosomes preferentially translate distinct subpools of mRNAs genome-wide. Mol Cell. 2017;67:71–83 e77. https://doi.org/10.1016/j.molcel.2017.05.021.
66. Simsek D, et al. The mammalian Ribo-interactome reveals ribosome functional diversity and heterogeneity. Cell. 2017;169:1051–1065 e1018. https://doi.org/10.1016/j.cell.2017.05.022.
67. Li D, Wang J. Ribosome heterogeneity in stem cells and development. J Cell Biol. 2020;219:e202001108. https://doi.org/10.1083/jcb.202001108.
68. Locati MD, et al. Expression of distinct maternal and somatic 5.8S, 18S, and 28S rRNA types during zebrafish development. RNA. 2017;23:1188–99. https://doi.org/10.1261/rna.061515.117.
69. Parks MM, et al. Variant ribosomal RNA alleles are conserved and exhibit tissue-specific expression. Sci Adv. 2018;4:eaao0665. https://doi.org/10.1126/sciadv.aao0665.
70. Wang M, Lemos B. Ribosomal DNA copy number amplification and loss in human cancers is linked to tumor genetic context, nucleolus activity, and proliferation. PLoS Genet. 2017;13:e1006994. https://doi.org/10.1371/journal.pgen.1006994.
71. Hafner SJ, et al. Ribosomal RNA 2'-O-methylation dynamics impact cell fate decisions. Dev Cell. 2023;58:1593–1609 e1599. https://doi.org/10.1016/j.devcel.2023.06.007.
72. Yoon A, et al. Impaired control of IRES-mediated translation in X-linked dyskeratosis congenita. Science. 2006;312:902–6. https://doi.org/10.1126/science.1123835.
73. Gupta V, Warner JR. Ribosome-omics of the human ribosome. RNA. 2014;20:1004–13. https://doi.org/10.1261/rna.043653.113.
74. Guimaraes JC, Zavolan M. Patterns of ribosomal protein expression specify normal and malignant human cells. Genome Biol. 2016;17:236. https://doi.org/10.1186/s13059-016-1104-z.
75. Ferretti MB, Ghalei H, Ward EA, Potts EL, Karbstein K. Rps26 directs mRNA-specific translation by recognition of Kozak sequence elements. Nat Struct Mol Biol. 2017;24:700–7. https://doi.org/10.1038/nsmb.3442.
76. Nguyen AT, et al. UBE2O remodels the proteome during terminal erythroid differentiation. Science. 2017;357:eaan0218. https://doi.org/10.1126/science.aan0218.
77. Higgins R, et al. The unfolded protein response triggers site-specific regulatory Ubiquitylation of 40S ribosomal proteins. Mol Cell. 2015;59:35–49. https://doi.org/10.1016/j.molcel.2015.04.026.
78. Monem PC, Arribere JA. A ubiquitin language communicates ribosomal distress. Semin Cell Dev Biol. 2024;154:131–7. https://doi.org/10.1016/j.semcdb.2023.03.009.
79. DaRosa PA, et al. UFM1 E3 ligase promotes recycling of 60S ribosomal subunits from the ER. Nature. 2024;627:445–52. https://doi.org/10.1038/s41586-024-07073-0.
80. Dopler A, et al. P-stalk ribosomes act as master regulators of cytokine-mediated processes. Cell. 2024;187:6981–6993 e6923. https://doi.org/10.1016/j.cell.2024.09.039.
81. Robertson N, et al. A disease-linked lncRNA mutation in RNase MRP inhibits ribosome synthesis. Nat Commun. 2022;13:649. https://doi.org/10.1038/s41467-022-28295-8.
82. MacInnes AW. The role of the ribosome in the regulation of longevity and lifespan extension. Wiley Interdiscip Rev RNA. 2016;7:198–212. https://doi.org/10.1002/wrna.1325.
83. Khajuria RK, et al. Ribosome levels selectively regulate translation and lineage commitment in human hematopoiesis. Cell. 2018;173:90–103 e119. https://doi.org/10.1016/j.cell.2018.02.036.
84. Kampen KR, et al. The ribosomal RPL10 R98S mutation drives IRES-dependent BCL-2 translation in T-ALL. Leukemia. 2019;33:319–32. https://doi.org/10.1038/s41375-018-0176-z.
85. Iskander D, et al. Single-cell profiling of human bone marrow progenitors reveals mechanisms of failing erythropoiesis in Diamond-Blackfan anemia. Sci Transl Med. 2021;13:eabf0113. https://doi.org/10.1126/scitranslmed.abf0113.

86. Boussaid I, et al. Integrated analyses of translatome and proteome identify the rules of translation selectivity in RPS14-deficient cells. Haematologica. 2021;106:746–58. https://doi.org/10.3324/haematol.2019.239970.
87. Ludwig LS, et al. Altered translation of GATA1 in Diamond-Blackfan anemia. Nat Med. 2014;20:748–53. https://doi.org/10.1038/nm.3557.
88. Mills EW, Wangen J, Green R, Ingolia NT. Dynamic regulation of a ribosome rescue pathway in erythroid cells and platelets. Cell Rep. 2016;17:1–10. https://doi.org/10.1016/j.celrep.2016.08.088.
89. Liakath-Ali K, et al. An evolutionarily conserved ribosome-rescue pathway maintains epidermal homeostasis. Nature. 2018;556:376–80. https://doi.org/10.1038/s41586-018-0032-3.
90. Dutt S, et al. Haploinsufficiency for ribosomal protein genes causes selective activation of p53 in human erythroid progenitor cells. Blood. 2011;117:2567–76. https://doi.org/10.1182/blood-2010-07-295238.
91. Moniz H, et al. Primary hematopoietic cells from DBA patients with mutations in RPL11 and RPS19 genes exhibit distinct erythroid phenotype in vitro. Cell Death Dis. 2012;3:e356. https://doi.org/10.1038/cddis.2012.88.
92. Ellis SR. Nucleolar stress in Diamond Blackfan anemia pathophysiology. Biochim Biophys Acta. 2014;1842:765–8. https://doi.org/10.1016/j.bbadis.2013.12.013.
93. Hannan KM, et al. Nuclear stabilization of p53 requires a functional nucleolar surveillance pathway. Cell Rep. 2022;41:111571. https://doi.org/10.1016/j.celrep.2022.111571.
94. Eastham MJ, et al. The induction of p53 correlates with defects in the production, but not the levels, of the small ribosomal subunit and stalled large ribosomal subunit biogenesis. Nucleic Acids Res. 2023;51:9397–414. https://doi.org/10.1093/nar/gkad637.
95. Dai MS, et al. Ribosomal protein L23 activates p53 by inhibiting MDM2 function in response to ribosomal perturbation but not to translation inhibition. Mol Cell Biol. 2004;24:7654–68. https://doi.org/10.1128/Mcb.24.17.7654 7668.2004.
96. Horn HF, Vousden KH. Cooperation between the ribosomal proteins L5 and L11 in the p53 pathway. Oncogene. 2008;27:5774–84. https://doi.org/10.1038/onc.2008.189.
97. Tagneres S, et al. SURF2 is a MDM2 antagonist in triggering the nucleolar stress response. Nat Commun. 2024;15:8404. https://doi.org/10.1038/s41467-024-52659-x.
98. McGowan KA, et al. Ribosomal mutations cause p53-mediated dark skin and pleiotropic effects. Nat Genet. 2008;40:963–70. https://doi.org/10.1038/ng.188.
99. Uechi T, et al. Deficiency of ribosomal protein S19 during early embryogenesis leads to reduction of erythrocytes in a zebrafish model of Diamond-Blackfan anemia. Hum Mol Genet. 2008;17:3204–11. https://doi.org/10.1093/hmg/ddn216.
100. Danilova N, Sakamoto KM, Lin S. Ribosomal protein S19 deficiency in zebrafish leads to developmental abnormalities and defective erythropoiesis through activation of p53 protein family. Blood. 2008;112:5228–37. https://doi.org/10.1182/blood-2008-01-132290.
101. Chakraborty A, Uechi T, Higa S, Torihara H, Kenmochi N. Loss of ribosomal protein L11 affects zebrafish embryonic development through a p53-dependent apoptotic response. PLoS One. 2009;4:e4152. https://doi.org/10.1371/journal.pone.0004152.
102. Falcon KT, et al. Dynamic regulation and requirement for ribosomal RNA transcription during mammalian development. Proc Natl Acad Sci USA. 2022;119:e2116974119. https://doi.org/10.1073/pnas.2116974119.
103. Kirwan M, et al. Dyskeratosis congenita and the DNA damage response. Br J Haematol. 2011;153:634–43. https://doi.org/10.1111/j.1365-2141.2011.08679.x.
104. Tourlakis ME, et al. In vivo senescence in the Sbds-deficient murine pancreas: cell-type specific consequences of translation insufficiency. PLoS Genet. 2015;11:e1005288. https://doi.org/10.1371/journal.pgen.1005288.
105. Frattini A, et al. Enhanced p53 levels are involved in the reduced mineralization capacity of osteoblasts derived from Shwachman-Diamond syndrome subjects. Int J Mol Sci. 2021;22:13331. https://doi.org/10.3390/ijms222413331.

106. Ulirsch JC, Verboon JM, Kazerounian S, et al. The genetic landscape of Diamond-Blackfan anemia. Am J Hum Genet. 2018;103:930–47.
107. Wlodarski MW, et al. Diagnosis, treatment, and surveillance of Diamond-Blackfan anaemia syndrome: international consensus statement. Lancet Haematol. 2024;11:e368–82. https://doi.org/10.1016/S2352-3026(24)00063-2.
108. Gripp KW, et al. Diamond-Blackfan anemia with mandibulofacial dystostosis is heterogeneous, including the novel DBA genes TSR2 and RPS28. Am J Med Genet A. 2014;164A:2240–9. https://doi.org/10.1002/ajmg.a.36633.
109. O'Donohue MF, et al. HEATR3 variants impair nuclear import of uL18 (RPL5) and drive Diamond-Blackfan anemia. Blood. 2022;139:3111–26. https://doi.org/10.1182/blood.2021011846.
110. Sankaran VG, et al. Exome sequencing identifies GATA1 mutations resulting in Diamond-Blackfan anemia. J Clin Invest. 2012;122:2439–43. https://doi.org/10.1172/JCI63597.
111. Kim AR, et al. Functional selectivity in cytokine signaling revealed through a pathogenic EPO mutation. Cell. 2017;168:1053–1064 e1015. https://doi.org/10.1016/j.cell.2017.02.026.
112. Toki T, et al. De novo mutations activating germline TP53 in an inherited bone-marrow-failure syndrome. Am J Hum Genet. 2018;103:440–7. https://doi.org/10.1016/j.ajhg.2018.07.020.
113. Da Costa L, Leblanc T, Mohandas N. Diamond-Blackfan anemia. Blood. 2020;136:1262–73. https://doi.org/10.1182/blood.2019000947.
114. Da Costa L, Narla A, Mohandas N. An update on the pathogenesis and diagnosis of Diamond-Blackfan anemia. F1000Res. 2018;7 https://doi.org/10.12688/f1000research.15542.1.
115. Da Costa L, et al. Molecular approaches to diagnose Diamond-Blackfan anemia: the EuroDBA experience. Eur J Med Genet. 2018;61:664–73. https://doi.org/10.1016/j.ejmg.2017.10.017.
116. Doherty L, et al. Ribosomal protein genes RPS10 and RPS26 are commonly mutated in Diamond-Blackfan anemia. Am J Hum Genet. 2010;86:222–8. https://doi.org/10.1016/j.ajhg.2009.12.015.
117. Farrar JE, et al. Abnormalities of the large ribosomal subunit protein, Rpl35a, in Diamond-Blackfan anemia. Blood. 2008;112:1582–92. https://doi.org/10.1182/blood-2008-02-140012.
118. Gazda HT, et al. Ribosomal protein S24 gene is mutated in Diamond-Blackfan anemia. Am J Hum Genet. 2006;79:1110–8. https://doi.org/10.1086/510020.
119. Gazda HT, et al. Frameshift mutation in p53 regulator RPL26 is associated with multiple physical abnormalities and a specific pre-ribosomal RNA processing defect in Diamond-blackfan anemia. Hum Mutat. 2012;33:1037–44. https://doi.org/10.1002/humu.22081.
120. Gazda HT, et al. Ribosomal protein L5 and L11 mutations are associated with cleft palate and abnormal thumbs in Diamond-Blackfan anemia patients. Am J Hum Genet. 2008;83:769–80. https://doi.org/10.1016/j.ajhg.2008.11.004.
121. Lezzerini M, et al. Ribosomal protein gene RPL9 variants can differentially impair ribosome function and cellular metabolism. Nucleic Acids Res. 2020;48:770–87. https://doi.org/10.1093/nar/gkz1042.
122. Mirabello L, et al. Whole-exome sequencing and functional studies identify RPS29 as a novel gene mutated in multicase Diamond-Blackfan anemia families. Blood. 2014;124:24–32. https://doi.org/10.1182/blood-2013-11-540278.
123. Wang R, et al. Loss of function mutations in RPL27 and RPS27 identified by whole-exome sequencing in Diamond-Blackfan anaemia. Br J Haematol. 2015;168:854–64. https://doi.org/10.1111/bjh.13229.
124. Wlodarski MW, et al. Recurring mutations in RPL15 are linked to hydrops fetalis and treatment independence in Diamond-Blackfan anemia. Haematologica. 2018;103:949–58. https://doi.org/10.3324/haematol.2017.177980.
125. Draptchinskaia N, et al. The gene encoding ribosomal protein S19 is mutated in Diamond-Blackfan anaemia. Nat Genet. 1999;21:169–75. https://doi.org/10.1038/5951.
126. Ohene-Abuakwa Y, Orfali KA, Marius C, Ball SE. Two-phase culture in Diamond Blackfan anemia: localization of erythroid defect. Blood. 2005;105:838–46. https://doi.org/10.1182/blood-2004-03-1016.

127. Aspesi A, et al. Dissecting the transcriptional phenotype of ribosomal protein deficiency: implications for Diamond-Blackfan Anemia. Gene. 2014;545:282–9. https://doi.org/10.1016/j.gene.2014.04.077.
128. Torihara H, et al. Erythropoiesis failure due to RPS19 deficiency is independent of an activated Tp53 response in a zebrafish model of Diamond-Blackfan anaemia. Br J Haematol. 2011;152:648–54. https://doi.org/10.1111/j.1365-2141.2010.08535.x.
129. Singh SA, et al. p53-independent cell cycle and erythroid differentiation defects in murine embryonic stem cells haploinsufficient for Diamond Blackfan anemia-proteins: RPS19 versus RPL5. PLoS One. 2014;9:e89098. https://doi.org/10.1371/journal.pone.0089098.
130. Gastou M, et al. The severe phenotype of Diamond-Blackfan anemia is modulated by heat shock protein 70. Blood Adv. 2017;1:1959–76. https://doi.org/10.1182/bloodadvances.2017008078.
131. Rio S, et al. Regulation of globin-heme balance in Diamond-Blackfan anemia by HSP70/GATA1. Blood. 2019;133:1358–70. https://doi.org/10.1182/blood-2018-09-875674.
132. Yang Z, et al. Delayed globin synthesis leads to excess heme and the macrocytic anemia of Diamond Blackfan anemia and del(5q) myelodysplastic syndrome. Sci Transl Med. 2016;8:338ra367. https://doi.org/10.1126/scitranslmed.aaf3006.
133. Doty RT, et al. Single-cell analyses demonstrate that a heme-GATA1 feedback loop regulates red cell differentiation. Blood. 2019;133:457–69. https://doi.org/10.1182/blood-2018-05-850412.
134. Heijnen HF, et al. Ribosomal protein mutations induce autophagy through S6 kinase inhibition of the insulin pathway. PLoS Genet. 2014;10:e1004371. https://doi.org/10.1371/journal.pgen.1004371.
135. Doulatov S, et al. Drug discovery for Diamond-Blackfan anemia using reprogrammed hematopoietic progenitors. Sci Transl Med. 2017;9 https://doi.org/10.1126/scitranslmed.aah5645.
136. Gonzalez-Menendez P, et al. Arginine metabolism regulates human erythroid differentiation through hypusination of eIF5A. Blood. 2023;141:2520–36. https://doi.org/10.1182/blood.2022017584.
137. Boocock GR, et al. Mutations in SBDS are associated with Shwachman-Diamond syndrome. Nat Genet. 2003;33:97–101. https://doi.org/10.1038/ng1062.
138. Warren AJ. Molecular basis of the human ribosomopathy Shwachman-Diamond syndrome. Adv Biol Regul. 2018;67:109–27. https://doi.org/10.1016/j.jbior.2017.09.002.
139. Nelson A, Myers K. In: Adam MP, et al., editors. GeneReviews((R)); 1993.
140. Dhanraj S, et al. Biallelic mutations in DNAJC21 cause Shwachman-Diamond syndrome. Blood. 2017;129:1557–62. https://doi.org/10.1182/blood-2016-08-735431.
141. Tummala H, et al. DNAJC21 mutations link a cancer-prone bone marrow failure syndrome to corruption in 60S ribosome subunit maturation. Am J Hum Genet. 2016;99:115–24. https://doi.org/10.1016/j.ajhg.2016.05.002.
142. Stepensky P, et al. Mutations in EFL1, an SBDS partner, are associated with infantile pancytopenia, exocrine pancreatic insufficiency and skeletal anomalies in aShwachman-Diamond like syndrome. J Med Genet. 2017;54:558–66. https://doi.org/10.1136/jmedgenet-2016-104366.
143. Tan S, et al. EFL1 mutations impair eIF6 release to cause Shwachman-Diamond syndrome. Blood. 2019;134:277–90. https://doi.org/10.1182/blood.2018893404.
144. Carapito R, et al. Mutations in signal recognition particle SRP54 cause syndromic neutropenia with Shwachman-Diamond-like features. J Clin Invest. 2017;127:4090–103. https://doi.org/10.1172/JCI92876.
145. Bellanne-Chantelot C, et al. Mutations in the SRP54 gene cause severe congenital neutropenia as well as Shwachman-Diamond-like syndrome. Blood. 2018;132:1318–31. https://doi.org/10.1182/blood-2017-12-820308.
146. Jaako P, et al. eIF6 rebinding dynamically couples ribosome maturation and translation. Nat Commun. 2022;13:1562. https://doi.org/10.1038/s41467-022-29214-7.
147. Donadieu J, et al. Classification of and risk factors for hematologic complications in a French national cohort of 102 patients with Shwachman-Diamond syndrome. Haematologica. 2012;97:1312–9. https://doi.org/10.3324/haematol.2011.057489.

148. In K, et al. Shwachman-Bodian-Diamond syndrome (SBDS) protein deficiency impairs translation re-initiation from C/EBPalpha and C/EBPbeta mRNAs. Nucleic Acids Res. 2016;44:4134–46. https://doi.org/10.1093/nar/gkw005.
149. Tourlakis ME, et al. Deficiency of Sbds in the mouse pancreas leads to features of Shwachman-Diamond syndrome, with loss of zymogen granules. Gastroenterology. 2012;143:481–92. https://doi.org/10.1053/j.gastro.2012.04.012.
150. Revy P, Kannengiesser C, Fischer A. Somatic genetic rescue in Mendelian haematopoietic diseases. Nat Rev Genet. 2019;20:582–98. https://doi.org/10.1038/s41576-019-0139-x.
151. Machado HE, et al. Convergent somatic evolution commences in utero in a germline ribosomopathy. Nat Commun. 2023;14:5092. https://doi.org/10.1038/s41467-023-40896-5.
152. Kennedy AL, et al. Distinct genetic pathways define pre-malignant versus compensatory clonal hematopoiesis in Shwachman-Diamond syndrome. Nat Commun. 2021;12:1334. https://doi.org/10.1038/s41467-021-21588-4.
153. Tan S, et al. Somatic genetic rescue of a germline ribosome assembly defect. Nat Commun. 2021;12:5044. https://doi.org/10.1038/s41467-021-24999-5.
154. Lee S, et al. Somatic uniparental disomy mitigates the most damaging EFL1 allele combination in Shwachman-Diamond syndrome. Blood. 2021;138:2117–28. https://doi.org/10.1182/blood.2021010913.
155. Parikh S, et al. Acquired copy number neutral loss of heterozygosity of chromosome 7 associated with clonal haematopoiesis in a patient with Shwachman-Diamond syndrome. Br J Haematol. 2012;159:480–2. https://doi.org/10.1111/bjh.12032.
156. Xia J, et al. Somatic mutations and clonal hematopoiesis in congenital neutropenia. Blood. 2018;131:408–16. https://doi.org/10.1182/blood-2017-08-801985.
157. Cull AH, Kent DG, Warren AJ. Emerging genetic technologies informing personalized medicine in SDS and other inherited bone marrow failure disorders. Blood. 2024;144:931–9. https://doi.org/10.1182/blood.2023019986.
158. Vulliamy T, et al. Mutations in the telomerase component NHP2 cause the premature ageing syndrome dyskeratosis congenita. Proc Natl Acad Sci USA. 2008;105:8073–8. https://doi.org/10.1073/pnas.0800042105.
159. Benyelles M, et al. Impaired telomere integrity and rRNA biogenesis in PARN-deficient patients and knock-out models. EMBO Mol Med. 2019;11:e10201. https://doi.org/10.15252/emmm.201810201.
160. Tummala H, et al. Poly(A)-specific ribonuclease deficiency impacts telomere biology and causes dyskeratosis congenita. J Clin Invest. 2015;125:2151–60. https://doi.org/10.1172/JCI78963.
161. Dokal I. Dyskeratosis congenita. Hematology Am Soc Hematol Educ Program. 2011;480-486:2011. https://doi.org/10.1182/asheducation-2011.1.480.
162. Dokal I, Vulliamy T, Mason P, Bessler M. Clinical utility gene card for: Dyskeratosis congenita – update 2015. Eur J Hum Genet. 2015;23 https://doi.org/10.1038/ejhg.2014.170.
163. Dokal I, Tummala H, Vulliamy T. Inherited bone marrow failure in the pediatric patient. Blood. 2022;140:556–70. https://doi.org/10.1182/blood.2020006481.
164. Touzot F, et al. Heterogeneous telomere defects in patients with severe forms of dyskeratosis congenita. J Allergy Clin Immunol. 2012;129:473–82., 482 e471–473. https://doi.org/10.1016/j.jaci.2011.09.043.
165. Wong JM, Collins K. Telomerase RNA level limits telomere maintenance in X-linked dyskeratosis congenita. Genes Dev. 2006;20:2848–58. https://doi.org/10.1101/gad.1476206.
166. Gu BW, et al. Impaired telomere maintenance and decreased canonical WNT signaling but Normal ribosome biogenesis in induced pluripotent stem cells from X-linked Dyskeratosis Congenita patients. PLoS One. 2015;10:e0127414. https://doi.org/10.1371/journal.pone.0127414.
167. McKusick VA, Eldridge R, Hostetler JA, Ruangwit U, Egeland JA, Dwarfism in the Amish. Ii. Cartilage-hair hypoplasia. Bull Johns Hopkins Hosp. 1965;116:285–326.

168. Ridanpaa M, et al. Mutations in the RNA component of RNase MRP cause a pleiotropic human disease, cartilage-hair hypoplasia. Cell. 2001;104:195–203. https://doi.org/10.1016/s0092-8674(01)00205-7.
169. Goldfarb KC, Cech TR. Targeted CRISPR disruption reveals a role for RNase MRP RNA in human preribosomal RNA processing. Genes Dev. 2017;31:59–71. https://doi.org/10.1101/gad.286963.116.
170. Thiel CT, Mortier G, Kaitila I, Reis A, Rauch A. Type and level of RMRP functional impairment predicts phenotype in the cartilage hair hypoplasia-anauxetic dysplasia spectrum. Am J Hum Genet. 2007;81:519–29. https://doi.org/10.1086/521034.
171. Kostjukovits S, et al. Decreased telomere length in children with cartilage-hair hypoplasia. J Med Genet. 2017;54:365–70. https://doi.org/10.1136/jmedgenet-2016-104279.
172. Marszalek-Kruk BA, Wojcicki P. Identification of three novel TCOF1 mutations in patients with Treacher Collins syndrome. Hum Genome Var. 2021;8:36. https://doi.org/10.1038/s41439-021-00168-4.
173. Marszalek-Kruk BA, Wojcicki P, Dowgierd K, Smigiel R. Treacher Collins syndrome: genetics, clinical features and management. Genes (Basel). 2021;12:1392. https://doi.org/10.3390/genes12091392.
174. Dauwerse JG, et al. Mutations in genes encoding subunits of RNA polymerases I and III cause Treacher Collins syndrome. Nat Genet. 2011;43:20–2. https://doi.org/10.1038/ng.724.
175. Sanchez E, et al. POLR1B and neural crest cell anomalies in Treacher Collins syndrome type 4. Genet Med. 2020;22:547–56. https://doi.org/10.1038/s41436-019-0669-9.
176. Jones NC, et al. Prevention of the neurocristopathy Treacher Collins syndrome through inhibition of p53 function. Nat Med. 2008;14:125–33. https://doi.org/10.1038/nm1725.
177. Narla A, Ebert BL. Ribosomopathies: human disorders of ribosome dysfunction. Blood. 2010;115:3196–205. https://doi.org/10.1182/blood-2009-10-178129.

Open Access This chapter is licensed under the terms of the Creative Commons Attribution 4.0 International License (http://creativecommons.org/licenses/by/4.0/), which permits use, sharing, adaptation, distribution and reproduction in any medium or format, as long as you give appropriate credit to the original author(s) and the source, provide a link to the Creative Commons license and indicate if changes were made.

The images or other third party material in this chapter are included in the chapter's Creative Commons license, unless indicated otherwise in a credit line to the material. If material is not included in the chapter's Creative Commons license and your intended use is not permitted by statutory regulation or exceeds the permitted use, you will need to obtain permission directly from the copyright holder.

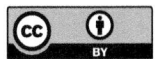

Chapter 20
Clinical Management of Diamond–Blackfan Anemia Syndromes and Other Inherited Ribosomal Disorders

Thierry Leblanc and Maurizio Miano

Introduction

The term ribosomopathy emerged in the medical literature in 2010 [1]. This is an expanding group of rare diseases associated with pathogenic variants in genes involved in ribosome biosynthesis and functions. This chapter will focus on the clinical management of inherited ribosomopathies associated with a hematological phenotype [2]. The pathology of ribosomopathies is fully detailed in another chapter in this book.

Ribosomopathies with Hematological Features

Inherited ribosomopathies associated with a hematological phenotype are listed in Table 20.1. Most of them are also classified as inherited bone marrow failure syndromes (IBMFs), and some are discussed elsewhere as Shwachman–Diamond syndrome (fully detailed in another chapter in this book) and telomere biology disorders (TBDs) (fully detailed in another chapter in this book).

Diamond–Blackfan anemia syndrome (DBAS) comprises true ribosomopathies and a small subgroup, newly named "DBA-other," not associated with ribosomal

---

CRMR Aplasies médullaires
CRMR Cytopénies Autoimmunes de l'enfant

T. Leblanc (✉)
Department of Pediatric Hematology and Immunology, Robert Debré Academic Hospital
GHU AP-HP Nord Université Paris Cité, Paris, France
e-mail: thierry.leblanc@aphp.fr

M. Miano
Hematology Unit, IRCCS Istituto Giannina Gaslini, Genoa, Italy

Table 20.1 Ribosomopathies with hematological phenotype

Disease	Genes	Transmission	Main hematological phenotypes	Main extra-hematological phenotypes
Diamond-Blackfan anemia syndrome	RPS7, RPS10, RPS15A, RPS17, **RPS19**, RPS20, RPS24, **RPS26**, RPS27, RPS28, RPS29 RL4, **RPL5**, RPL8, RPL9, **RPL11**, RPL15, RPL17, RPL18, RPL26, RPL27, RPL31, RPL35, RPL35A TSR2 HEATR3	AD X-linked AR	Hydrops fetalis (rare) Erythroblastopenia and severe anemia in an infant (classical phenotype) Mild macrocytic anemia isolated or associated to mild leuconeutropenia. Platelets counts more often normal; transient thrombocytosis possible in infants Isolated macrocytosis Normal blood counts (previously reported as silent phenotype) Severe hematological toxicity (BMF) post chemotherapy HM: Mostly MDS and AML	Growth retardation Congenital anomalies: Most frequent: Thumbs, cleft palate, hearth and kidney malformations Immunodeficiency (CVD type) Solid tumors: High-risk for osteosarcoma and colorectal cancer
Shwachman-diamond syndrome	**SBDS** EFL1, DNAJC21, SRP54,	AR	Neutropenia associated or not to other cytopenias BMF HM: Mostly MDS and AML	Growth retardation Pancreatic insufficiency Immune deficiency (CVD type)
Telomeropathies	DKC1 PARN, NHP2, NOP10	X-linked AD or AR	Pancytopenia, BMF HM: MDS/AML, lymphomas	Abnormal skin pigmentation, dystrophy Of the nails, premature canities, oral leukoplakia Pulmonary fibrosis Liver diseases Immune deficiency (B and T) Solid tumors
Cartilage-hair hypoplasia	**RMRP**	AR	Macrocytic and hyporegenerative anemia (may be severe requiring transfusion support) HM: NHL (mostly DLBCL), HL, leukemias	Severe disproportionate (short-limb) short stature Joint hypermobility Fine and silky hair Hirschsprung disease Impaired spermatogenesis Immune deficiency (B and T) Augmented risk for cancer

AD autosomic dominant, *AML* acute myeloblastic leukemia, *AR* autosomic recessive, *BMF* bone marrow failure, *CVD* common variable deficiency, *HM* hematological malignancies, *MDS* myelodysplastic syndrome, *NHL* non-Hodgkin lymphomas protein genes or genes directly involved in ribogenesis [3]. DBA-other is associated with either specific variants in *GATA1*, the consequence of which is the expression of GATA1s but the absence of full-length GATA1 [4], or *TP53* gain-of-function mutation [5, 6]. Both diseases may present with erythroblastopenia or hyporegenerative anemia and have altered pathways directly connected to DBAS.

Regarding TBD, only a few of the involved genes are associated with a defect of rRNA processing or ribosomal biosynthesis, and whether ribosome biogenesis impairment can contribute to the clinical phenotype and aggravate it remains to be defined [2]. The clinical management of patients affected with TBD is actually not different for this subgroup.

Cartilage-hair hypoplasia (CHH) is a true ribosomopathy, and the majority of patients present with hypo-regenerative anemia, which may be severe in a few of them.

Treacher Collins syndrome (TCS) may mimic the DBAS extra-hematological phenotype but is not associated with any hematological phenotype.

Clinical Management of Diamond–Blackfan Anemia Syndrome

DBAS is a rare disease, with an estimated incidence of five to seven cases/million live births. International guidelines for the diagnosis, treatment, and surveillance of patients with Diamond–Blackfan anemia syndrome (DBAS) have been recently published [3]. The designation "syndrome" underscores that patients with DBAS may present without anemia.

DBAS-Positive Diagnosis

DBAS diagnosis implies the association of a pathogenic or likely pathogenic variant in one of the DBAS genes and a known DBAS phenotype. Current consensus is that a pathogenic variant is sufficient to diagnose DBAS [3]. This allows the inclusion of patients previously classified as "silent phenotype," as we know now that such patients may eventually present with anemia, hypogammaglobulinemia, myelodysplastic syndrome (MDS), or DBAS-related cancer when they get older.

Currently, a pathogenic variant may be identified in up to 90% of patients; patients without variants are candidates for whole exome or whole genome sequencing. Other biological features are supportive (Table 20.2).

The typical clinical presentation is an infant with severe non-regenerative anemia and isolated erythroblastopenia at the bone marrow (BM) evaluation; other hematological phenotypes are listed in Table 20.1. More than half of the patients have congenital abnormalities, which may be very diverse, the most frequent being craniofacial dysmorphisms (cleft lip or palate) and radial ray (thumb), cardiac, or urogenital anomalies. More than one anomaly occurs in approximately 25% of patients.

Table 20.2 DBAS diagnosis

Diagnostic criteria

Pathogenic or likely pathogenic[a] variant in a bona fide DBAS gene
OR
Hematologic features suggestive of DBAS:
  Blood: Macrocytic anemia with reticulocytopenia (0 to 20 G/L)[b]
  BM: Isolated erythroblastopenia at BMA analysis: No dysplasia or dyserythropoiesis, no ring sideroblasts (Perls coloration), no significant decrease in other lineages[c]
AND: Exclusion of known differential diagnoses

Typical findings (not mandatory for diagnosis)
Age at anemia diagnosis less than 1 year Elevated eADA activity (prior first transfusion; in non-transfused patients and/or parents)[d] Elevated HbF (reliably assessed in patients >6 months of age) Positive family history or unexplained history of anemia during infancy or childhood Congenital abnormalities reported in DBAS Abnormal rRNA processing in patient cells[e]

Adapted from ref. [3]

[a]: according to the ACMG/AMP classification; [b]: some anemic patients have not so severe reticulocytopenia; mild leuconeutropenia may be present; severe neutropenia possible in patients with *RPL35a* mutation; rare cases of thrombocytosis in infants (transient); platelets counts mostly normal, milt thrombocytopenia possible especially in patients with severe iron overload; [c]: some dyserythropoietic features may be present in patients with *GATA1* mutation; BM may be poor at biopsy in adult patients nevertheless pancytopenia is very rare out of clonal evolution; [d]: in a patient with recent transfusions, eADA activity may be evaluated only after 3 months without transfusion; [e]: only in specialized labs; mostly used for variant classification

BM bone marrow, *BMA* BM aspiration, *eADA* erythrocyte deaminase

Developmental delay is rare in patients with large deletions (contiguous gene syndrome) [3].

Nevertheless, expensive knowledge on new phenotypes and larger availability of genetic tests allow a diagnosis of DBAS in more and more children of any age and also in adults. Patients may present without significant anemia. Clinical nonclassical presentations include congenital anomalies and polymalformative syndrome without significant anemia, failure to thrive, immunodeficiency (common variable deficiency type), hematological malignancies without a history of anemia, and solid tumors with a significantly augmented risk of osteosarcoma and colorectal cancer. To note, DBAS patients exhibit unexpected hematological toxicity after chemotherapy for solid tumors or hematological malignancies.

To date, genotype/phenotype correlations are limited and of little clinical value. Most of them concern congenital anomalies, e.g., frequency of thumb anomaly in patients with mutations within *RPL11* and *RPL5*. Overall, patients with mutations in *RPL* genes have more congenital anomalies than those with *RPS* variants. Regarding hematopoietic phenotype, it has been said that patients with *RPL* mutations may present with mild hematological features; on the contrary, *RPS19* patients are less often therapeutically independent. No evidence of correlation with cancer risk is currently established [3].

DBAS-Differential Diagnosis

Acquired Erythroblastopenia

In children, the most frequent causes of erythroblastopenia in DBAS are transient childhood erythroblastopenia (TCE) and parvovirus B19–induced aplastic crisis in children with chronic hemolytic anemia (typically spherocytosis).

TCE pathology is still poorly understood. TCE is a rare disease, and its incidence seems to be decreasing. At diagnosis, children are mostly in the 1–4-year range; there is no familial history and no congenital anomalies, and MCV, eADA, and fetal Hb are normal. Most of the children need one or two transfusions, but the outcome is always good [7].

Other causes of acquired erythroblastopenias, like drugs or autoimmune disease, including pure red cell aplasia (PRCA), are rare in children but may be discussed in adulthood.

In adult patients, the main differential diagnosis is myelodysplastic syndrome (MDS), including the 5q deletion syndrome, classified as an acquired ribosomopathy (deletion of *RPS14*). One difficulty is that DBAS syndrome may evolve to MDS. In an adult patient, DBAS without clonal evolution must be suspected if the patient is young for MDS (less than 55 years), if the red cell lineage is the most affected one, and if there is no prominent dysplasia, no cytogenetic abnormality, and no pathogenic variant in myeloid genes. This presentation deserves a genetic test in order to look for IBMF gene variants. In a patient with frank MDS or acute myeloid leukemia (AML), DBAS should be discussed when a past history of anemia is available, typically in a patient with short stature and congenital anomalies, and when MDS occurred at a young age.

Inherited Erythroblastopenia

Some inherited erythroblastopenias are now classified as DBAS phenocopies. These include deficiency of adenosine deaminase 2 (DADA2) syndrome [8] and erythropoietin (EPO) deficiency [9]. Both may be present with isolated severe anemia and erythroblastopenia in an infant. *ADA2/CECR1* and *EPO* genes are currently included in DBAS diagnostic panels. Hematopoietic stem cell transplantation (HSCT) is urgent in DADA syndrome, as these children may have immunodeficiency and severe autoinflammatory syndrome. On the contrary, HSCT is contraindicated in patients with EPO deficiency, who actually respond to EPO administration.

IBMFs may be discussed in some patients, especially when congenital anomalies (part of both DBAS and Fanconi anemia phenotypes, for instance) are present or when more than one lineage is affected. Nevertheless, in other IBMFs, there is no frank dissociation seen in DBAS among lineages, i.e., severe anemia, requiring transfusion support, and mild neutropenia with, most frequently, normal platelet counts. Specific diagnostic tests may be required in some patients.

Treacher Collins syndrome, another ribosomopathy, shares some extra-hematological presentations with DBAS. Actually, two DBAS genes (*RPS28* and *TSR2*) were identified in a cohort of TCS patients without mutation in *TCOF1* and other genes involved in TCS [10]. But TCS patients do not have a hematological phenotype, and fetal Hb and eADA are normal.

Last, other red cell diseases associated with central anemia, like congenital dyserythropoietic anemia, congenital sideroblastic anemia, or Pearson syndrome, may be discussed in some patients but are easy to distinguish in bone marrow film analysis. The exception is GATA1 syndrome, which includes different entities; DBAS associated with *GATA1* variants may present with dyserythropoiesis and are currently classified as DBA-other [3]. To note, early evolution to MDS, associated with monosomy 7, has been reported in one DBA-other patient with *GATA1* variant [4].

DBAS Treatment

As of 2024, the three therapeutic approaches in DBAS remain red cell transfusion support, corticosteroid therapy, and HSCT [3]. No drug has been demonstrated to be able to correct anemia. Gene therapy, currently focusing on *RPS19*-mutated cases, is coming but not yet available.

Transfusion Support

Indications and Practice

Transfusion is the only option in children before the age of 1 year. The current recommendation is to maintain hemoglobin level above 9–10 g/dL in order to allow normal child development and a good quality of life [3]. To note, recent data in thalassemic patients support the need for maintaining satisfactory Hb levels, with a direct link between the threshold used for transfusion and survival [11]. Many patients will require lifelong red blood cell (RBC) transfusions, and transfusion support must be adapted to age and activities: A higher Hb nadir may be needed in some patients to ensure a good quality of life. Of note, some patients with DBAS and persistent reticulocytosis may require regular transfusions at intervals of 2–3 months. Others, with only mild anemia (hemoglobin >10 g/dL), may need transfusions only occasionally, for example during intercurrent viral infections. Finally, pregnant women with DBAS should be maintained at a hemoglobin level above 10.5 g/dL [12]. Patients presenting with hydrops are rare and may need in utero transfusion; this is associated specifically with variants in *RPL15* but has also been reported for patients with mutations within *RPS19* [13, 14]. DBAS should be included in the etiological diagnosis of hydrops.

Chelation Therapy

Iron overload is, with cancer, the leading cause of death in non-transplanted DBAS patients. DBAS is not an iron-loading anemia, and iron overload is mainly due to transfusions. Iron overload is reported to develop more rapidly and be more severe in DBAS than in other red cell diseases with transfusion support, and this may be due to the lack of erythron in the bone marrow and the non-utilization of iron for red cell production [15]. Non-transferrin bound iron (NTBI) is also reported to be especially high, and this may also explain the incidence of early and severe cardiac and pancreatic iron loading seen in DBAS patients.

Indicators of iron overload are serum ferritin levels (SFLs), associated with elevated transferrin saturation and liver iron concentration (LIC), measured by magnetic resonance imaging (MRI). SLF has low accuracy in measuring the total iron burden and is affected by infection and inflammation. So MRI must be performed in any patient at the first evaluation, as soon as possible in children in whom this may require general anesthesia if done before the age of 5–6 years, and repeated every 12–18 months according to iron overload [3]. Nevertheless, SFL evolution, associated with an LIC result, allows us to properly follow up with the patient. SFL must be evaluated just before a transfusion and, at best, in the same lab.

Current indication to start chelation in DBAS patients is an evidence of iron overload: ferritin >500 ng/ml, transferrin saturation > 60%, or elevated LIC (> 3 mg/g) [3]. In children, this usually corresponds to ten to 15 transfusions and the first steroid test.

Before the age of 2 years, only deferoxamine (DFO), at a reduced dose (maximum: 30 mg/kg/d in children <3 years), may be used; after 3 years, the dose is standard (50–60 mg/kg/d). Deferasirox (DFX) at a standard dose (14–28 mg/kg/d) may be used in older children (> 2 years) and in adults. The use of deferiprone (DFP) should be considered with caution because of an established high risk of agranulocytosis in DBAS patients (up to 10%), which, nevertheless, usually has a standard course [16, 17]. DFP should be prescribed as a third line only or in patients with severe cardiac iron overload, in association with DFO. Maximal DFP dose in DBAS patients is 75 mg/kg/d, and education, monitoring of neutrophil counts, and an emergency plan are warranted [3].

The goals of chelation therapy are to maintain SFL in the 300–500 ng/ml range, LIC < 3 mg/g, and cardiac T2* > 20–25 ms [3]. In DBAS patients, this implies the frequent use of a combination of two chelators in patients with severe iron overload. To note, control of NTBI implies, at best, giving a chelator any day, and this may also be achieved with such combinations, e.g., 5 days with DFO and 2 days with DFX. Chelation therapy must be evaluated every 3–4 months, within a dedicated consultation, in order to adapt the dose (increase or decrease) and evaluate chelators' toxicity, at least yearly, and the clinical impact of hemochromatosis. To note, all chelating agents are more toxic for low SFL, and one must be aware of hyperchelation consequences, e.g., tubulopathy, hypophosphoremia, and lithiasis in a patient on DFX. Nevertheless, in a patient with low SFL (but >300 ng/ml) and high LIC, chelation must be pursued at lower doses and with intensified follow-up.

Note that, even in therapeutically independent patients, phlebotomies cannot be used: DBAS patients cannot cope with erythropoietic stress, and even small-volume, spaced-apart phlebotomies are poorly tolerated. On the other hand, phlebotomies can be useful after transplantation.

Other Associated Measures in Transfused Patients

Every transfused patient should be vaccinated against hepatitis B and regularly monitored for hepatitis B, hepatitis C, and HIV.

Corticosteroid Therapy

Corticosteroids (steroids) have been successfully used in treating DBAS for more than 70 years. Both prednisone and prednisolone can be used. Steroids should be tested in any transfusion-dependent patient. In children, the test is done after 1 year of age and, optimally, after live vaccine immunizations (measles, mumps, rubella, and varicella) [3]. Steroid administration modalities are given in Fig. 20.1. In responding patients, significant reticulocytosis (usually >100 G/L) is observed at D10/D15 (like after iron administration in iron deficiency anemia) and hemoglobin is thereafter stable or increasing, allowing progressive tapering. The maximum long-term maintenance dose should not exceed 0.3 mg/kg/d (10–15 mg/d in adults) and should, at best, be less than 0.15 mg/kg/d [3].

Patients may be classified into different profiles based on their response to steroids:

- Primary refractory patients: no rise in reticulocytes (20–30% of patients).
- Clinically nonresponding patients: responds initially, but loss of response was noticed during tapering, at dose >0.3 mg/kg/d.
- Poorly responding patients: effective partial response but relatively high-dose requirement, e.g., 0.25/0.30 mg/kg/d. These patients frequently associate persistent anemia and steroid toxicity, and transfusion support should be discussed.
- Good-responsive patients: good response, with subnormal or normal Hb level (possibly, persistent macrocytosis) and very low dose requirement (< 0.15 mg/kg/d).

In responding pediatric patients, steroid therapy may be temporarily stopped (for 2–3 years) before puberty to optimize growth [3].

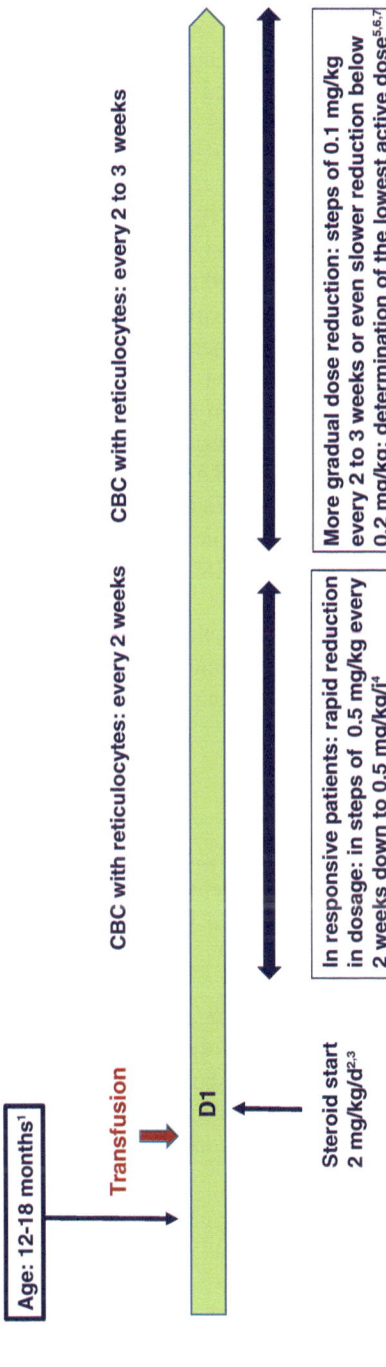

Fig. 20.1 Steroid treatment in DBAS patients

1: in children with failure to thrive and no severe iron overload, test may be delayed up to 15–18 months in order to optimize growth

2: steroids may be started either 1 day or 2 weeks after the last transfusion according to local practices

3: maximal dose (children and adult): 80 mg/d4: in non-responsive patients same dose for 2 weeks more. If no response: the patient is classified as primary corticoresistant. Stop steroids within 1 week.

A second test may be tempted especially before HSCT

5: possible decrease 1 mg by 1 mg; active dose may be as low as less than 0.10 mg/kg/d in "true" steroid-sensitive patients

6: when the lowest efficient dose is determined: it is possible to give twice the dose every other day (children); further passive weaning is possible: non-growth-adaptation of dose. 40% of DBAS patients remain on steroids life long

7: patients who, during tapering, have a decrease in reticulocytes and Hb at dose >0.3 mg/kg/d are classified as non-steroid-sensitive patients. Steroids must be stopped within 1 week and the patient should be placed back on transfusion support

Hematopoietic Stem Cell Transplantation

Allogeneic HSCT is the only way to achieve the cure of anemia in steroid nonresponding patients, and prevent clonal evolution. An analysis from Germany and France, done on 70 HSCT patients (1985–2017) and comparing match-sibling donor (MSD) or match-unrelated donor (MUD) found comparable results for the 5-year overall survival at 91% and 92% respectively, with a similar chronic graft-versus-host disease-free survival at 89% and 83% [18]. To note, age and the HSCT era were prognostic, with better results in children under the age of 10 years and transplants done after 2000. In the European Society for Blood and Marrow Transplantation (EBMT) survey on 104 transplants (1985–2016), the 3-year event-free survival is 84%, again with similar outcomes for sibling and unrelated donors [19]. Comparable results have been achieved by other groups [3]. Given these improvements, the 2024 guidelines recommend HSCT, at best, under the age of 5 years from MSD or 10/10 human leukocyte antigen (HLA) MUD for children who are transfusion-dependent [3]. To note, DBAS must be excluded from MSD, and this is not easy if there is no identified variant in DBAS genes. In such cases, the workup must include clinical examination, complete blood count (CBC) with reticulocytes, fetal Hb, and eADA activity evaluation; some teams may also consider transplant with a 10/10 MUD. Other indications and HSCT modalities are given in Table 20.3.

A currently unresolved point is the risk of post-transplant increase in solid tumor incidence, as established for patients with Fanconi anemia. Some authors suggest starting systematic colonoscopies in transplanted patients earlier [20].

Other Agents

The amino acid leucine is able to induce an erythroid response in a very small proportion of DBAS patients who are transfusion-dependent [21]. The clinical benefit is more marked with respect to the general status and linear growth in children, making this drug routinely used by some physicians. Studies with leucine for steroid-responsive DBAS are underway.

Erythropoietin and other erythropoietic stimulating agents, like sotatercept, as an immunosuppressive therapy (rituximab or cyclosporine) are ineffective. Metoclopramide, acting via prolactin stimulation, has shown very limited and irregular responses [22, 23]. Eltrombopag does not seem to be of clinical benefit in DBAS and is associated with thrombocytosis [24]. Eltrombopag should not be used outside of a clinical trial.

Table 20.3 Recommendations for allogeneic HSCT in DBAS

Pre-transplant evaluation	
Age	For non-steroid responsive patients: consider transplant before the age of 10 years and at best within 2–5 years of age. After 10 years of age: HSCT may be discussed considering the burden of transfusion and chelation, and organ functions. In adults, HSCT is usually non considered for transfusion dependency only but may be discussed on a case-per case basis
Iron overload	Assessment with liver and cardiac MRI. The goal is to control iron overload before HSCT: SFL < 1000 ng/ml, no severe liver (LIC closed to 3 mg/g and not exceeding 7 mg/g) and no cardiac iron overload.
Indications in order of increasing emergency and clinical necessity	
	Transfusion support in patients non-responding to steroids
	Non-manageable iron overload (chelation failure, severe toxicity)
	Transfusion support and alloimmunization to red cells
	Other severe cytopenia(s)[a], severe immunodeficiency or both
	MDS or AML
Donor choice from most to less optimal	
	MSD after exclusion of DBAS (clinical examination, complete BCC with reticulocytes, fetal Hb, eADA activity, and genetic testing[b]
	MUD: 10/10 as per molecular testing
	HLA-mismatched unrelated or familial donor (including haplo-identical donors): Only for patients with clonal evolution or within a clinical trial
Stem cell source	
	Bone marrow (any donor)
	Cord blood (non DBAS sibling donor)
	NB: Avoid unmanipulated peripheral blood stem cells
Conditioning regimen	
	Myeloablative: Busulfan or treosulfan (± thiotepa) combined with fludarabine
	NB: Avoid irradiation
GVG disease prophylaxis	
	Standard, i.e., calcineurin inhibitors + methotrexate or mycophenolate mofetil + serotherapy (also for MSD)
Specific post-transplants considerations	
	Intensify cancer screening. Consider phlebotomies in patients with persistent iron overload

Adapted from reference [3]

[a]: mostly: severe neutropenia in *RPL35a*-mutated patient; pancytopenia is very rare in DBAS patients outside of clonal evolution; [b]: may be difficult when no genetic variant is identified: 10/10 MUD is discussed by some teams in such cases

DBAS Diamond Blackfan Anemia Syndrome, *eADA* erythrocyte deaminase, *HSCT* hematopoietic stem cell transplantation, *LIC* liver iron concentration, *MRI* magnetic resonance imaging, *MSD* match-sibling donor, *MUD* match-unrelated donor, *SFL* serum ferritin levels

Surveillance in DBAS Patients

Hematological Outcomes in DBAS

Clinical remission, i.e., therapeutic independence, may be achieved in up to 20% of DBAS patients, the chance being most important in patients on steroids than for those on transfusion: 33% and 4%, respectively, in a study from the French registry [25]. In such patients, anemia may recur, either transiently (viral infection or drug) or chronically, especially when the patient gets older.

Mild leuconeutropenia is frequent, especially in adult patients, but is not severe and without clinical impact in *RPL35a* patients. Platelet counts are mostly normal. Thrombocytopenia may be present in some patients, including those with severe iron overload, but in a patient with previous normal counts, thrombocytopenia is a warning event and suggests clonal evolution. Severe pancytopenia and true aplastic anemia features are not part of the DBAS phenotype in clonal evolution. Nevertheless, if performed, BM biopsy may show poor cellularity.

DBAS patients are at a very high risk of clonal evolution and MDS or AML [3, 26]. Reported data on MDS presentation in DBAS are currently scarce. MDS in DBAS occurs earlier than in the general population. From our experiment, the karyotype is often complex and includes *TP53* alterations. Chemotherapy may be associated with severe hematological toxicity, and the prognosis is poor. Hematopoietic stem cell transplantation (HSCT) is the only option to cure the patient.

To date, there is no consensus on regular BM screening evaluation, but any significant change in CBC suggests considering BM evaluation.

Cancer Risk and Surveillance in DBAS

DBAS is a cancer-prone disease. In the first report of the US registry, the observed-to-expected ratio (O/E) for all cancers combined was 5.4 [26]. The spectrum of observed cancer is large, but DBAS patients are specifically at a very high risk of osteosarcoma in children and adolescents (O/E: 42.4) and colorectal cancer in adults (O/E: 44.7) [27]. The recent international guidelines recommend colorectal cancer screening in patients with DBAS, starting at the age of 20 years, with follow-up every 5 years. There is no consensus on post-HSCT colonoscopy timing, but starting before the age of 20 years is reasonable. International workshops are currently devoted to analyze cancer incidence and management in DBAS patients.

Other Outcomes

Outside of hematology and cancer phenotype, DBAS patients may present with many clinical situations [3]. Children with DBAS must be closely followed up for growth. Therapeutic interventions may include a temporary stop of steroids and growth hormone administration [3]. DBAS patients may present with immunodeficiency (decreased B/NK lymphocyte counts and immunoglobulins (Igs)), and this warrants immune parameter monitoring [3]. In adolescents and adults, genetic counseling and family planning must be offered. It should be noted that, whatever the phenotype of the affected parent or the first affected child, no prediction in terms of severity can be made for the next offspring [3]. Pregnancies in DBAS women are at high risk. Due to placental vasculopathy, prophylaxis with acetylsalicylic acid may be considered [3, 12]. A comprehensive long-term surveillance program is given in the recent international guidelines [3].

> DBAS is a complex and very heterogeneous disease, and patients must be cared for by expert teams. Transfusion support and iron chelation have to be optimal. Indications for HSCT are currently expanding. Future challenges include knowledge expansion on cancer in DBAS patients (clinical profile, screening, and treatment modalities) and the development of new therapeutic approaches (targeted therapies and gene therapy).

Clinical Management of Cartilage-Hair Hypoplasia

Clinical Presentation and Diagnosis

Cartilage-hair hypoplasia (CHH) is a very rare congenital disorder outside of the Amish (prevalence: 1–2/1000) and Finnish (1/23,000) populations; fewer than 1000 patients are known [28, 29].The phenotype associates with metaphyseal dysplasia, characterized by growth retardation, hypoplastic hair, Hirschsprung disease, immunodeficiency, cancer predisposition, and anemia. CHH is secondary to bi-allelic mutations (autosomal recessive transmission) in the ribonuclease mitochondrial RNA processing (*RMRP*).

Hematological involvement consists of mild macrocytic anemia, secondary to defective erythropoiesis, which is present in 70% of cases during early infancy and, in most cases, resolves spontaneously. However, in 6% of patients, anemia is persistent, severe, and transfusion-dependent, resembling DBAS [30, 31]. In addition, cases of autoimmune hemolytic anemia (AIHA) have also been reported and are secondary to the impairment of the immune system, which is often part of the clinical phenotype [29, 32]. The immunological defect of CHH is highly variable, ranging from mere laboratory abnormalities to severe hypogammaglobulinemia and/or combined immunodeficiency/immune dysregulation. In particular, patients may show defects of T cell count and function and B cell maturation impairment, with low production of immunoglobulins [33–35].

Overall, the risk of undergoing chronic infection (such as respiratory infections, bronchiectasis, and chronic viral infections) has been reported in 35–65% of cases [29]. Fatal varicella infection has also been reported, but in most cases, the infection can run uncomplicated. Hirschsprung disease is present in about 8% of patients during the newborn period, but other gastrointestinal issues can occur later in life, such as chronic diarrhea, malabsorption, and poor weight gain [29]. Patients also show a higher risk of developing cancer, in particular lymphomas [36].

Patient Care and Surveillance

CHH is usually managed only with supportive treatments. Monitoring of growth, cognitive assessment, and pubertal development should be performed annually throughout adolescence. The use of specific growth curves and regular X-ray examination of lower extremities and spine are recommended. Immunological status should be evaluated during follow-up to monitor the evolution of immunodeficiency/immune dysregulation over the years, and in addition, specific pulmonary assessment should be regularly performed to watch over respiratory tract infections and bronchiectasis. According to the Ig levels and the frequency of infective complications, the administration of regular intravenous immunoglobulin infusions is recommended. Patients should undergo a regular hematological follow-up, tailored to the specific phenotype. Complete blood count should be evaluated over time in all cases, and monitoring/treatment of iron overload should be offered to all patients who require regular transfusions [28]. Sirolimus has been shown to be useful in improving anemia in one patient [32].

HSCT represents the only curative option for CHH patients and should be offered to those with transfusion-dependent erythroid failure and/or with severe immunodeficiency associated with chronic infections [37]. Although HSCT does not correct the skeletal abnormalities, it can be helpful in reducing the infection load, correcting anemia, and improving the failure to thrive.

Patients should undergo the procedure preferably before the onset of severe infections and organ complications, which are reported to have a negative impact on outcomes. The use of reduced-intensity conditioning (RIC) regimen has been reported in patients with severe combined deficiency phenotype in order to reduce toxicity: Despite a higher incidence of mixed chimerism, encouraging results have been reported [38].

> CHH is a very rare disease. Only a few patients have a severe hematological phenotype. HSCT corrects both severe anemia and immunodeficiency and should be discussed on a case-by-case basis.

References

1. Narla A, Ebert BL. Ribosomopathies: human disorders of ribosome dysfunction. Blood. 2010;115(16):3196–205.
2. Da Costa L, Mohandas N, David-NGuyen L, et al. Diamond-Blackfan anemia, the archetype of ribosomopathy: how distinct is it from the other constitutional ribosomopathies? Blood Cells Mol Dis. 2024;106:102838.
3. Wlodarski MW, Vlachos A, Farrar JE, et al. Diagnosis, treatment, and surveillance of Diamond-Blackfan anaemia syndrome: international consensus statement. Lancet Haematol. 2024;11(5):e368–82.
4. Parrella S, Aspesi A, Quarello P, et al. Loss of GATA-1 full length as a cause of Diamond-Blackfan anemia phenotype. Pediatr Blood Cancer. 2014;61(7):1319–21.
5. Toki T, Yoshida K, Wang R, et al. De novo mutations activating germline TP53 in an inherited bone-marrow-failure syndrome. Am J Hum Genet. 2018;103(3):440–7.
6. Fedorova D, Ovsyannikova G, Kurnikova M, et al. De novo TP53 germline activating mutations in two patients with the phenotype mimicking Diamond-Blackfan anemia. Pediatr Blood Cancer. 2022;69(4):e29558.
7. van den Akker M, Dror Y, Odame I. Transient erythroblastopenia of childhood is an underdiagnosed and self-limiting disease. Acta Paediatr. 2014;103(7):e288–94.
8. Lee PY. Vasculopathy, immunodeficiency, and bone marrow failure: the intriguing syndrome caused by deficiency of adenosine deaminase 2. Front Pediatr. 2018;6:282.
9. Kim AR, Ulirsch JC, Wilmes S, et al. Functional selectivity in cytokine signaling revealed through a pathogenic EPO mutation. Cell. 2017;168(6):1053–1064.e15.
10. Gripp KW, Curry C, Olney AH, et al. Diamond-Blackfan anemia with mandibulofacial dystostosis is heterogeneous, including the novel DBA genes TSR2 and RPS28. Am J Med Genet A. 2014;164A(9):2240–9.
11. Musallam KM, Barella S, Origa R, et al. Pretransfusion hemoglobin level and mortality in adults with transfusion-dependent β-thalassemia. Blood. 2024;143(10):930–2.
12. Faivre L, Meerpohl J, Da Costa L, et al. High-risk pregnancies in Diamond-Blackfan anemia: a survey of 64 pregnancies from the French and German registries. Haematologica. 2006;91(4):530–3.
13. Wlodarski MW, Da Costa L, O'Donohue M-F, et al. Recurring mutations in RPL15 are linked to hydrops fetalis and treatment independence in Diamond-Blackfan anemia. Haematologica. 2018;103(6):949–58.
14. Da Costa L, Chanoz-Poulard G, Simansour M, et al. First de novo mutation in RPS19 gene as the cause of hydrops fetalis in Diamond–Blackfan anemia. Am J Hematol. 2013;88(4):340–1.
15. Porter JB, Walter PB, Neumayr LD, et al. Mechanisms of plasma non-transferrin bound iron generation: insights from comparing transfused Diamond-blackfan anaemia with sickle cell and thalassaemia patients. Br J Haematol. 2014;167(5):692–6.
16. Tricta F, Uetrecht J, Galanello R, et al. Deferiprone-induced agranulocytosis: 20 years of clinical observations. Am J Hematol. 2016;91(10):1026–31.
17. Lecornec N, Castex M-P, Réguerre Y, et al. Agranulocytosis in patients with Diamond-Blackfan anaemia (DBA) treated with deferiprone for post-transfusion iron overload: a retrospective study of the French DBA cohort. Br J Haematol. 2022;199(2):285–8.
18. Strahm B, Loewecke F, Niemeyer CM, et al. Favorable outcomes of hematopoietic stem cell transplantation in children and adolescents with Diamond-Blackfan anemia. Blood Adv. 2020;4(8):1760–9.

19. Miano M, Eikema D-J, de la Fuente J, et al. Stem cell transplantation for Diamond-Blackfan anemia. A retrospective study on behalf of the severe aplastic anemia working party of the European Blood and Marrow Transplantation Group (EBMT). Transplant Cell Ther. 2021;27(3):274.e1–5.
20. Lipton JM, Molmenti CLS, Hussain M, et al. Colorectal cancer screening and surveillance strategy for patients with Diamond Blackfan anemia: preliminary recommendations from the Diamond Blackfan anemia registry. Pediatr Blood Cancer. 2021;68(8):e28984.
21. Vlachos A, Atsidaftos E, Lababidi ML, et al. L-leucine improves anemia and growth in patients with transfusion-dependent Diamond-Blackfan anemia: results from a multicenter pilot phase I/II study from the Diamond-Blackfan anemia registry. Pediatr Blood Cancer. 2020;67(12):e28748.
22. Abkowitz JL, Schaison G, Boulad F, et al. Response of Diamond-Blackfan anemia to metoclopramide: evidence for a role for prolactin in erythropoiesis. Blood. 2002;100(8):2687–91.
23. Leblanc TM, Da Costa L, Marie I, Demolis P, Tchernia G. Metoclopramide treatment in DBA patients: no complete response in a French prospective study. Blood. 2007;109(5):2266–7.
24. Duncan BB, Lotter JL, Superata J, et al. Treatment of refractory/relapsed Diamond-Blackfan anaemia with eltrombopag. Br J Haematol. 2024;204(5):2077–85.
25. Willig TN, Niemeyer CM, Leblanc T, et al. Identification of new prognosis factors from the clinical and epidemiologic analysis of a registry of 229 Diamond-Blackfan anemia patients. DBA group of Société d'Hématologie et d'Immunologie Pédiatrique (SHIP), Gesellshaft für Pädiatrische Onkologie und Hämatologie (GPOH), and the European Society for Pediatric Hematology and Immunology (ESPHI). Pediatr Res. 1999;46(5):553–61.
26. Vlachos A, Rosenberg PS, Atsidaftos E, Alter BP, Lipton JM. Incidence of neoplasia in Diamond Blackfan anemia: a report from the Diamond-Blackfan anemia registry. Blood. 2012;119(16):3815–9.
27. Vlachos A, Rosenberg PS, Atsidaftos E, et al. Increased risk of colon cancer and osteogenic sarcoma in Diamond-Blackfan anemia. Blood. 2018;132(20):2205–8.
28. Mäkitie O, Vakkilainen S. Cartilage-hair hypoplasia–anauxetic dysplasia spectrum disorders. In: GeneReviews®. Seattle: University of Washington; 1993.
29. Mäkitie O, Kaitila I. Cartilage-hair hypoplasia–clinical manifestations in 108 Finnish patients. Eur J Pediatr. 1993;152(3):211–7.
30. Williams MS, Ettinger RS, Hermanns P, et al. The natural history of severe anemia in cartilage-hair hypoplasia. Am J Med Genet A. 2005;138(1):35–40.
31. Taskinen M, Toiviainen-Salo S, Lohi J, et al. Hypoplastic anemia in cartilage-hair hypoplasia-balancing between iron overload and chelation. J Pediatr. 2013;162(4):844–9.
32. Del Borrello G, Miano M, Micalizzi C, et al. Sirolimus restores erythropoiesis and controls immune dysregulation in a child with cartilage-hair hypoplasia: a case report. Front Immunol. 2022;13:893000.
33. Vakkilainen S, Mäkitie R, Klemetti P, et al. A wide spectrum of autoimmune manifestations and other symptoms suggesting immune dysregulation in patients with cartilage-hair hypoplasia. Front Immunol. 2018;9:2468.
34. Vakkilainen S, Taskinen M, Mäkitie O. Immunodeficiency in cartilage-hair hypoplasia: pathogenesis, clinical course and management. Scand J Immunol. 2020;92(4):e12913.
35. Kostjukovits S, Klemetti P, Valta H, et al. Analysis of clinical and immunologic phenotype in a large cohort of children and adults with cartilage-hair hypoplasia. J Allergy Clin Immunol. 2017;140(2):612–614.e5.
36. Kukkola H-L, Utriainen P, Huttunen P, et al. Lymphomas in cartilage-hair hypoplasia – a case series of 16 patients reveals advanced stage DLBCL as the most common form. Front Immunol. 2022;13:1004694.
37. Bordon V, Gennery AR, Slatter MA, et al. Clinical and immunologic outcome of patients with cartilage hair hypoplasia after hematopoietic stem cell transplantation. Blood. 2010;116(1):27–35.
38. Fitch T, Bleesing J, Marsh RA, Chandra S. Reduced intensity conditioning allogeneic transplant for SCID associated with cartilage hair hypoplasia. J Clin Immunol. 2022;42(8):1604–7.

Open Access This chapter is licensed under the terms of the Creative Commons Attribution 4.0 International License (http://creativecommons.org/licenses/by/4.0/), which permits use, sharing, adaptation, distribution and reproduction in any medium or format, as long as you give appropriate credit to the original author(s) and the source, provide a link to the Creative Commons license and indicate if changes were made.

The images or other third party material in this chapter are included in the chapter's Creative Commons license, unless indicated otherwise in a credit line to the material. If material is not included in the chapter's Creative Commons license and your intended use is not permitted by statutory regulation or exceeds the permitted use, you will need to obtain permission directly from the copyright holder.

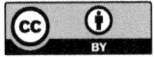

Chapter 21
Chronic Neutropenias

Francesca Fioredda and Helen A. Papadaki

The term chronic neutropenia (Np) encompasses a group of disorders related to a persistent reduction or absence of mature neutrophils in the circulation. The absolute neutrophil count (ANC) threshold to define "neutropenia" is different according to age and ethnicity, but in general, values above 1.5×10^9/L and 1.8×10^9/L are considered abnormal for Caucasian children aged more than 1 year and adults, respectively [1–3].

The diagnostic approach to neutropenia, according to the recent international guidelines, suggests the exclusion of (i) neutropenias considered more a condition rather than a disease like *ACKR1/DARC*-associated neutropenia (ADAN), formerly known as ethnic neutropenia, and (ii) drug-related and postinfectious neutropenias, which are the two most common forms in adults and children (Fig. 21.1) [4–6]. Subsequent steps of investigation across the diagnostic algorithm are directed (Table 21.1) [6] toward two main categories, which are the congenital and the acquired forms (Table 21.2) [6]. In addition, a new provisional category named likely acquired neutropenia has been added to the first two. They will be discussed later in detail [6].

F. Fioredda (✉)
Hematology Unit-IRCCS Istituto Giannina Gaslini, Genoa, Italy
e-mail: francescafioredda@gaslini.org

H. A. Papadaki
Department of Hematology & Hemopoiesis Research Laboratory, School of Medicine University of Crete, Greece and University Hospital of Heraklion, Heraklion, Greece

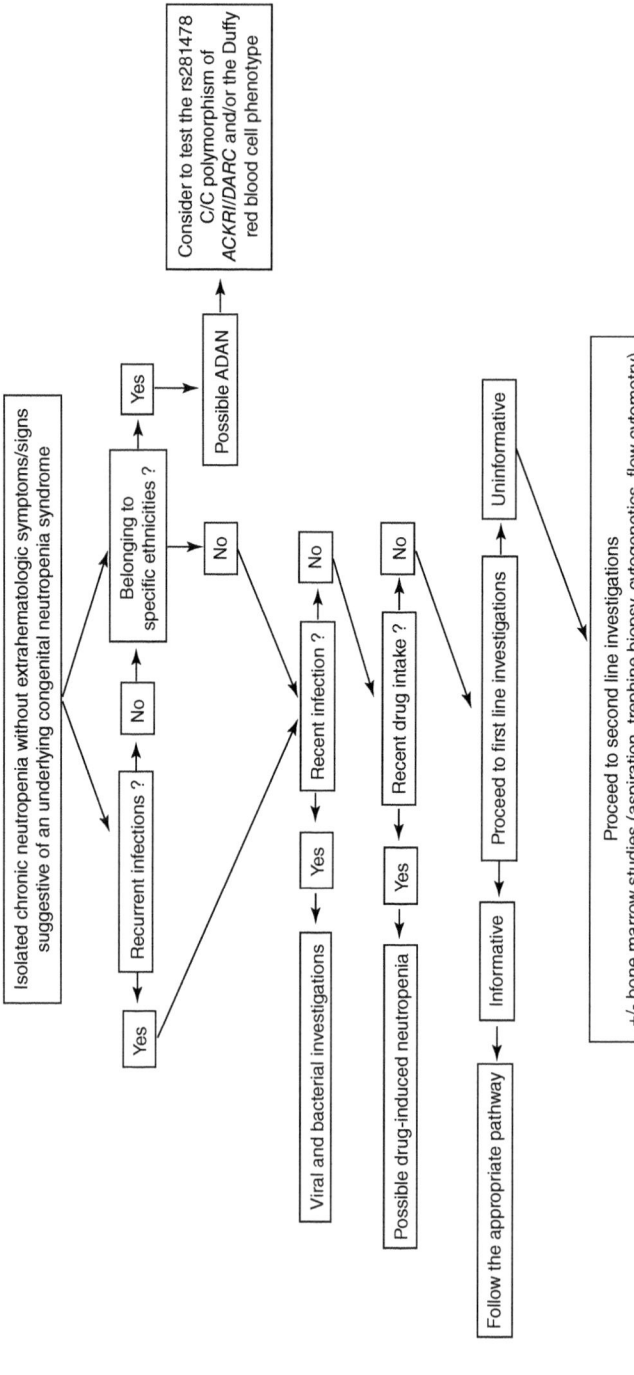

Fig. 21.1 Diagnostic algorithm according to international guidelines [6]

Table 21.1 First- and second-line investigations according to international guidelines [6]

First-line investigations	CBCs; PB smear; biochemistry tests, including liver and kidney function, immunoglobulin levels, CRP, vitamin B12, and folate; flow cytometric analysis of PB lymphocyte subsets; virology antibody screening (i.e., HepB, HepC, HIV, EBV, CMV, and parvovirus); indirect antineutrophil antibodies (GIFT, GAT, and others); thyroid hormones (FT3, FT4, and TSH); antithyroid antibodies (anti-TG and anti-TPO) Additional investigation in children: flow cytometric analysis of TCR-α/β--positive double-negative (CD4− and CD8−) CD3 PB lymphocytes Additional investigations in adults: antiphospholipid and anticardiolipin antibodies, flow cytometric analysis of LGL/TCR clonality in PB lymphocytes, serum ferritin, RF, ANA, ENA, ds-DNA, and ESR
Second-line investigations	CBCs in family members, serial blood counts twice a week over a period of 6 weeks to exclude CyN, copper; ceruloplasmin, anti-tTG-IgA, deamidated gliadin peptide antibodies IgA/IgG and pancreatic isoamylase Additional investigation in children: RF, ANA, ENA, and ds-DNA

AML acute myeloid leukemia, *ANA* antinuclear antibodies, *anti-TG* antithyroglobulin, *anti-TPO* antithyroid peroxidase, *CBC* complete blood count, *CMV* cytomegalovirus, *CyN* cyclic neutropenia, *ds-DNA* double-stranded DNA, *tTG* tissue transglutaminase antibodies, *EBV* Epstein–Barr virus, *ENA* extractable nuclear antigen, *ESR* erythrocyte sedimentation rate, *GAT* granulocyte agglutination test, *Hep* hepatitis, *HIV* human immunodeficiency virus, *GIFT* granulocyte immunofluorescence test, *LGL* large granular lymphocytes, *MDS* myelodysplastic syndrome, *PB* peripheral blood, *RF* rheumatoid factor, *TCR* T cell receptor

Table 21.2 Classification of neutropenia according to international guidelines [6]

Congenital	Acquired	Likely acquired

Isolated
Associated with various extra-hematologic manifestations
Associated with immunodeficiency/immune dysregulation
Associated with metabolic disorders and nutritional deficiency
Associated with bone marrow failure
	Primary or idiopathic
	   Antibody-mediated
	   Non-antibody-mediated
	Secondary due to
	   Hypersplenism
	   Infections
	   Autoimmune diseases
	   Nutritional deficiencies
	   Hematologic diseases
	   Drug-induced
		Late-onset/long-lasting Nps with/without antibodies against neutrophils

Congenital Neutropenia

Congenital neutropenias (CNs) are innate disorders, with variable modes of inheritance and with a prevalence of 3–8 cases per million inhabitants [7, 8]. The "classical congenital form" is due to a maturation impairment of the myeloid precursors or a deficient output of mature elements from the bone marrow (BM) to the bloodstream due to different mechanisms [9].

Congenital neutropenia may be isolated or associated with a number of extrahematologic signs. The two most frequently involved genes in CN are *ELANE* for the isolated neutropenia and *HAX1*, which is generally associated with neurological symptoms, neurodevelopment delay, and ovarian failure, as recently described [9, 10]. *ELANE* is the most common gene related to congenital neutropenia in North American and European countries, while *HAX1* is more frequently seen in Eastern countries due to a high degree of consanguinity [11, 12].

Both *ELANE*- and *HAX1*-related neutropenias are due to the block of neutrophil maturation and increased apoptosis of the myeloid precursors at the stage of promyelocyte [8]. Other genes generate neutropenia through increased promyelocyte apoptosis (i.e., *SRP54, TCIRG1, SEC61A1, EIF2AK, CSFR3R, GFI1,* and *JAGN1*), but neutropenia may also be due to alternative mechanisms, including ribosomal defect (*RPS7,10,15,19,* etc. and *GATA1, TSR2, HEATR3,* etc.), mitochondrial failure (*AK2* and *TAZ*), granule-processing synthesis (*VPS45* and *VPS13*), or the retention of mature elements within the bone marrow (*CXCR4* and *CXCR2*) [6, 8, 12–16]. Many neutropenias are part of syndromes such as glycogen storage disease 1 (*SLC37A/G6PT1*), Shwachman–Diamond syndrome (*SBDS, EFL1, and DNAJC21*), and *G6PC3* disease [6, 17–19].

In spite of the active research in this field, almost one-third of the patients are still gene-orphans [6–8]. The most recent identified genes are the monoallelic variants of *CLPB* [20], mutations in *DBF4* [21], *SRPA/SRP19* [22], and biallelic loss-of-function mutation of *CXCR2* [23], which cause neutropenia because of mitochondrial dysfunction, defect in DNA transcription, defect in protein processing, intracellular trafficking, neutrophils' homeostasis, and impaired neutrophil egression from the bone marrow.

Infections are the most common clinical manifestation, usually affecting patients with the highest degree of neutropenia and occurring very early in life [6, 7].

The site and the type of infections could drive the suspicion of a congenital neutropenia diagnosis. The umbilical cord, skin, internal ear, mouth, and lungs are frequent sites of infections, with variable degrees of severity. Sepsis is an event that may result in increased lethality [6–8]. According to the Severe Congenital Neutropenia International Registry (SCNIR), lethal sepsis has a cumulative incidence of 5–18% after 15 years of granulocyte colony-stimulating factor (G-CSF), depending on the required dose [24].

Transformation into myelodysplastic syndrome (MDS)/acute leukemia (AL) is another expected event, at least in a portion of patients, due to the intrinsic propensity of the disorders and the potential G-CSF pressure on the bone marrow [6–8]. According to the SCNIR data, MDS/AL cumulative incidence has been assessed at 22–30% after 15 years of G-CSF with an increased risk in subjects treated with doses higher than 8 mcg/kg/day [24]. G-CSF, introduced in clinical practice in the 1990s, in spite of its proliferative pressure, has been of paramount importance in fighting infections, preventing fatal complications, and substantially improving the prognosis of the affected subjects [6–8, 25].

G-CSF standard dose is considered to be 5 mcg/kg/day, which is sufficient to protect the majority of patients from infections; a small subgroup (around 5–10%) is defined nonresponders due to scarce or absent ANC increase, injecting G-CSF doses even above 20 mcg/kg/day [25].

Therapies, other than G-CSF, have been shown to be effective only in specific disorders. This is the case of mavorixafor in warts, hypogammaglobulinemia, infections, and myelokathexis (WHIM) (a disease due to CXCR4 variants) and empagliflozin in Glycogenosis IB and G6PC3 neutropenias [26, 27]. On the contrary, drugs like nicotinamide and sivelestat were shown to be only partially effective in managing "classical" congenital neutropenias [28, 29]. Pegfilgrastim, the long-life G-CSF, is considered a possible alternative in neutropenic patients with scarce/low compliance to traditional daily injections of G-CSF [30]. Gene therapy for congenital neutropenia is a potential future alternative approach, which is currently under investigation at the experimental preclinical level.

Presently, the only curative therapy is hematopoietic stem cell transplantation (HSCT), which, unfortunately, carries an intrinsic risk of mortality estimated at a rate of 17%, based on data coming from the largest cohort of severe CN-transplanted patients ever collected [31].

The choice of whether to perform HSCT or not must be carefully evaluated. This procedure is clearly indicated in case of MDS/AL, in neutropenic subjects carrying variants with an intrinsic high risk of transformation, or in case of an inability to control the disorder with very high doses of G-CSF (i.e., >20 mcg/kg). Other elements to consider with respect to HSCT are the availability of a healthy HLA-identical family donor and the expertise of the reference center [32].

Acquired Neutropenias

Acquired forms of neutropenias include primary or idiopathic and secondary neutropenias that are usually associated with other specific disorders [6].

In primary idiopathic forms, neutropenia is a predominant, often isolated feature, which can either be antibody- (antineutrophil) (as in primary autoimmune and alloimmune neutropenias) or non-antibody-mediated (as in idiopathic neutropenia of infancy and chronic idiopathic neutropenia (CIN) in adults, also known as idiopathic cytopenia of undetermined significance—neutropenia (ICUS-N)).

Secondary neutropenias may be associated with a number of diseases, i.e., hypersplenism, infections (viral, like human immunodeficiency virus (HIV), HCV, HBV, cytomegalovirus (CMV), Epstein–Barr virus (EBV), influenza, and SARS-CoV-2; bacterial, including salmonella, brucella, rickettsia, mycobacterium, and mycoplasma; parasitic, like plasmodium spp. and visceral leishmaniasis; and fungal, like histoplasmosis), autoimmune diseases (thyroid diseases, systemic lupus erythematosus, rheumatoid arthritis, and Sjogren's syndrome), nutritional deficiencies (B12, folic acid, iron, and copper deficiencies, and caloric malnutrition), immune-dysregulation disorders (e.g., common variable immunodeficiency), hematologic diseases (aplastic anemia and myeloid or lymphoid malignancies, including large granular lymphocytic leukemia), and drug-induced.

Children

The most common forms of acquired neutropenias in infancy are primary autoimmune neutropenia (pAIN) and idiopathic neutropenia (IN). It is generally accepted that they are the same disease with the discriminatory presence of specific antibodies against neutrophils in the first, which are not detected in the second due to the suboptimal sensitivity of antineutrophil antibody assays [33–35].

Primary autoimmune and idiopathic neutropenias usually arise within the first year of life, have a mild clinical course, and tend to resolve 24–36 months after their appearance in almost 90% of cases [34]. Severe infections account only for a minor portion of affected subjects (10–12%), and for this reason, no continuative treatment with G-CSF is needed [36].

On-demand G-CSF therapy could be necessary when infections persist in spite of antibiotic therapy. The reasons why these neutropenias appear, persist, and spontaneously remit are not completely known; a role may be played by the immaturity of the immune system in the first years of life, but this hypothesis would need further confirmation [34, 35].

Recently, two categories of neutropenia, which belong neither to the primary autoimmune nor to the idiopathic forms of infancy and not even to secondary neutropenias, have been described. Their main features are the following: duration of neutropenia longer than the typical 24–36 months (long-lasting neutropenia (LLNp)) or "late appearance," which is a rise after the usual age of 3 years (late-onset neutropenia (LONp)) [37, 38]. LLNp and LONp may sometimes be diagnosed by chance due to the very mild clinical phenotype and do not usually show remission. Antineutrophil antibodies can or cannot be detected. A recent study showed that these forms of neutropenia have a limited infection risk, some distinct immunological features (leukopenia and lymphopenia with decreased B and NK cells), a tendency to develop autoimmune symptoms/signs over time, and in about 10% of subjects, an underlying genetic background related to immune-dysregulation/deficiency disorders [39].

These neutropenias were considered a new provisional category named "likely acquired neutropenias" because of the underlying genetic background observed in a proportion of subjects [6, 39]. These findings have clinical relevance since they suggest that the diagnostic workup and management of NPs lasting longer than the typical time frame and appearing in late childhood and adolescence should be fairly different and more immune-genetic-oriented compared to the typical pAIN diagnosed in early infancy or remitting within the expected time [37, 38].

Adults

In contrast to children, primary AIN is extremely rare in adults, and therefore, a thorough investigation and close follow-up is mandatory to exclude a latent autoimmune or immune-dysregulation disorder in these patients. According to the authors' experience, the non-antibody-mediated chronic idiopathic neutropenia (CIN) is the most common diagnosis in adults with unexplained neutropenia proceeding to the outpatient hematology clinic after a baseline evaluation from their internists. The usual profile of CIN adult patients includes middle-aged women who display an uncomplicated course without infections.

The pathophysiologic mechanisms associated with CIN involve increased apoptosis of the granulocytic progenitor cells within an inhibitory bone marrow (BM) microenvironment, consisting of myelosuppressive oligoclonal T-lymphocytes, activated monocytes with upregulation of the toll-like receptor–4 signaling, and mesenchymal stem cells with altered properties [40–44]. All these cells collectively produce proinflammatory mediators, such as transforming growth factor (TGF)-β1, tumor necrosis factor (TNF)-α, interferon (IFN)-γ, Fas-ligand, interleukin(IL)-1β, and IL-6, which further contribute to the inflammatory BM microenvironment [45–47].

Despite the progress in the clarification of the pathophysiologic mechanisms associated with CIN, the underlying pathogenesis remains obscure. This is due to the fact that under the diagnosis of CIN, different disease entities apparently exist. In favor of this hypothesis is a recent whole exome sequencing (WES) study in adult patients with CIN, which showed that a constitutional/congenital background may be found in some patients [48]. Specifically, the WES analysis showed ten pathogenic/likely pathogenic variants in ten out of 16 studied patients. These variants included a heterozygous mutation in *G6PC3* that, in homozygosity, is associated with congenital neutropenia, mutations in *FANCM* and *CTC1, genes* associated with BM failure syndromes, and genes related to immune deficiency and dysregulation, such as *DCLRE1C, ORAI1, SPINK5, MEFV, PSMG2, IRF7,* and *PEPD.* An average number of 4.5 variants of undetermined significance (VUS) per patient was also identified in genes related to congenital neutropenias (*HAX1, VPS13B,* and *LYST*), BM failure (*GATA2, SAMD9,* and *CXCR4*), or immunodeficiency (*TCF3*) syndromes. Definitely, more studies are required to investigate the precise role of these variants in the pathogenesis of CIN.

In contrast to patients with congenital neutropenias, patients with CIN have a low propensity to transform to myelodysplastic syndrome (MDS)/acute myeloid leukemia (AML). However, the application of next-generation sequencing (NGS) for the analysis of genes commonly mutated in myeloid malignancies has shown that CIN patients with clonal hematopoiesis (CH) have a relative risk for transformation of 31.24 compared to non-clonal patients [49]. The risk is higher in patients with mutations in *IDH1/2*; in RNA-splicing genes, such as *SRSF2* and *ZRSR2*; and in combined mutations implicating age-related clonal hemopoiesis genes (*DNMT3,*

ASXL1, and *TET2*) [49, 50]. A variant allele frequency (VAF) of the mutant clones higher than 10% is an additional risk factor for MDS/AML transformation [49, 50]. Based on these findings and also given that the absence of CH in CIN patients is associated with a high negative predictive value (0.99) for the development of MDS/AML, the inclusion of an NGS myeloid panel is highly recommended for the investigation of CIN patients [6, 49]. It is also recommended that CIN patients with CH, particularly with high VAF (>10%) mutations and young (the frequency of age-related CH is low than in older subjects) subjects, need to have a closer follow-up for the early identification of peripheral blood (PB) changes denoting MDS/AML transformation.

References

1. Common Terminology Criteria for Adverse Events CTCAE version 5.0 Nov 2017 at https://ctep.cancer.gov/protocoldevelopment/electronic_applications/ctc.htm#ctc_50.
2. Dinauer MC, Newburger PE, Borregaard N. The phagocyte system and disorders of granulopoiesis and granulocyte function. In: Orkin SH, Fisher DE, Look AT, Lux SE, Nathan DG, editors. Nathan and OsKi's hematology of infancy and childhood. 8th ed. Philadelphia: Elsevier Saunders Company; 2015. p. 773–850.
3. Valent P. Low blood counts: immune mediated, idiopathic, or myelodysplasia. Hematology Am Soc Hematol Educ Program. 2012;2012:485–91.
4. Shoenfeld Y, Alkan ML, Asaly A, Carmeli Y, Katz M. Benign familial leukopenia and neutropenia in different ethnic groups. Eur J Haematol. 1988;41(3):273–7.
5. Atallah-Yunes SM, Ready A, Newburger PE. Benign ethnic neutropenia. Blood Rev. 2019;37:S0268-960X(19)30024-4.
6. Fioredda F, Skokowa J, Tamary H, et al. The European guidelines on diagnosis and management of neutropenia in adults and children: a consensus between the European Hematology Association and the EuNet-INNOCHRON COST Action. Hema. 2023;7:e872.
7. Donadieu J, Beaupain B, Fenneteau O, et al. Congenital neutropenia in the era of genomics: classification, diagnosis, and natural history. Br J Haematol. 2017;179:557–74.
8. Skokowa J, Dale DC, Touw IP, Zeidler C, Welte K. Severe congenital neutropenias. Nat Rev Dis Primers. 2017;3:17032.
9. Klein C, Grudzien M, Appaswamy M, et al. HAX1 deficiency causes autosomal recessive severe congenital neutropenia (Kostmann disease). Nat Genet. 2007;39:86–92.
10. Pogozhykh D, Yilmaz Karapinar D, Klimiankou M, et al. HAX1-related congenital neutropenia: long-term observation in paediatric and adult patients enrolled in the European branch of the Severe Chronic Neutropenia International Registry (SCNIR). Br J Haematol. 2023;202:393–411.
11. Alizadeh Z, Fazlollahi MR, Houshmand M, et al. Different pattern of gene mutations in Iranian patients with severe congenital neutropenia (including 2 new mutations). Iran J Allergy Asthma Immunol. 2013;12:86–92.
12. Lebel A, Yacobovich J, Krasnov T, et al. Genetic analysis and clinical picture of severe congenital neutropenia in Israel. Pediatr Blood Cancer. 2015;62:103–8.
13. Glaubach T, Minella AC, Corey SJ. Cellular stress pathways in pediatric bone marrow failure syndromes: many roads lead to neutropenia. Pediatr Res. 2014;75:189–95.
14. Boxer LA, Newburger PE. A molecular classification of congenital neutropenia syndromes. Pediatr Blood Cancer. 2007;49:609–14.
15. Klein C. Congenital neutropenia. Hematology Am Soc Hematol Educ Program. 2009;2009:344–50.

16. Tangye SG, Al-Herz W, Bousfiha A, et al. Human inborn errors of immunity: 2022 update on the classification from the International Union of Immunological Societies Expert Committee. J Clin Immunol. 2022;42:1473–507.
17. OMIM® Online Mendelian Inheritance in Man® Updated January 10, 2022. https://www.omim.org/.
18. Boztug K, Appaswamy G, Ashikov A, et al. A syndrome with congenital neutropenia and mutations in G6PC3. N Engl J Med. 2009;360:32–43.
19. Thompson AS, Giri N, Gianferante DM, Jones K, et al. Shwachman Diamond syndrome: narrow genotypic spectrum and variable clinical features. Pediatr Res. 2022;92:1671–80.
20. Warren JT, Cupo RR, Wattanasirakul P, Spencer DH, et al. Heterozygous variants of CLPB are a cause of severe congenital neutropenia. Blood. 2022;139:779–91.
21. Willemsen M, Barber JS, Nieuwenhove EV, Staels F, et al. Homozygous DBF4 mutation as a cause of severe congenital neutropenia. J Allergy Clin Immunol. 2023;152:266–77.
22. Linder MI, Mizoguchi Y, Hesse S, Csaba G, et al. Human genetic defects in SRP19 and SRPRA cause severe congenital neutropenia with distinctive proteome changes. Blood. 2023;141:645–58.
23. Marin-Esteban V, Youn J, Beaupain B, et al. Biallelic CXCR2 loss-of-function mutations define a distinct congenital neutropenia entity. Haematologica. 2022;107:765–9.
24. Rosenberg PS, Zeidler C, Bolyard AA, et al. Stable long term risk of leukaemia in patients with severe congenital neutropenia maintained on G-CSF therapy. Br J Haematol. 2010;150:196–9.
25. Dale DC. How I manage neutropenia in children. Br J Haematol. 2017;178:351–63.
26. Dale DC, Firkin F, Bolyard AA, Kelley M, et al. Results of a phase 2 trial of an oral CXCR4 antagonist, mavorixafor, for treatment of WHIM syndrome. Blood. 2020;136(26):2994–3003.
27. Grunert SC, Derks TGJ, Adrian K, et al. Efficacy and safety of empagliflozin in glycogen storage disease type Ib: data from an international questionnaire. Genet Med. 2022;24:1781–8.
28. Nayak RC, Trump LR, Aronow BJ, Myers K, et al. Pathogenesis of ELANE-mutant severe neutropenia revealed by induced pluripotent stem cells. J Clin Invest. 2015;125:3103–16.
29. Deordieva E, Shvets O, Voronin K, Maschan A, et al. Nicotinamide (vitamin B3) treatment improves response to G-CSF in severe congenital neutropenia patients. Br J Haematol. 2021;192:788–92.
30. Fioredda F, Lanza T, Gallicola F, et al. Long-term use of pegfilgrastim in children with severe congenital neutropenia: clinical and pharmacokinetic data. Blood. 2016;128:2178–81.
31. Fioredda F, Iacobelli S, van Biezen A, et al. Stem cell transplantation in severe congenital neutropenia: an analysis from the European Society for Blood and Marrow Transplantation. Blood. 2015;126:1885–92.
32. Peffault de Latour R, Peters C, Gibson B, et al. Recommendations on hematopoietic stem cell transplantation for inherited bone marrow failure syndromes. Bone Marrow Transplant. 2015;50:1168–72.
33. Bux J, Behrens G, Jaeger G, Welte K. Diagnosis and clinical course of autoimmune neutropenia in infancy: analysis of 240 cases. Blood. 1998;91:181–6.
34. Farruggia P, Fioredda F, Puccio G, et al. Autoimmune neutropenia of infancy: data from the Italian Neutropenia Registry. Am J Hematol. 2015;90:E221–2.
35. Farruggia P, Fioredda F, Puccio G, et al. Idiopathic neutropenia of infancy: data from the Italian Neutropenia Registry. Am J Hematol. 2019;94:216–22.
36. Fioredda F, Onofrillo D, Farruggia P, et al. Diagnosis and management of neutropenia in children: the approach of the Study Group on Neutropenia and Marrow Failure Syndromes of the Pediatric Italian Hemato-Oncology Association (Associazione Italiana Emato-Oncologia Pediatrica – AIEOP). Pediatr Blood Cancer. 2022;69:e29599.
37. Fioredda F, Dufour C, Höglund P, et al. Autoimmune neutropenias: update on clinical and biological features in children and adults. Haemasphere. 2022;7:e814. https://www.ncbi.nlm.nih.gov/pmc/articles/PMC9771305/.
38. Fioredda F, Rotulo GA, Farruggia P, et al. Late-onset and long-lasting autoimmune neutropenia: an analysis from the Italian Neutropenia Registry. Blood Adv. 2020;4:5644–9.

39. Fioredda F, Beccaria A, Casartelli P, et al. Late-onset and long-lasting neutropenias in the young: a new entity anticipating immune-dysregulation disorders. Am J Haematol. 2024;99:534.
40. Papadaki HA, Eliopoulos AG, Kosteas T, Gemetzi C, Damianaki A, Koutala H, et al. Impaired granulocytopoiesis in patients with chronic idiopathic neutropenia is associated with increased apoptosis of bone marrow myeloid progenitor cells. Blood. 2003;101(7):2591–600.
41. Papadaki HA, Stamatopoulos K, Damianaki A, Gemetzi C, Anagnostopoulos A, Papadaki T, et al. Activated T-lymphocytes with myelosuppressive properties in patients with chronic idiopathic neutropenia. Br J Haematol. 2005;128(6):863–76.
42. Velegraki M, Koutala H, Tsatsanis C, Papadaki HA. Increased levels of the high mobility group box 1 protein sustain the inflammatory bone marrow microenvironment in patients with chronic idiopathic neutropenia via activation of toll-like receptor 4. J Clin Immunol. 2012;32(2):312–22.
43. Bizymi N, Velegraki M, Damianaki A, Koutala H, Papadaki HA. Altered monocyte subsets in patients with chronic idiopathic neutropenia. J Clin Immunol. 2019;39(8):852–4.
44. Stavroulaki E, Kastrinaki MC, Pontikoglou C, Eliopoulos D, Damianaki A, Mavroudi I, et al. Mesenchymal stem cells contribute to the abnormal bone marrow microenvironment in patients with chronic idiopathic neutropenia by overproduction of transforming growth factor-β1. Stem Cells Dev. 2011;20(8):1309–18.
45. Koumaki V, Damianaki A, Ximeri M, Pontikoglou C, Axioti F, Spanoudakis M, et al. Pro-inflammatory bone marrow milieu in patients with chronic idiopathic neutropenia is associated with impaired local production of interleukin-10. Br J Haematol. 2006;135(4):570–3.
46. Papadaki HA, Giouremou K, Eliopoulos GD. Low frequency of myeloid progenitor cells in chronic idiopathic neutropenia of adults may be related to increased production of TGF-β1 by bone marrow stromal cells. Eur J Haematol. 1999;63(3):154–62.
47. Papadaki HA, Chatzivassili A, Stefanaki K, Koumaki V, Kanavaros P, Eliopoulos GD. Morphologically defined myeloid cell compartments, lymphocyte subpopulations, and histological findings of bone marrow in patients with nonimmune chronic idiopathic neutropenia of adults. Am J Hematol. 2000;79:563–70.
48. Tsaknakis G, Grossi A, Rusmini M, Ceccherini I, Uva P, Miano M, et al. Heterogeneous genetic landscape of chronic idiopathic neutropenia revealed by whole exome sequencing. Blood. 2023;142(Supplement 1):931.
49. Tsaknakis G, Gallì A, Papadakis S, et al. Incidence and prognosis of clonal hematopoiesis in patients with chronic idiopathic neutropenia. Blood. 2021;138:1249–57.
50. Malcovati L, Gallì A, Travaglino E, et al. Clinical significance of somatic mutation in unexplained blood cytopenia. Blood. 2017;129:3371–8.

Open Access This chapter is licensed under the terms of the Creative Commons Attribution 4.0 International License (http://creativecommons.org/licenses/by/4.0/), which permits use, sharing, adaptation, distribution and reproduction in any medium or format, as long as you give appropriate credit to the original author(s) and the source, provide a link to the Creative Commons license and indicate if changes were made.

The images or other third party material in this chapter are included in the chapter's Creative Commons license, unless indicated otherwise in a credit line to the material. If material is not included in the chapter's Creative Commons license and your intended use is not permitted by statutory regulation or exceeds the permitted use, you will need to obtain permission directly from the copyright holder.

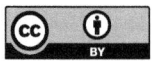

Chapter 22
Amegakaryocytic Thrombocytopenia

Chokri Ben Lamine, Thierry Leblanc, Mahmoud Aljurf,
and Jean-Hugues Dalle

Introduction

Congenital amegakaryocytic thrombocytopenia (CAMT) is a rare, autosomal recessive, inherited bone marrow failure (IBMF) disorder defined by a significant reduction or complete absence of megakaryocytes in the bone marrow. This diagnosis should be considered mostly in infants or toddlers presenting with early onset of bruising or bleeding caused by nonimmune thrombocytopenia, especially in the absence of physical abnormalities. Confirmation of the diagnosis relies on laboratory and clinical evaluations, including peripheral blood analysis, bone marrow examination, measurement of platelet volume, serum thrombopoietin (TPO) levels, and genetic analysis identifying mutations in the c-MPL gene. Mild cases of thrombocytopenia might escape early detection, leading to delayed diagnosis. However, to date, all reported cases have been identified prior to adulthood [1–3].

Molecular Pathogenesis

CAMT is caused by mutations in the c-MPL gene, which encodes the thrombopoietin (TPO) receptor. These mutations result in an abnormal receptor that lacks the capacity to bind TPO, leading to impaired megakaryopoiesis despite significantly

---

C. B. Lamine (✉) · M. Aljurf
Department of Hematology, Stem Cell Transplant & Cellular Therapy, Cancer Centre of Excellence, King Faisal Specialist Hospital & Research Centre, Riyadh, Saudi Arabia
e-mail: bcben@kfshrc.edu.sa

T. Leblanc · J.-H. Dalle
Department of Pediatric Hematology and Immunology, Robert Debré Academic Hospital, GHU AP-HP Nord Université Paris Cité, Paris, France

elevated serum TPO levels [1, 4–10]. While the TPO signaling pathway is critical for megakaryopoiesis, it is not as singularly essential as erythropoietin is for erythropoiesis. Alternative pathways involving cytokines, such as interleukin-3 (IL-3), interleukin-6 (IL-6), and stem cell factor (SCF), can partially sustain megakaryocyte production. This residual megakaryopoiesis, observed in some CAMT patients, aligns with animal studies showing that mice deficient in TPO or its receptor (MPL) retain some megakaryopoiesis through these compensatory mechanisms [2, 11–13].

The TPO receptor belongs to the cytokine receptor superfamily, with roles extending beyond megakaryopoiesis to the maintenance of hematopoietic stem cell (HSC) homeostasis. Its expression on the CD34+ progenitor cells, bone marrow, spleen, and fetal liver underlines its pivotal function in overall hematopoietic health. Consequently, mutations in c-MPL can lead to marrow failure with pancytopenia due to the disruption of HSC quiescence and renewal [11–13].

Since the first mutation in c-MPL was identified by Kenji Ihara in 1999, more than 36 mutations have been reported. Genotype–phenotype correlation studies suggest that null mutations are associated with severe early thrombocytopenia and rapid progression to pancytopenia (CAMT-I), whereas missense mutations may result in transient improvement in platelet counts during childhood, followed by delayed progression to aplastic anemia (CAMT-II) [7–9, 14–16]. Most CAMT cases are attributed to homozygous or compound heterozygous c-MPL mutations. Truncating mutations typically result in defective TPO receptor presentation on the cell surface, rendering cells unresponsive to TPO [17, 18].

Clinical Manifestation and Diagnosis

The clinical presentation of CAMT is highly variable, with severe hemorrhagic symptoms commonly occurring during the neonatal period. Cases with fetal hemorrhage have been reported [19]. Newborns may develop life-threatening central nervous system (CNS) hemorrhages during childbirth. Infants and young children often present with bleeding symptoms, including petechiae, ecchymoses, and mucosal bleeding, even before achieving independent mobility. These hemorrhages can occur in unusual locations, and the severity ranges from mild purpura to life-threatening events. However, no specific hemorrhagic manifestation is pathognomonic for CAMT.

Clinical features may initially mimic conditions such as neonatal alloimmune thrombocytopenia or idiopathic thrombocytopenic purpura (ITP). Diagnosis requires persistent thrombocytopenia, absent or severely reduced bone marrow megakaryocytes, markedly elevated serum TPO levels, and progression to bone marrow failure (BMF). Confirmatory genetic testing identifies c-MPL mutations, as no other genes have yet been implicated in CAMT [3, 20].

A subset of patients presents with morphologic amegakaryocytosis without *c-MPL* mutations, termed CAMT Type III. These patients exhibit amegakaryocytic features and elevated TPO levels, suggesting alternative genetic or epigenetic etiologies. Milder cases of thrombocytopenia may evade detection during early childhood but are invariably diagnosed before adulthood.

The natural progression of CAMT involves worsening, with a median progression to pancytopenia by 39 months in 68% of cases reported up to 2011. The projected median age for the development of aplastic anemia is 5 years, with over 90% of cases progressing by age 13 [3, 21].

CAMT can be categorized into three clinical subtypes based on disease progression:

1. *Type I*: persistent severe thrombocytopenia ($<50 \times 10^9$/L) progressing to pancytopenia within 2 years
2. *Type II*: transient improvement in platelet counts (up to ~50×10^9/L), followed by pancytopenia around 5 years
3. *Type III*: ineffective megakaryopoiesis associated with amegakaryocytosis and elevated TPO levels without identified c-MPL mutations.

The malignant transformation is rare compared to other inherited bone marrow failure syndromes, possibly due to the protective role of hematopoietic stem cell transplantation (HSCT) in preventing leukemic evolution.

Although congenital abnormalities are not commonly part of the CAMT phenotype, some cases have reported associated malformations, including cardiac septal defects, ocular anomalies, and cerebral abnormalities, such as cortical dysplasia, lissencephaly, hypoplastic cerebellar vermis, and enlarged cisterna magna [6].

When CAMT presents with typical clinical features and amegakaryocytosis, the differential diagnosis is narrow. Conditions to exclude include the following:

- *Thrombocytopenia with Absent Radii (TAR) Syndrome*: Characterized by bilateral and symmetric radial hypoplasia with preserved thumbs.
- *Inherited Bone Marrow Failure Syndromes (IBMFs)*: Include Fanconi anemia, dyskeratosis congenita, Shwachman–Diamond syndrome, and telomeropathies. These typically involve additional cytopenias or physical anomalies, unlike isolated thrombocytopenia seen in CAMT. In infants with BMF, MECOM syndrome is the main differential diagnosis; SAMD9/SAMD9L syndrome and severe forms of telomeropathies (Hoyeraal–Hreidarsson syndrome) may also present with early (<2 years) BMF.
- *Wiskott–Aldrich Syndrome*: Distinguished by microthrombocytes (low mean platelet volume (MPV)) and associated immune deficiency and skin manifestations, whereas MPV is normal in CAMT.
- *Other Congenital Thrombocytopenias (CT)*: Blood and bone marrow film analysis associated with genetic analysis allow correct diagnosis. Among CT, megakaryocytes may be reduced in patients with RUSAT/MECOM syndrome, TAR syndrome, and IBMF associated with *THPO* variants.

Rarely, neonatal alloimmune amegakaryocytosis has been reported, but these cases are infrequent in recent literature. Additionally, some neonates suspected of CAMT have been found to carry chromosomal abnormalities, such as 22q11.2 deletions (DiGeorge syndrome), or mutations in genes associated with Noonan syndrome.

This comprehensive diagnostic framework underscores the importance of integrating clinical, laboratory, and genetic findings to distinguish CAMT from other thrombocytopenic disorders and ensure timely and accurate diagnosis.

Laboratory Features

Thrombocytopenia in CAMT is typically profound, with a median platelet count of approximately $17 \times 10^9/L$ at the time of diagnosis, ranging between 4 and $96 \times 10^9/L$ [15]. Platelet size and morphology are normal, as reflected by a normal mean platelet volume (MPV) and normal appearance on peripheral blood films [24]. The expression of platelet surface glycoproteins is also preserved, which helps distinguish CAMT from conditions like Wiskott–Aldrich syndrome [9]. At the time of diagnosis, other hematopoietic lineages remain unaffected, with no evidence of concurrent cytopenias.

Bone marrow examination in CAMT typically reveals a normocellular marrow, with either absent or markedly reduced megakaryocytes, while other hematopoietic lineages appear normal. When megakaryocytes are present, they are often small and immature in morphology. However, a single bone marrow evaluation may not always demonstrate the characteristic findings, as megakaryocytes can occasionally appear normal during the early stages of disease [24]. Therefore, repeat bone marrow aspirations may be necessary when CAMT is strongly suspected but when initial findings are inconclusive [15].

Serum thrombopoietin (TPO) levels in CAMT are consistently and markedly elevated, often significantly higher (10- to 50-fold) than those observed in other conditions associated with reduced megakaryopoiesis, regardless of etiology. Elevated TPO levels provide an important diagnostic clue, supporting the diagnosis of CAMT when paired with clinical and histopathological findings.

Although additional diagnostic tools have been proposed, they are not currently routine in clinical practice [15]. The definitive diagnosis of CAMT rests on identifying severe isolated thrombocytopenia with normal platelet size, a marked reduction or absence of megakaryocytes in the bone marrow, and elevated serum TPO levels. Genetic testing for mutations in the *c-MPL* gene remains the gold standard for diagnosis, with sequencing of the entire coding region providing the highest diagnostic yield. This comprehensive approach ensures accurate differentiation of CAMT from other causes of thrombocytopenia and informs timely therapeutic decisions. To our knowledge, no case of somatic genetic rescue has been reported.

Treatment and Supportive Care

Supportive Care

Treatment options for CAMT remain highly limited, as patients typically show no response to therapies such as immunoglobulins, corticosteroids, splenectomy, or androgens. Moreover, to date, TPO receptor agonists have demonstrated no clinical benefit in managing CAMT. Supportive care primarily involves long-term transfusions of blood products, tailored to mitigate hemorrhagic risks and improve quality of life.

Key principles for transfusion management include the following:

- Use of irradiated, leukocyte-depleted, and compatible blood products to reduce alloimmunization risk.
- Restriction of platelet transfusions to cases with clinical bleeding; prophylactic transfusions based solely on platelet counts are discouraged.
- Tranexamic acid may be useful in patients with active bleeding [20].

Given the risk of clonal evolution and potential malignant transformation, annual bone marrow examination, including cytogenetic monitoring, is essential. For patients progressing to pancytopenia, prophylactic antimicrobial therapy—targeting bacterial and fungal infections—should be considered to reduce severe infections that may impair eligibility for future curative therapies, such as HSCT.

Hematopoietic Stem Cell Transplantation (HSCT)

HSCT remains the only curative treatment for CAMT, offering the potential to restore normal hematopoiesis. Recent retrospective data from the European Society for Blood and Marrow Transplantation (EBMT) demonstrate its efficacy, although outcomes depend on several critical factors [22, 23].

- Efficacy: In a cohort of 63 patients undergoing HSCT (1987–2013), the 5-year overall survival (OS) rate was 76.6%, regardless of donor type or stem cell source. Transplant-related mortality (TRM) was approximately 13% at 3 years.
- Donor Selection: Forty percent of transplants were from HLA-matched sibling donors, while another 40% utilized unrelated donors. Seventeen percent employed unrelated cord blood. Although OS was comparable across donor types, sibling donors and bone marrow grafts showed trends toward better outcomes and lower TRM.
- Age of Transplantation: Median age at HSCT was 7 years. Early transplantation during childhood, ideally before significant pancytopenia or transfusion-associated complications, improves outcomes. However, transplantation before 1 year of age is avoided due to excessive toxicity in infancy.

Indication

HSCT should be considered in any child with severe thrombocytopenia (requiring transfusion), BMF, or evidence of clonal evolution.

Stem Cell Source and Dose

Bone marrow is the preferred stem cell source in CAMT patients, consistent with data from other IBMF syndromes, such as Fanconi anemia and acquired aplastic anemia. Bone marrow offers lower risks of chronic graft-versus-host disease (cGvHD) compared to peripheral blood stem cells. Recommended cell doses are as follows:

- Bone marrow: $>3 \times 10^8$ total nucleated cells/kg recipient body weight
- Cord blood: $>3 \times 10^7$ total nucleated cells/kg recipient body weight (pre-freezing) [25]

Conditioning and GvHD Prophylaxis

- Conditioning Regimen: Myeloablative conditioning is standard, with regimens excluding total body irradiation (TBI) to reduce long-term toxicities.
- GvHD Prevention: Prophylaxis with cyclosporin A (CSA) and methotrexate is recommended. CSA is gradually tapered and discontinued within 6–12 months post- HSCT, assuming no evidence of chronic GvHD. Pretransplantation serotherapy (antithymocyte globulin or alemtuzumab) is indicated for unrelated donor transplants to prevent graft rejection, though it is not routinely used in sibling donor transplants due to higher infection-related TRM.

Challenges and Risks

Patients with CAMT face a higher risk of transplant-related complications, including the following:

- Graft Rejection: 17% of patients require a second or third HSCT for primary graft failure.
- Transplant-Related Mortality: Contributing factors include prior infections, prolonged aplasia, and iron overload secondary to transfusions.

Alternative donor HSCT (e.g., haploidentical or unrelated cord blood) should only be performed at specialized centers due to higher risks of graft failure and TRM. These cases should also be reported to international registries to enhance the collective understanding of outcomes in rare diseases like CAMT.

This structured approach to treatment and supportive care highlights the central role of HSCT as a curative strategy, emphasizing the importance of early intervention, careful donor selection, and optimized transplant protocols to maximize outcomes.

References

1. Ballmaier M, Germeshausen M. Congenital amegakaryocytic thrombocytopenia: clinical presentation, diagnosis, and treatment. Semin Thromb Hemost. 2011;37(6):673–81.
2. Geddis AE. Congenital amegakaryocytic thrombocytopenia. Pediatr Blood Cancer. 2011;57(2):199–203.
3. Drachman JG. Inherited thrombocytopenia: when a low platelet count does not mean ITP. Blood. 2004;103(2):390–8.
4. Ihara K, Ishii E, Eguchi M, et al. Identification of mutations in the c-mpl gene in congenital amegakaryocytic thrombocytopenia. Proc Natl Acad Sci USA. 1999;96(6):3132–6.
5. Savoia A, Dufour C, Locatelli F, et al. Congenital amegakaryocytic thrombocytopenia: clinical and biological consequences of five novel mutations. Haematologica. 2007;92(9):1186–93.
6. King S, Germeshausen M, Strauss G, Welte K, Ballmaier M. Congenital amegakaryocytic thrombocytopenia: a retrospective clinical analysis of 20 patients. Br J Haematol. 2005;131(5):636–44.
7. Passos-Coelho JL, Sebastiao M, Gameiro P, et al. Congenital amegakaryocytic thrombocytopenia—report of a new c-mpl gene missense mutation. Am J Hematol. 2007;82(3):240–1.
8. Rose MJ, Nicol KK, Skeens MA, Gross TG, Kerlin BA. Congenital amegakaryocytic thrombocytopenia: the diagnostic importance of combining pathology with molecular genetics. Pediatr Blood Cancer. 2008;50(6):1263–5.
9. Ballmaier M, Germeshausen M. Advances in the understanding of congenital amegakaryocytic thrombocytopenia. Br J Haematol. 2009;146(1):3–16.
10. Varghese LN, Zhang JG, Young SN, et al. Functional characterization of c-Mpl ectodomain mutations that underlie congenital amegakaryocytic thrombocytopenia. Growth Factors. 2014;32(1):18–26.
11. Kaushansky K. The molecular mechanisms that control thrombopoiesis. J Clin Invest. 2005;115(12):3339–47.
12. Kobayashi M, Laver JH, Kato T, Miyazaki H, Ogawa M. Thrombopoietin supports proliferation of human primitive hematopoietic cells in synergy with steel factor and/or interleukin-3. Blood. 1996;88(2):429–36.
13. Yoshihara H, Arai F, Hosokawa K, et al. Thrombopoietin/MPL signaling regulates hematopoietic stem cell quiescence and interaction with the osteoblastic niche. Cell Stem Cell. 2007;1(6):685–97.
14. Freedman MH, Estrov Z. Congenital amegakaryocytic thrombocytopenia: an intrinsic hematopoietic stem cell defect. Am J Pediatr Hematol Oncol. 1990;12(2):225–30.
15. Stoddart MT, Connor P, Germeshausen M, Ballmaier M, Steward CG. Congenital amegakaryocytic thrombocytopenia (CAMT) presenting as severe pancytopenia in the first month of life. Pediatr Blood Cancer. 2013;60(9):E94–6.

16. Muraoka K, Ishii E, Ihara K, et al. Successful bone marrow transplantation in a patient with c-mpl-mutated congenital amegakaryocytic thrombocytopenia from a carrier donor. Pediatr Transplant. 2005;9(1):101–3.
17. Ballmaier M, Germeshausen M, Schulze H, et al. c-Mpl mutations are the cause of congenital amegakaryocytic thrombocytopenia. Blood. 2001;97(1):139–46.
18. Alter BP. Diagnosis, genetics, and management of inherited bone marrow failure syndromes. Hematology Am Soc Hematol Educ Program. 2007;2007:29–39.
19. Gano D, et al. Fetal intracranial hemorrhage due to uniparental disomy and unmasked MPL-related thrombocytopenia. Prenat Diagn. 2025. https://doi.org/10.1002/pd.6737.
20. Tirthani E, et al. Congenital amegakaryocytic thrombocytopenia. In: StatPearls [Internet]. Treasure Island: StatPearls Publishing; 2024.
21. Christensen RD, Wiedmeier SE, Yaish HM. A neonate with congenital amegakaryocytic thrombocytopenia associated with a chromosomal microdeletion at 21q22.11 including the gene RUNX1. J Perinatol. 2013;33(3):242–4.
22. Eapen M, et al. Effect of stem cell source on outcomes after unrelated donor transplantation in severe aplastic anemia. Blood. 2011;118(9):2618–21.
23. Peffault de Latour R, et al. Allogeneic hematopoietic stem cell transplantation in Fanconi anemia: the European Group for Blood and Marrow Transplantation experience. Blood. 2013;122(26):4279–86.
24. Henter JI, et al. Diagnostic guidelines for hemophagocytic lymphohistiocytosis: report of the histiocyte society. Pediatr Blood Cancer. 2008;50(6):1247–55.
25. Bacigalupo A, et al. Conditioning regimen for alternative donor transplants in acquired severe aplastic anemia. Haematologica. 2010;95(6):976–82.

Open Access This chapter is licensed under the terms of the Creative Commons Attribution 4.0 International License (http://creativecommons.org/licenses/by/4.0/), which permits use, sharing, adaptation, distribution and reproduction in any medium or format, as long as you give appropriate credit to the original author(s) and the source, provide a link to the Creative Commons license and indicate if changes were made.

The images or other third party material in this chapter are included in the chapter's Creative Commons license, unless indicated otherwise in a credit line to the material. If material is not included in the chapter's Creative Commons license and your intended use is not permitted by statutory regulation or exceeds the permitted use, you will need to obtain permission directly from the copyright holder.

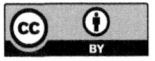

Chapter 23
Newly Recognized Inherited Bone Marrow Failure Syndromes

Alfadil Haroon, Marcin W. Wlodarski, Régis Peffault de Latour, and Mahmoud Aljurf

Introduction

Inherited bone marrow failure syndromes (IBMFSs) include both inherited and acquired disorders, which result in inadequate hematopoiesis and an increased predisposition to myeloid neoplasms. The classical IBMFSs include Fanconi anemia, severe congenital neutropenia, dyskeratosis congenita (telomere biology disorders), and Diamond–Blackfan anemia (DBA), which have been extensively characterized [1–3]. The advent of next-generation sequencing (NGS) technology has significantly expanded our understanding of IBMFS, revealing novel genetic etiologies beyond the previously established classifications (Table 23.1) [4]. Recent genomic studies have identified several emerging IBMFS entities caused by germline mutations in multiple genes, including Myb-like SWIRM and MPN domains 1 (MYSM1), ERCC6L2, MECOM, DNAJC21, alcohol dehydrogenase 5 (ADH5)/aldehyde dehydrogenase 2 (ALDH2), sterile alpha motif domain–containing (SAMD9/SAMD9-like (SAMD9L)) genes, TP53, and oncostatin M (OSM) [3–10]. These newly discovered entities typically present with early-onset cytopenias and show variable risks of progression to myeloid malignancies. This chapter examines these newly identified IBMFSs, focusing on their genetic characteristics, clinical manifestations, and treatment approaches (Table 23.1).

A. Haroon (✉) · M. Aljurf
Department of Hematology, Stem Cell Transplant & Cellular Therapy, Cancer Centre of Excellence, King Faisal Specialist Hospital & Research Centre, Riyadh, Saudi Arabia
e-mail: halfadil@kfshrc.edu.sa

M. W. Wlodarski
St. Jude Children's Research Hospital, Memphis, TN, USA

R. Peffault de Latour
Hematology and Transplant Unit, Saint-Louis Hospital, AP-HP and Université Paris Cité, Paris, France

Table 23.1 Disease summary

Gene	Disease nomenclature (OMIM #)	Inheritance (type of mutations)	Risk for MDS/AML
MYSM1	MYSM1 deficiency. OMIM: Bone marrow failure syndrome 4 (BMFS4, #618116)	AR (loss-of-function)	Low to moderate
ERCC6L	ERCC6L2 syndrome. OMIM: Bone marrow failure syndrome 2 (BMFS2, #615715)	AR (loss-of-function)	Very high, TP53-mutated MDS/AML
MECOM	MECOM syndrome. OMIM: Radioulnar synostosis with amegakaryocytic thrombocytopenia type 2 (RUSAT2, #616738)	AD (loss-of-function)	Relatively rare (~5%)
ADH5/ ALDH2	AMED syndrome, Aldehyde degradation deficiency syndrome. OMIM: Bone marrow failure syndrome 7 (#619151)	Digenic: biallelic ADH5 + ALDH2 E504K allele (loss-of-function)	Significant (MDS/AML)
SAMD9 SAMD9L	SAMD9 and SAMD9L syndromes. OMIM: SAMD9 (#164017), SAMD9L (#159550)	AD (gain-of-function)	Monosomy 7 common Advanced MDS and AML rare
DNAJC21	DNAJC21 syndrome. OMIM: Bone marrow failure syndrome 3 (BMFS3, #617052	AR (loss-of-function)	Undefined
TP53	TP53 activation syndrome (OMIM not yet assigned)	AD (TP53: loss-of-function) (MDM4: gain-of-function)	Undefined (only bone marrow failure thus far)
OSM	Oncostatin M-Related BMF. (OMIM not yet assigned)	AR (loss-of-function)	Risk of MDS progression documented

Abbreviations: *AD* autosomal dominant, *AR* autosomal recessive, *MDS* myelodysplastic syndrome, *AML* acute myeloid leukemia

MYSM1 Deficiency

Disease classification: MYSM1 deficiency is now officially classified as bone marrow failure syndrome 4 (BMFS4, OMIM #618116).

Myb-like SWIRM and MPN domains (MYSM1) are located on chromosome 1p32.1 and encode an 829-amino acid protein that functions as a chromatin-binding transcriptional regulator involved in histone H2AK119ub deubiquitination and the termination of DNA damage responses [5, 6]. The targeted deletion of murine MYSM1 causes severe hematopoietic defects, blocking B cell development and impairing stem cell maintenance, differentiation, and NK cell function [7–9]. There is evidence that MYSM1 deficiency results in ribosomal stress that triggers p53-mediated bone marrow failure (BMF) [10]. In 2013, biallelic loss-of-function mutations in MYSM1 were described for the first time in one family, with siblings presenting with anemia and facial dysmorphism [11]. To date, at least 12 cases have been reported [11–18]. Anemia was present in 12 (100%) cases, thrombocytopenia in four (33.3%), leukopenia in five (41.5%), and pancytopenia, accompanied by immune deficiencies such as B- and NK cell abnormalities and low IgM and IgG levels, in ten (83.3%). Some patients exhibited hypocellular bone marrow and myelodysplastic features, with dysplastic erythropoiesis and pseudo–Pelger–Huet anomaly (bahrami/klein). Non-hematologic features included developmental abnormalities like microcephaly, dysmorphic features, and neurodevelopmental delays. Infections included respiratory tract infections, with some patients requiring hematopoietic stem cell transplantation (HSCT) for treatment. Allogeneic HSCT was reported in three patients at the ages of 23 months, 42 months, and 6 years, conditioned with fludarabine, treosulfan, and alemtuzumab for the first two patients and fludarabine-based reduced intensity conditioning (RIC) for the last one [15, 19]. A patient with the homozygous c.1967A>G; p.His656Arg (H656R) MYSM1 variant showed spontaneous somatic genetic rescue (SGR), where one of the mutated alleles was reverted to the wild type in the patient's multipotent hematopoietic stem cell (HSC) compartment and resulted in hematopoietic improvement [20]. This supports the concept that in vivo gene therapy or targeted correction in HSC for disorders like MYSM1 can lead to competitive advantage of corrected cells and clinical improvement.

ERCC6L2-Associated Bone Marrow Failure Syndrome

Disease classification: ERCC6L2-associated bone marrow failure is officially classified as "bone marrow failure syndrome 2" (BMFS2, OMIM #615715).

ERCC6L2, located on chromosome 9q22.32, is an ATP-dependent DNA translocase, important in various processes, including DNA repair via the NHEJ pathway, recombination, translocation, and chromatin remodeling. Biallelic loss-of-function mutations of ERCC6L2 predispose individuals to BMF, myeloid malignancies, and neurological dysfunction [21–24]. Several reports have described biallelic germline ERCC6L2 variants manifesting with pancytopenia and hypocellular bone marrow, with or without dysplastic features [25, 26]. These carry a high risk of progression to acute myeloid leukemia (AML) or myelodysplastic syndrome (MDS), and cases have also been associated with TP53 mutations and monosomy 7 [27, 28]. Non-hematologic manifestations include microcephaly in ~5% of cases, neuropsychiatric manifestations (including developmental delay) in ~10%, and solid tumors in single cases (<5%), although exact percentages may vary across studies [29]. Additional features in single cases include failure to thrive, muscle ache, delayed eruption and replacement of teeth with adult teeth, arteriovenous malformations, leukoplakia, low birth weight, and short stature [21, 30]. To date, at least 52 cases across 35 families have been reported [31, 32]. The median age at initial diagnosis of bone marrow failure was 12 (range 2–57) years, while median age at presentation of MDS/AML was 29 (range 12–65) years [31]. ERCC6L2 mutations strongly predispose to TP53-mediated clonal evolution and progression to MDS/

AML. Indicators of disease progression included an increasing TP53 variant allele frequency, dysplasia of the megakaryocyte and/or the erythroid lineage, and erythroid predominance in bone marrow morphology [31]. Somatic TP53 mutations were present in 83% of patients at the BMF stage and 100% of patients with MDS/AML. A case series of 11 patients (authors' unpublished data) with ERCC6L2 mutations included eight patients with BMF, two with hypoplastic MDS, and one with MDS/AML. The median age was 14 years (range 6–37). Presentations included bleeding in 45% (5/11), anemia in 27% (3/11), and neurological symptoms in 9% (1/11), while two were asymptomatic. Eight patients had normal cytogenetics, one patient had monosomy 7, and two showed somatic TP53 mutations. Three patients underwent MSD HSCT, while two were transplanted from an matched unrelated donor (MUD) and one from a haploidentical donor [26]. The presence of germline ERCC6L2 mutations substantially increases the risk of clonal evolution and progression to leukemia, highlighting the need for careful follow-up [29]. Progression to high-risk leukemia or MDS or cases of transfusion dependency indicated the need for HSCT [24, 33]. Notably, patients with TP53-mutated MDS/AML had a dismal overall survival rate of 19% and a survival rate after HSCT of 28% [31]. In contrast, HSCT performed at an early stage of the disease (in patients presenting with BMF only) resulted in favorable outcomes, with >80% survival. Timing of HSCT has to be carefully balanced, and HSCT has to be optimally performed before patients develop TP53-driven MDS/AML.

MECOM-Related Bone Marrow Failure Syndrome

Disease classification: radioulnar synostosis with amegakaryocytic thrombocytopenia type 2 (RUSAT2, OMIM #616738).

The MECOM gene (MDS1 and EVI1 complex locus), located on chromosome 3q26.2 and comprising 24 exons, encodes multiple protein isoforms through alternative splicing, including MDS1, EVI1, and MDS1-EVI1 (also known as PRDM3) [34, 35]. MECOM gene functions as a transcriptional regulator important for hematopoiesis, apoptosis, development, and cell differentiation and proliferation [36, 37]. Mutations in MECOM can inhibit the transcriptional activity by changing the structural stability of zinc finger motifs and impairing the DNA-binding function of the C-terminal domain of the EVI1 protein [38, 39]. MECOM is also a critical transcription factor in hematopoiesis, which controls hematopoietic stem and progenitor cells (HSPC) homeostasis and myeloid differentiation through transcription factor interactions, such as GATA1, RUNX1, and SPI1 [40–43]. The first patient with severe thrombocytopenia associated with MECOM mutation who developed pancytopenia was reported in 2012 [44]. To date, more than 80 cases have been documented [45]. Most MECOM pathogenic variants are heterozygous, de novo, and include missense (56 [68.3%] cases), deletion (seven [8.5%] cases), splice-site (seven [8.5%] cases), frameshift (six [7.3%] cases), and nonsense (six [7.3%] cases) mutations [44, 45]. The hematologic features include single- or multi-lineage cytopenia, BMF, leukemia, MDS, and B cell deficiency. About half of the patients have radioulnar synostosis, thus leading to the designated disease name "radioulnar synostosis with amegakaryocytic thrombocytopenia type 2" (RUSAT2) [46–49]. Cytopenia or BMF was present in 80% of patients, with the onset at birth or during infancy, and some cases were so severe that they caused intrauterine death or necessitated early HSCT. There were rare instances of spontaneous improvement (~5%). Among non-hematologic features, the most common is radioulnar synostosis (54%), followed by digit anomalies (38%), hearing loss (20%), and congenital heart defects (18%). Polyhydramnios, hydrops fetalis, or prematurity were observed in 13%. Other infrequent manifestations included neurodevelopmental anomalies, skeletal abnormalities, clubfoot, renal defects, facial dysmorphisms, cleft palate, and gynecomastia. Hematologic malignancies were rare (~5% of cases: three MDS and one AML), and 50% of the patients had undergone HSCT for severe BMF [24, 46, 49–56].

AMED Syndrome (ADH5/ALDH2 Deficiency)

Disease classification: AMED syndrome, digenic; aldehyde degradation deficiency syndrome; and bone marrow failure syndrome 7 (OMIM #619151).

AMED syndrome is caused by homozygous or compound heterozygous mutations in the ADH5 gene (chr 4q), combined with at least one copy of the ALDH2 E504K allele (rs671) on chromosome 12q24. This represents a digenic inheritance pattern, where mutations in two distinct genes are both necessary to cause the disease.

Alcohol dehydrogenase 5 (ADH5, formaldehyde dehydrogenase, or glutathione-dependent formaldehyde dehydrogenase) is a primary enzyme responsible for metabolizing formaldehyde into formate in a glutathione-dependent manner. The main function of aldehyde dehydrogenase 2 (ALDH2) is to detoxify acetaldehyde, but it is also important for detoxification. The ALDH2 E504K variant (rs671) is common in East Asian populations (~40% in Japan) and causes adverse reactions after alcohol consumption, including flushing, headache, nausea, and palpitations [57, 58]. Formaldehyde exposure causes chromosomal aneuploidy, especially in chromosomes 5, 7, and 8, which is a common abnormality in AML [59]. In mice, exposure to formaldehyde leads to hematopoietic toxicity that results in bone marrow stem and progenitor cell damage, myeloid growth inhibition through oxidative stress, apoptosis, and altered colony-stimulating factor receptor signaling [60]. When both ADH5 and ALDH2 enzymes are deficient, endogenous formaldehyde accumulates to levels that overwhelm the DNA repair capacity. This causes significant DNA damage, including interstrand cross-links (ICLs) and oxidative lesions, which particularly affects rapidly dividing cells like hematopoietic stem cells. AMED syndrome was first reported in 2020 by Oka et al., who described ten Japanese patients with a previously unclassified syndrome characterized by aplastic anemia, mental retardation, and dwarfism (leading to the acronym AMED) [61]. All affected individuals carried biallelic mutations in ADH5 combined with the ALDH2 E504K variant as the causative genetic defect. To date, at least 18 cases have been reported: MDS: six patients (33%), AA with MDS features or progressing to MDS or AML: five patients (28%), BMF not otherwise specified: three patients (17%), AML: two patients (11%), macrocytosis only: one patient (6%), and not determined: four patients (22%). Reported syndromic features were short stature: 12 patients (67%), microcephaly: eight patients (44%), craniofacial anomalies (nasal ridge, micrognathia, and dolichocephaly): five patients (28%), intellectual disability/motor delay: ten patients (56%), ASD/ADHD: one patient, skin pigmentation anomalies/café au lait/vitiligo: eight patients (44%), toe/limb deformities: five patients (28%), endocrinal disorders (e.g., hypothyroidism, adrenal hypoplasia, and puberty issues): five patients (28%), and other problems (e.g., agenesis of corpus callosum, cardiomyopathy, and EB-HLH): four patients (22%). Eight of 11 patients (73%) with available cytogenetic data had a gain of chromosome 1q. Other recurrent abnormalities were monosomy 7, trisomy 8, and alterations involving chromosome 21p. Among 18 reported cases, eight patients underwent HSCT (two died following HSCT); additionally, two patients died from disease complications unrelated to transplantation [61–63].

SAMD9 and SAMD9L-Associated Bone Marrow Failure Syndromes

Disease classification: SAMD9-related disorder (#164017): most severe cases referred to as MIRAGE syndrome (Myelodysplasia, Infection, Restriction of growth, Adrenal hypoplasia, Genital phenotypes, and Enteropathy) and SAMD9L-related disorders (#159550): previously, ataxia-pancytopenia (ATXPC) syndrome, SAMD9L-associated autoinflammatory disease (SAAD), and spinocerebellar ataxia 49 (SCA49).

Sterile alpha motif domain–containing (SAMD9 and SAMD9-like) genes are two interferon-regulated genes located adjacent to each other on chromosome 7q21.2. SAMD9 and SAMD9L encode large cytoplasmic proteins that play roles in inhibiting cell proliferation, regulating endosomal transport, and mediating antiviral defense [64].

Their contribution to human disease was definitively established in 2016 with the discovery of germline variants in these genes. Germline heterozygous gain-of-function (GOF) mutations in the SAMD9L gene were identified as the underlying cause of ATXPC [65], while GOF mutations in the SAMD9 gene were initially identified in infants presenting with a severe syndromic disease termed MIRAGE syndrome (Myelodysplasia, Infection, Restriction of growth, Adrenal hypoplasia, Genital phenotypes, and Enteropathy) [66, 67]. Since their initial discovery, many cases were reported with the unifying phenotype of cytopenia and MDS, but not all of them had the neurological phenotypes (SAMD9L) or syndromic features

(SAMD9) [24, 68–71]. This suggests that a more inclusive disease name, "SAMD9/9L syndromes," is most appropriate. Based on comprehensive registry data from St. Jude with 243 published patients and 62 additional unpublished cases, a total of 305 individuals with SAMD9/9L syndromes have been documented to date [72]. The vast majority (92%) of mutations are missense that enhance the natural growth-inhibitory function of these proteins, while a subset of SAMD9L patients with early-onset autoinflammatory disease carries frameshift-truncating variants that also confer GOF effects [64, 68, 73]. Functionally, these mutations can cause enhanced translational repression and accelerated cell death. However, the exact pathomechanism linking these mutations to bone marrow failure remains under investigation.

A hallmark of SAMD9/9L syndromes is the presence of somatic genetic rescue (SGR) in at least two-thirds of patients [28]. This phenomenon represents an attempt by hematopoietic cells to overcome the growth-inhibitory effects of mutant SAMD9/9L. Three types of SGR are recurrent in these patients: (i) monosomy 7, where chromosome 7 carrying the mutant SAMD9/9L allele is lost (monosomy 7 can be transient and spontaneously disappear); (ii) somatic SAMD9/9L mutations, which act as loss-of-function and counteract the pathogenic effect of germline variants; and (iii) uniparental disomy 7q (UPD7q), which causes duplication of the wild-type allele in hematopoietic cells. Importantly, SGR events can facilitate long-term remission, with stable remissions documented up to 20 years after diagnosis [74]. Approximately 50% of patients have syndromic features, which can affect virtually any organ system (with neurology prominent in SAMD9L syndrome and endocrinal/gastrointestinal/urogenital issues common in SAMD9). The unifying feature is hematologic dysfunction, ranging from isolated thrombocytopenia to severe pancytopenia. The bone marrow typically shows hypocellularity, with dysplastic features consistent with refractory cytopenia of childhood and resembling classical BMF syndromes. In pediatric cohorts, SAMD9/9L mutations constitute 8–18.6% of BMF and MDS cases. MDS with monosomy 7 is a common presentation, with 21% of pediatric monosomy 7 MDS cases attributable to SAMD9/9L mutations. Progression to advanced MDS or AML occurs in a subset of patients. Adult-onset hematologic manifestations are rare (nine adults reported to date), suggesting a unique age-related risk profile, where SAMD9/9L-associated hematologic risk is the highest in childhood but is negligible in adults. This is most likely due to successful SGR events arising during childhood in hematopoiesis.

The outcome depends on the severity of the disease. In a large consortium study by Sahoo et al., among 42 SAMD9/9L cases, the 5-year overall survival was 84% for SAMD9 and 93% for SAMD9L patients. Karyotype emerged as the key prognostic factor, with 5-year overall survival of 95% for normal karyotype versus 76% for monosomy 7. Among 29 patients undergoing HSCT, 5-year overall survival was 93% for those with normal karyotype versus 77% for those with monosomy 7. Of note, since monosomy 7 clones can disappear completely in young children with SAMD9/9L disease, management of patients with monosomy 7 has to be individually tailored. Young children (≤ 5 years) with stable counts may undergo close monitoring rather than immediate transplant, given the possibility of transient monosomy 7. HSCT is indicated when patients develop progressive immunodeficiency or worsening cytopenia or acquire secondary MDS/AML-type driver mutations, while older children and adults with monosomy 7 typically proceed directly to transplant [2, 28].

DNAJC21: Ribosomopathy-Associated Bone Marrow Failure

Disease classification: bone marrow failure syndrome 3 (OMIM #617052).

DNAJC21 is broadly expressed and encodes a 531-amino-acid protein with a conserved DnaJ chaperone domain, a central coiled-coil region, and two zinc finger motifs [75]. The large 60S ribosomal subunit undergoes its final maturation in DNAJC21, and this process involves PA2G4, a nuclear-cytoplasmic shuttling factor that transports the pre-60S subunit to the cytoplasm [76]. Germline biallelic mutations in the DnaJ heat shock protein family (Hsp40) member C21 (DNAJC21) gene were discovered in Shwachman–Diamond syndrome (SDS) patients lacking SBDS mutations [77]. Mutations that impair ribosome biogenesis cause nucleolar stress, which leads to the activation of the p53 pathway, resulting in apoptosis or reduced proliferation of hematopoietic progenitor cells and marrow failure [78]. Studies on lymphoblastoid cell lines derived from patients suggested that DNAJC21 plays a role in rRNA biogenesis and 60S ribosome maturation, similar to SBDS. As a result, there is a decrease in the interaction between HSPA8, ZNF622, and PA2G4, which eventually causes cell death in individuals with DNAJC21 deficiency [77]. In a zebrafish model, supplementation with exogenous nucleosides restored neutrophil counts, linking nucleotide imbalance to neutrophil differentiation in DNAJC21-mutant SDS [79]. Tummala et al. discovered three patients with homozygous variants in DNAJC21 after whole exome sequencing (WES) screening of 28 unrelated patients with BMF and syndromic features in 2016 [77]. The hematologic features include cytopenia affecting one or more lineages and hypocellular bone marrow. Growth retardation resembling EH, developmental delays, and skeletal abnormalities are observed as non-hematologic features. Some features, such as exocrine dysfunction, mimic classical Shwachman–Diamond syndrome presentation, while others, like skin, dental, and retinal abnormalities, overlap with telomeropathies, reflecting phenotypic variability in related genetic disorders [80]. The management includes supportive transfusions, growth factors, and prophylactic antimicrobial therapies. Patients with severe or progressive disease may benefit from allogeneic HSCT. Long-term close monitoring is required due to the potential (yet undefined) risk of progression to MDS.

TP53 Germline Activation Syndrome

Disease classification: TP53 IBFMS due to germline gain-of-function TP53 mutations (OMIM not yet assigned).

TP53 activation syndrome represents a new and unique group of IBMFSs, caused either by germline gain-of-function mutations in the TP53 gene or germline loss-of-function mutations in the MDM4 gene (causing TP53 hyperactivation) [81–83]. Unlike the well-known Li–Fraumeni syndrome, which results from loss-of-function mutations in TP53 that predispose to cancer development, TP53 activation syndrome is characterized by augmented p53 activity that leads to a distinct clinical phenotype dominated by bone marrow failure.

TP53: Thus far, five patients have been reported with germline gain-of-function TP53 mutations, which specifically affect the C-terminal domain of the p53 protein. These mutations are de novo, truncating, and result in shortened and constitutively active p53 protein with augmented transcriptional capabilities. Clinically, patients present in early infancy with severe red cell aplasia requiring transfusions and have a recognized phenocopy of Diamond–Blackfan anemia (DBA) syndrome. Beyond hematologic manifestations, patients exhibit hypogammaglobulinemia and severe growth retardation, and some have microcephaly. Neurological issues include developmental delay, intellectual disability, and seizures. Additional features may include reticular skin pigmentation, dental anomalies, and hypogonadism. Despite phenotypic similarities to dyskeratosis congenita, telomere lengths typically remain normal. Treatment responses vary, with some demonstrating corticosteroid responsiveness, while others show a spontaneous improvement of anemia.

MDM4: Germline MDM4 loss-of-function mutations have been described in several patients with a similar marrow failure phenotype. MDM4 normally functions as a negative regulator of p53; thus, the loss of MDM4 function results in a hyperactive TP53 state. To date, seven (one reported [82] and six unpublished from M. Wlodarski and F. Beier groups) unrelated individuals with various MDM4 mutations, including frameshift, nonsense, splice-site, and missense variants, have been reported. They presented with a spectrum of hematologic manifestations ranging from isolated neutropenia to red cell aplasia, pancytopenia, and hypocellular marrow; one developed MDS. The syndrome can present from infancy to the fifth decade with variable penetrance. Key features include bone marrow hypocellularity with dysplastic changes, variable cytopenias, and in some cases, shortened telomeres and liver dysfunction. In summary, loss-of-function TP53 mutations and loss-of-function MDM4 mutations represent a novel syndrome where excessive p53 activity causes bone marrow failure.

OSM-Related Bone Marrow Failure Syndrome

Disease classification: oncostatin M-Related BMF syndrome (OMIM not yet assigned).

Oncostatin M (OSM) is an IL-6-family cytokine produced by immune cells, regulating hematopoiesis by stimulating hematopoietic stem and progenitor cells as well as stromal cells. OSM signals through OSMR glycoprotein 130 (gp130) and leukemia inhibitory factor (LIFR) gp130, regulating hematopoietic progenitor proliferation and differentiation [84]. Patient frameshift mutation disrupts OSM's FxxK motif, impairing signaling and hindering hematopoietic progenitor differentiation, causing bone marrow failure [85]. OSM deficiency due to homozygous mutations in OSM was identified as a cause of BMF that can progress into MDS [85, 86]. The homozygous OSM variant results in a frameshift that abolishes OSM's C-terminal FxxK motif and replaces it with a neopeptide that significantly alters OSM's interaction with cytokines and abolishes signal transduction [85]. In zebrafish models, OSM/OSMR's capacity to promote erythroid progenitor proliferation as well as differentiation into neutrophils has been demonstrated [85]. Patients with OSM deficiency exhibit disrupted bone marrow microenvironments, leading to neutrophil, erythrocyte, and platelet abnormalities [85], with documented cases of childhood MDS [86]. The first report presented three sisters from a consanguineous Moroccan family, carrying the c.507_508insG OSM mutation, who were diagnosed with pancytopenia during infancy (3–6 months). One of them experienced progressive cytopenias requiring blood transfusions. The bone marrow studies revealed dyserythropoiesis and dysgranulopoiesis, together with ineffective hematopoiesis [85]. In the same year, three female patients from two consanguineous Saudi families harboring homozygous Gln97Ter mutation were reported [86]. They were diagnosed with thrombocytopenia, anemia, or pancytopenia between ages 5–25 years and had variable reduction of bone marrow progenitors and hypo/normocellular bone marrow. The adult patient progressed to MDS with t(10;13) translocation and underwent HSCT at the age of 40 years. Remarkably, the other two patients showed a response to eltrombopag and danazol with an increase in counts.

References

1. Revy P, Kannengiesser C, Bertuch AA. Genetics of human telomere biology disorders. Nat Rev Genet. 2023;24(2):86–108.
2. Erlacher M, et al. Spontaneous remission and loss of monosomy 7: a window of opportunity for young children with SAMD9L syndrome. Haematologica. 2024;109(2):422–30.
3. Skokowa J, et al. Severe congenital neutropenias. Nat Rev Dis Primers. 2017;3:17032.
4. Feurstein S. Emerging bone marrow failure syndromes- new pieces to an unsolved puzzle. Front Oncol. 2023;13:1128533.
5. Zhu P, et al. A histone H2A deubiquitinase complex coordinating histone acetylation and H1 dissociation in transcriptional regulation. Mol Cell. 2007;27(4):609–21.

6. Mathias B, et al. MYSM1 attenuates DNA damage signals triggered by physiologic and genotoxic DNA breaks. J Allergy Clin Immunol. 2024;153(4):1113–1124.e7.
7. Jiang XX, et al. Control of B cell development by the histone H2A deubiquitinase MYSM1. Immunity. 2011;35(6):883–96.
8. Wang T, et al. The control of hematopoietic stem cell maintenance, self-renewal, and differentiation by Mysm1-mediated epigenetic regulation. Blood. 2013;122(16):2812–22.
9. Nandakumar V, et al. Epigenetic control of natural killer cell maturation by histone H2A deubiquitinase, MYSM1. Proc Natl Acad Sci USA. 2013;110(41):E3927–36.
10. Belle JI, et al. MYSM1 maintains ribosomal protein gene expression in hematopoietic stem cells to prevent hematopoietic dysfunction. JCI Insight. 2020;5(13):e125690.
11. Alsultan A, et al. MYSM1 is mutated in a family with transient transfusion-dependent anemia, mild thrombocytopenia, and low NK- and B-cell counts. Blood. 2013;122(23):3844–5.
12. Li N, et al. Further delineation of bone marrow failure syndrome caused by novel compound heterozygous variants of MYSM1. Gene. 2020;757:144938.
13. Zhan X, et al. A novel compound heterozygous mutation of MYSM1 gene in a patient with bone marrow failure syndrome 4. Br J Biomed Sci. 2021;78(4):239–43.
14. Le Guen T, et al. An in vivo genetic reversion highlights the crucial role of Myb-Like, SWIRM, and MPN domains 1 (MYSM1) in human hematopoiesis and lymphocyte differentiation. J Allergy Clin Immunol. 2015;136(6):1619–1626.e5.
15. Bahrami E, et al. Myb-like, SWIRM, and MPN domains 1 (MYSM1) deficiency: genotoxic stress-associated bone marrow failure and developmental aberrations. J Allergy Clin Immunol. 2017;140(4):1112–9.
16. Nanda A, et al. Neutrophilic panniculitis in a child with MYSM1 deficiency. Pediatr Dermatol. 2019;36(2):258–9.
17. Mantravadi V, et al. Immunological findings and clinical outcomes of infants with positive newborn screening for severe combined immunodeficiency from a Tertiary Care Center in the U.S. Front Immunol. 2021;12:734096.
18. Sakovich IS, et al. Clinical course and family history of adult patient with novel MYSM1 variant. J Clin Immunol. 2023;44(1):9.
19. Barhoom D, et al. Successful allogeneic stem cell transplantation with fludarabine-based reduced intensity conditioning in bone marrow failure syndrome 4. Pediatr Transplant. 2021;25(7):e14089.
20. de Tocqueville S, et al. Long-term assessment of haematological recovery following somatic genetic rescue in a MYSM1-deficient patient: implications for in vivo gene therapy. Br J Haematol. 2024;205(6):2349–54.
21. Tummala H, et al. ERCC6L2 mutations link a distinct bone-marrow-failure syndrome to DNA repair and mitochondrial function. Am J Hum Genet. 2014;94(2):246–56.
22. Douglas SPM, et al. ERCC6L2 defines a novel entity within inherited acute myeloid leukemia. Blood. 2019;133(25):2724–8.
23. Flaus A, et al. Identification of multiple distinct Snf2 subfamilies with conserved structural motifs. Nucleic Acids Res. 2006;34(10):2887–905.
24. Bluteau O, et al. A landscape of germ line mutations in a cohort of inherited bone marrow failure patients. Blood. 2018;131(7):717–32.
25. Hakkarainen M, et al. The clinical picture of ERCC6L2 disease: from bone marrow failure to acute leukemia. Blood. 2023;141(23):2853–66.
26. Haroon A, et al. First description of new variant of germline ERCC6L2 mutations causing bone marrow failure, a single center report of 11 cases in 7 families. Blood. 2024;144:5706.
27. Hakkarainen M, et al. Multinational study on the clinical and genetic features of the ERCC6L2-disease. Blood. 2021;138:864.
28. Sahoo SS, et al. Clinical evolution, genetic landscape and trajectories of clonal hematopoiesis in SAMD9/SAMD9L syndromes. Nat Med. 2021;27(10):1806–17.
29. Shabanova I, et al. ERCC6L2-associated inherited bone marrow failure syndrome. Mol Genet Genomic Med. 2018;6(3):463–8.

30. Zhang S, et al. A nonsense mutation in the DNA repair factor Hebo causes mild bone marrow failure and microcephaly. J Exp Med. 2016;213(6):1011–28.
31. Hakkarainen M, et al. The clinical picture of ERCC6L2 disease: from bone marrow failure to acute leukemia. Blood J Am Soc Hematol. 2023;141(23):2853–66.
32. Wlodarski MW. ERCC6L2 syndrome: attack of the TP53 clones. Blood. 2023;141(23):2788–9.
33. Boutakoglou E, et al. Identification of GFI1 mutations in adult patients with congenital neutropenia. Ann Hematol. 2022;101(12):2771–3.
34. Fears S, et al. Intergenic splicing of MDS1 and EVI1 occurs in normal tissues as well as in myeloid leukemia and produces a new member of the PR domain family. Proc Natl Acad Sci USA. 1996;93(4):1642–7.
35. Glass C, et al. The role of EVI1 in myeloid malignancies. Blood Cells Mol Dis. 2014;53(1–2):67–76.
36. Voit RA, Sankaran VG. MECOM deficiency: from bone marrow failure to impaired B-cell development. J Clin Immunol. 2023;43(6):1052–66.
37. Baldazzi C, et al. Complex chromosomal rearrangements leading to MECOM overexpression are recurrent in myeloid malignancies with various 3q abnormalities. Genes Chromosomes Cancer. 2016;55(4):375–88.
38. Delwel R, et al. Four of the seven zinc fingers of the Evi-1 myeloid-transforming gene are required for sequence-specific binding to GA(C/T)AAGA(T/C)AAGATAA. Mol Cell Biol. 1993;13(7):4291–300.
39. Glass C, et al. Global identification of EVI1 target genes in acute myeloid leukemia. PLoS One. 2013;8(6):e67134.
40. Kataoka K, et al. Evi1 is essential for hematopoietic stem cell self-renewal, and its expression marks hematopoietic cells with long-term multilineage repopulating activity. J Exp Med. 2011;208(12):2403–16.
41. Laricchia-Robbio L, et al. Point mutations in two EVI1 Zn fingers abolish EVI1-GATA1 interaction and allow erythroid differentiation of murine bone marrow cells. Mol Cell Biol. 2006;26(20):7658–66.
42. Laricchia-Robbio L, et al. EVI1 impairs myelopoiesis by deregulation of PU.1 function. Cancer Res. 2009;69(4):1633–42.
43. Senyuk V, et al. Repression of RUNX1 activity by EVI1: a new role of EVI1 in leukemogenesis. Cancer Res. 2007;67(12):5658–66.
44. Nielsen M, et al. Deletion of the 3q26 region including the EVI1 and MDS1 genes in a neonate with congenital thrombocytopenia and subsequent aplastic anaemia. J Med Genet. 2012;49(9):598–600.
45. Li J, et al. A novel MECOM gene variant causes severe thrombocytopenia in a neonate: a case report and review of the literature. J Med Case Rep. 2025;19(1):147.
46. Lord SV, et al. A MECOM variant in an African American child with radioulnar synostosis and thrombocytopenia. Clin Dysmorphol. 2018;27(1):9–11.
47. Osumi T, et al. Somatic MECOM mosaicism in a patient with congenital bone marrow failure without a radial abnormality. Pediatr Blood Cancer. 2018;65(6):e26959.
48. Walne A, et al. Expanding the phenotypic and genetic spectrum of radioulnar synostosis associated hematological disease. Haematologica. 2018;103(7):e284–7.
49. Loganathan A, Munirathnam D, Ravikumar T. A novel mutation in the MECOM gene causing radioulnar synostosis with amegakaryocytic thrombocytopenia (RUSAT-2) in an infant. Pediatr Blood Cancer. 2019;66(4):e27574.
50. Niihori T, et al. Mutations in MECOM, encoding oncoprotein EVI1, cause radioulnar synostosis with amegakaryocytic thrombocytopenia. Am J Hum Genet. 2015;97(6):848–54.
51. Ripperger T, et al. MDS1 and EVI1 complex locus (MECOM): a novel candidate gene for hereditary hematological malignancies. Haematologica. 2018;103(2):e55–8.
52. Al-Abboh H, Zahra A, Adekile A. A novel MECOM variant associated with congenital amegakaryocytic thrombocytopenia and radioulnar synostosis. Pediatr Blood Cancer. 2022;69(12):e29761.

53. Germeshausen M, et al. MECOM-associated syndrome: a heterogeneous inherited bone marrow failure syndrome with amegakaryocytic thrombocytopenia. Blood Adv. 2018;2(6):586–96.
54. Weizmann D, et al. New MECOM variant in a child with severe neonatal cytopenias spontaneously resolving. Pediatr Blood Cancer. 2020;67(5):e28215.
55. van der Veken LT, et al. Lethal neonatal bone marrow failure syndrome with multiple congenital abnormalities, including limb defects, due to a constitutional deletion of 3' MECOM. Haematologica. 2018;103(4):e173–6.
56. Bouman A, et al. Congenital thrombocytopenia in a neonate with an interstitial microdeletion of 3q26.2q26.31. Am J Med Genet A. 2016;170a(2):504–9.
57. Edenberg HJ, McClintick JN. Alcohol dehydrogenases, aldehyde dehydrogenases, and alcohol use disorders: a critical review. Alcohol Clin Exp Res. 2018;42(12):2281–97.
58. Matsumura Y, et al. Gene therapy correction of aldehyde dehydrogenase 2 deficiency. Mol Ther Methods Clin Dev. 2019;15:72–82.
59. Zhang L, et al. Occupational exposure to formaldehyde, hematotoxicity, and leukemia-specific chromosome changes in cultured myeloid progenitor cells. Cancer Epidemiol Biomarkers Prev. 2010;19(1):80–8.
60. Wei C, et al. Formaldehyde induces toxicity in mouse bone marrow and hematopoietic stem/progenitor cells and enhances benzene-induced adverse effects. Arch Toxicol. 2017;91(2):921–33.
61. Oka Y, et al. Digenic mutations in ALDH2 and ADH5 impair formaldehyde clearance and cause a multisystem disorder, AMeD syndrome. Sci Adv. 2020;6(51):eabd7197.
62. Dingler FA, et al. Two aldehyde clearance systems are essential to prevent lethal formaldehyde accumulation in mice and humans. Mol Cell. 2020;80(6):996–1012.e9.
63. Matsumoto M, et al. Characteristic phenotypes of ADH5/ALDH2 deficiency during childhood. Eur J Med Genet. 2024;69:104939.
64. Nagamachi A, et al. Haploinsufficiency of SAMD9L, an endosome fusion facilitator, causes myeloid malignancies in mice mimicking human diseases with monosomy 7. Cancer Cell. 2013;24(3):305–17.
65. Chen DH, et al. Ataxia-pancytopenia syndrome is caused by missense mutations in SAMD9L. Am J Hum Genet. 2016;98(6):1146–58.
66. Narumi S, et al. SAMD9 mutations cause a novel multisystem disorder, MIRAGE syndrome, and are associated with loss of chromosome 7. Nat Genet. 2016;48(7):792–7.
67. Buonocore F, et al. Somatic mutations and progressive monosomy modify SAMD9-related phenotypes in humans. J Clin Invest. 2017;127(5):1700–13.
68. Tesi B, et al. Gain-of-function SAMD9L mutations cause a syndrome of cytopenia, immunodeficiency, MDS, and neurological symptoms. Blood. 2017;129(16):2266–79.
69. Gorcenco S, et al. Ataxia-pancytopenia syndrome with SAMD9L mutations. Neurol Genet. 2017;3(5):e183.
70. Schwartz JR, et al. The genomic landscape of pediatric myelodysplastic syndromes. Nat Commun. 2017;8(1):1557.
71. Ahmed IA, et al. Outcomes of hematopoietic cell transplantation in patients with germline SAMD9/SAMD9L mutations. Biol Blood Marrow Transplant. 2019;25(11):2186–96.
72. Sahoo SS, Erlacher M, Wlodarski MW. Genetic and clinical spectrum of SAMD9 and SAMD9L syndromes: from variant interpretation to patient management. Blood. 2025;145(5):475–85.
73. Nagata Y, et al. Germline loss-of-function SAMD9 and SAMD9L alterations in adult myelodysplastic syndromes. Blood. 2018;132(21):2309–13.
74. Pastor VB, et al. Constitutional SAMD9L mutations cause familial myelodysplastic syndrome and transient monosomy 7. Haematologica. 2018;103(3):427–37.
75. Meyer AE, Hoover LA, Craig EA. The cytosolic J-protein, Jjj1, and Rei1 function in the removal of the pre-60 S subunit factor Arx1. J Biol Chem. 2010;285(2):961–8.
76. Dhanraj S, et al. Biallelic mutations in DNAJC21 cause Shwachman-Diamond syndrome. Blood. 2017;129(11):1557–62.
77. Tummala H, et al. DNAJC21 mutations link a cancer-prone bone marrow failure syndrome to corruption in 60S ribosome subunit maturation. Am J Hum Genet. 2016;99(1):115–24.

78. Bursac S, et al. Activation of the tumor suppressor p53 upon impairment of ribosome biogenesis. Biochim Biophys Acta. 2014;1842(6):817–30.
79. Ketharnathan S, et al. Loss of Dnajc21 leads to cytopenia and altered nucleotide metabolism in zebrafish. Leukemia. 2024;38(10):2115–26.
80. D'Amours G, et al. Refining the phenotype associated with biallelic DNAJC21 mutations. Clin Genet. 2018;94(2):252–8.
81. Toki T, et al. De novo mutations activating germline TP53 in an inherited bone-marrow-failure syndrome. Am J Hum Genet. 2018;103(3):440–7.
82. Toufektchan E, et al. Germline mutation of MDM4, a major p53 regulator, in a familial syndrome of defective telomere maintenance. Sci Adv. 2020;6(15):eaay3511.
83. Kumar RD, et al. The germline p53 activation syndrome: a new patient further refines the clinical phenotype. Am J Med Genet A. 2022;188(7):2204–8.
84. Sims NA, Lévesque JP. Oncostatin M: dual regulator of the skeletal and hematopoietic systems. Curr Osteoporos Rep. 2024;22(1):80–95.
85. Garrigue A, et al. Human oncostatin M deficiency underlies an inherited severe bone marrow failure syndrome. J Clin Invest. 2025;135(6):e180981.
86. Alfalah AH, et al. Biallelic OSM deficiency presents with juvenile myelodysplastic syndrome and response to treatment. J Clin Invest. 2025;135(9):e192422.

Open Access This chapter is licensed under the terms of the Creative Commons Attribution 4.0 International License (http://creativecommons.org/licenses/by/4.0/), which permits use, sharing, adaptation, distribution and reproduction in any medium or format, as long as you give appropriate credit to the original author(s) and the source, provide a link to the Creative Commons license and indicate if changes were made.

The images or other third party material in this chapter are included in the chapter's Creative Commons license, unless indicated otherwise in a credit line to the material. If material is not included in the chapter's Creative Commons license and your intended use is not permitted by statutory regulation or exceeds the permitted use, you will need to obtain permission directly from the copyright holder.

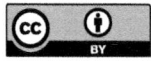

Part VIII
Challenges in Global Management

Chapter 24
Managing Bone Marrow Failure in Countries with Restricted Resources

Raheel Iftikhar, Carmem Bonfim, Moosa Patel, Hazza Alzahrani, Adetola Kassim, and Mahmoud Aljurf

Introduction

The management of aplastic anemia (AA) in restricted-resource settings is challenging due to the nonavailability of specialized diagnostic services, impaired referral systems, limited transplant centers, and out-of-pocket healthcare spending, Moreover, the health sector is affected by urban–rural disparities in healthcare facilities and an imbalance in the workforce, with insufficient doctors, nurses, and paramedics in the rural peripheral areas. Consequently, the management strategies must be tailored according to the available diagnostic and therapeutic resources for a disease that will turn rapidly fatal if left untreated. This chapter will focus on the special considerations for AA management in resource-constrained settings.

R. Iftikhar (✉)
Armed Forces Bone Marrow Transplant Center, Rawalpindi, Pakistan

C. Bonfim
Division of Pediatric Transplantation and Cellular Therapy, Duke University, Durham, NC, USA

M. Patel
Department of Clinical Hematology, Faculty of Health Sciences, School of Clinical Medicine, University of the Witwatersrand, Johannesburg, South Africa

H. Alzahrani · M. Aljurf
Department of Hematology, Stem Cell Transplant & Cellular Therapy, Cancer Centre of Excellence, King Faisal Specialist Hospital & Research Centre, Riyadh, Saudi Arabia

A. Kassim
Department of Medicine, Division of Hematology/Oncology, Vanderbilt University Medical Center, Nashville, TN, USA

Epidemiology and Pathogenesis

The incidence of AA is higher in Asia as compared to the USA and Europe [1], with variable rates between different Asian countries (7.4/million in China, 3.7–5.0/million in Thailand [2], 4.8/million in Malaysia [3], 6.8/million in India [4], 3.9/million in Thailand, 5.16/million in Korea, and 6–7/million in Pakistan) [5]. Developing countries have a younger median age of presentation: 22 years in Nigeria [6], 25 years in India [7], 25.4 years in South Africa [8], and 20 years in Pakistan, with 87% of the patients younger than 40 years [5]. As compared to developed countries [9], more males seem to be reported in the developing countries, with a male-to-female ratio of 3.4:1 in Malaysia [3], 2.3:1 in India [7], 1.7:1 in South Africa [8], and 2.8:1 in Pakistan [10]. Higher male presentation could be due to social bias, where males have more and faster access to healthcare in developing countries [5].

Table 24.1 summarizes the demographics, clinical features, and care considerations of AA patients presenting in countries with restricted resources.

Table 24.1 Demographics, clinical features, and care considerations

Patterns of presentation:
Overall younger median age
Higher proportion of male patients presenting with aplastic anemia
Etiology:
Higher prevalence of hepatitis B virus (HBV) and hepatitis C virus (HCV) infection in some Asian countries
Family history of blood disorders or inherited syndromes
Higher proportion of inherited BMF syndrome as a result of marital consanguinity
Exposure to pesticides and industrial contaminants
Drug-induced bone marrow failure due to the usage of herbal and alternative remedies
Treatment challenges:
Delayed referral, resulting in frequent infections and multiple transfusions, before presentation to a specialized care center
Limited access to genomic testing to ascertain the possibility of inherited bone marrow failure syndromes
Scarcity of standardized transfusion services and supportive care facilities
Financial barriers, limiting the availability of specific treatments

Etiology

Various studies suggest a genetic predisposition as the cause of the high incidence of AA among Asian populations. A study by McCahon et al. reported a higher incidence of AA in children of East/Southeast Asian descent (6.9/million/year) and South Asian descent (7.3/million/year) as compared to those of white/mixed ethnic descent (1.7/million/year). The study concluded that the increased incidence of AA is mainly related to genetic predisposition among Asian children [11] and that the environmental factors seem to be of less relevance [11]. It has been reported that one-third of the Asian population lacks aldehyde dehydrogenase, an important enzyme involved in alcohol metabolism. This deficiency leads to the accumulation of acetaldehyde, which causes irreversible DNA damage to the hematopoietic stem cells and, eventually, AA [12]. Other causes include single-nucleotide polymorphisms (SNPs) of the Fas/FasL system. A significantly higher incidence of deletion of genes involved in detoxifying enzymes glutathione S-transferase M1 (GSTM1) and glutathione S-transferase T1 (GSTT1) was reported in the Korean population. Other exposures, including to pesticides [13] (carbamates, DDT, organophosphate, etc.) [14], arsenic, and unsafe drinking water [15], were also associated with a higher AA incidence.

Diagnosis of AA in Resource-Constrained Settings

In developing countries with restricted access to specialized hematology centers and limited availability of genetic testing, a careful investigation of personal and family history, along with a thorough physical examination, is essential to rule out disorders such as megaloblastic anemia, hypoplastic myelodysplasia (MDS), hypoplastic acute myeloid leukemia (AML), paroxysmal nocturnal hemoglobinuria (PNH), large granular lymphocytic leukemia (LGL), lymphoma infiltrating marrow, mycobacterial infections, and anorexia nervosa. History of anemia, MDS, acute leukemia, or dysmorphic features among siblings and first-degree relatives should raise the suspicion of underlying constitutional bone marrow failure (BMF) [16]. In addition, a history of drug intake, exposure to toxins, recent infection, pregnancy, and autoimmune disorders are relevant in assessing the underlying cause of AA. Due to resource constraints, the selection of patients for genetic testing may be based on detailed investigation of clinical and family history and physical examination [17]. Figure 24.1 provides a diagnostic algorithm of AA in resource-constrained settings.

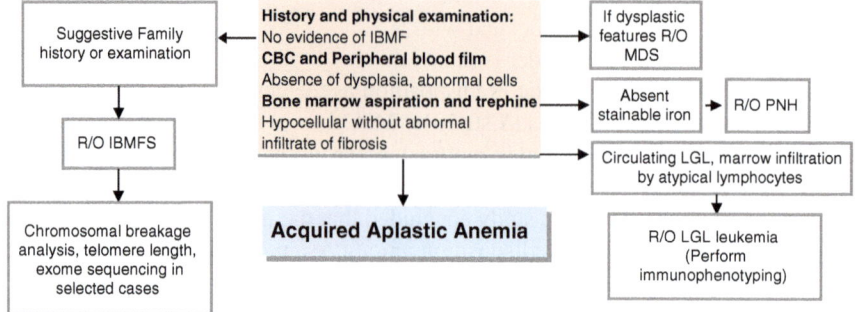

Fig. 24.1 Diagnostic algorithm of AA in resource-constrained settings. *Key*: H/O: history of, R/O: rule out, SOB: shortness of breath, IBMFS: inherited bone marrow failure syndrome, PNH: paroxysmal nocturnal hemoglobinuria and LGL: large granular lymphocytic leukemia

Issues Related to the Overall Management

Healthcare delivery is often compromised in countries with restricted resources due to a lack of proper referral pathways, absence of specialized diagnostic services, sociocultural values, and above all, financial barriers to treatment [18]. Significant urban–rural disparities in healthcare services exist, with lower numbers of medical and paramedical personnel in the peripheral areas.

Moreover, the irradiation of blood products is almost nonexistent, and directed family donation of blood products is widely practiced. The presence of the above challenges leads to two significant consequences: the acquisition of multiple infections and excessive transfusions, leading to significant alloimmunization and transfusion iron overload [19]. Moreover, the lack of adequate supportive care and transfusion services, financial constraints, limited access to horse antithymocyte globulin (hATG) and eltrombopag, limited numbers of transplantation centers, prolonged waiting time before hematopoietic stem cell transplantation (HSCT), absence of matched unrelated donor (MUD) registries, and experience with alternate donor transplant contribute to poor treatment outcomes [20].

Issues Related to Supportive Care

In resource-limited settings, the aim should be to reduce the risk of infection- and bleeding-related deaths through adequate prophylaxis and timely intervention [19]. Patients should take adequate hygienic precautions, which can be an issue in developing countries, and be advised to avoid exposure to construction sites, potted plants, garbage, and compost to reduce the risk of mold infections, especially aspergillosis. Patients should be counseled regarding handwashing; avoiding the use of dry fruits, unwashed fruits, and uncooked vegetables; and other appropriate dietary restrictions [21]. Regular oral care with saline rinses, chlorhexidine mouthwash, and nystatin oral suspension is advisable. In addition, meticulous general body care with daily baths and good toilet hygiene is recommended. Antibacterial and antifungal prophylaxis should be considered for patients with very severe AA (VSAA) and selected high-risk patients after immunosuppressive therapy (IST) or HSCT. A mold-active azole is preferred (posaconazole, voriconazole, and isavuconazole). Fluconazole is a useful alternative in the absence of the above drugs and low incidence of mold infections should be used for prophylaxis [22].

Transfusion is recommended for patients with hemoglobin <70 g/L and platelets <10 × 10^9/L. We recommend platelet transfusions if the count is <5 × 10^9/L in asymptomatic young patients and <10 × 10^9/L in case of any signs of bleeding. The transfusion guidelines provided here are general recommendations tailored for settings with limited resources and may not apply universally. Transfusion thresholds, particularly for platelets and hemoglobin, should always be individualized based on the patient's clinical condition, bleeding risk, and local healthcare standards. Decisions should be made by qualified healthcare professionals considering patient-specific factors, and these guidelines should not replace formal medical advice. Institutions with access to comprehensive transfusion support and monitoring may follow different transfusion protocols to optimize patient outcomes.

There are few reports on the use of adjuvant granulocyte transfusion in patients with severe infections due to neutropenia from the USA [23] and India [24]. There is no evidence to support the use of erythropoietin or granulocyte colony-stimulating factor (G-CSF) in AA patients, and their routine use is not recommended [25].

Immunosuppressive Therapy (IST)

While high response rates have been reported with IST by using hATG plus cyclosporine (CsA) +/− eltrombopag, particularly in young patients [26], in most developing countries, access to hATG is limited, and responses to rabbit ATG (rATG) are disappointing [8]. A substantial proportion of the patients do not survive immediate cytopenia resulting from ATG administration, and others do not survive long enough to witness the response following ATG-based combination treatments. Moreover, the prohibitive cost of hATG and eltrombopag limits their use in resource-constrained settings.

Single-agent CsA has been used with variable success and can be useful in selected patients with non-severe aplastic anemia (NSAA), PNH clone, lack of donor availability, and lack of resources for triple IST. A study by Maschan et al. in pediatric patients showed an overall response rate (complete response (CR) + partial response (PR)) of 45% with CsA monotherapy [27]. In another study of CsA monotherapy use in 57 patients from India, the overall response rate (ORR) was

19.6% at 6 months; the median age was 37 years (range: 6–81 years) [28]. A study from Pakistan on a large cohort of 513 AA patients showed an ORR of 30.2% (CR 12.3% and PR 17.9%) with the use of CsA monotherapy. Higher responses were seen in patients with less severe disease (54% in NSAA, 28% in severe aplastic anemia (SAA), and 9% in VSAA patients). These data suggest that CsA monotherapy can be used for selected patients with NSAA if there is no access to hATG/eltrombopag [29].

Addition of other immunosuppressive agents (mycophenolate mofetil (MMF) and sirolimus) did not improve the response rates [30, 31].

Eltrombopag monotherapy may benefit certain patients with renal dysfunction or active infection, who require immunosuppressive therapy. Again, the prohibitive cost of eltrombopag limits its availability; however, it has the great advantage of simplicity and relative safety in administration compared to ATG in less experienced centers. In pediatric patients, the addition of eltrombopag to the IST did not improve the outcomes [32].

Use of Androgen Therapy

Androgens have historically been used for both inherited and acquired bone marrow failure syndromes but rarely analyzed prospectively for their efficacy and safety. The use of androgens enhances the responsiveness of pluripotent, erythroid, and committed granulocyte progenitors, leading to a clinical response in BMF syndromes [33]. The first report about the possible effectiveness of androgens was regarding the spontaneous remission in two boys upon achieving puberty [34]. This was followed by several publications supporting the role of anabolic steroids in BMF syndromes [35, 36]. A recently published European Society for Blood and Marrow Transplantation (EBMT) study across 82 centers documented 3 months of complete and partial remission rates of 6% and 29% in acquired aplastic anemia [37]. The safety profile was manageable. In restricted-resource settings with limited access to modern treatments and clinical trials, androgens may be useful in selected groups of patients, with a higher response probability. These include patients with mild-to-moderate cytopenia, higher residual cellularity, toxin-induced BMF, and early improvement in counts after androgen initiation [38]. Androgen therapy may also be considered for older SAA patients with a lack of donor options for hematopoietic stem cell transplantation (HSCT) and patients with renal failure precluding the use of CsA or thrombopoietin (TPO) mimetics [38].

Hematopoietic Stem Cell Transplantation

A meta-analysis of 15 studies comparing HSCT with IST for patients with AA has shown the superiority of first-line matched related donor (MRD)–HSCT over IST [39]. The cost of triple IST exceeds the cost of an MRD-HSCT in developing countries and should be the first-line treatment in patients ≤50 years of age with SAA/VSAA if MRD is available. For patients between 40 and 50 years without MRD and those >50 years of age with MRD, the frontline treatment should be individualized based on the transplant risk factors, performance status, comorbidities, disease severity, genetic markers, and probability of responding to immunosuppressive therapy [40]. At present, haploidentical transplant remains the only practical alternative donor option for HSCT in countries with restricted resources. Various risk factors are associated with poor HSCT outcomes, including increasing age, longer disease duration, higher transfusion burden, active infection, comorbidities, and disease severity at presentation. As mentioned earlier, many of these risk factors are highly prevalent in developing countries. In addition, the center's experience with mismatched and alternate donor transplants and the availability of essential drugs and blood components should guide the treatment decision. Figure 24.2 shows the proposed treatment algorithm for acquired SAA.

MRD availability may reach more than 50% in many developing countries due to the large family size; hence, MRD constitutes the primary donor source in developing countries. While matched unrelated donor (MUD) and umbilical cord blood (UCB) transplants are available in most developed countries, they are mostly unavailable in most resource-constrained countries. The reasons are the lower likelihood of finding a suitable donor in the international unrelated donor registries due to underrepresentation of some ethnic groups in donor registries, the high cost and complicated logistics of transporting stem cell product, the delay in finding a suitable HLA match, the lack of expertise for MUD transplantation in most centers, and

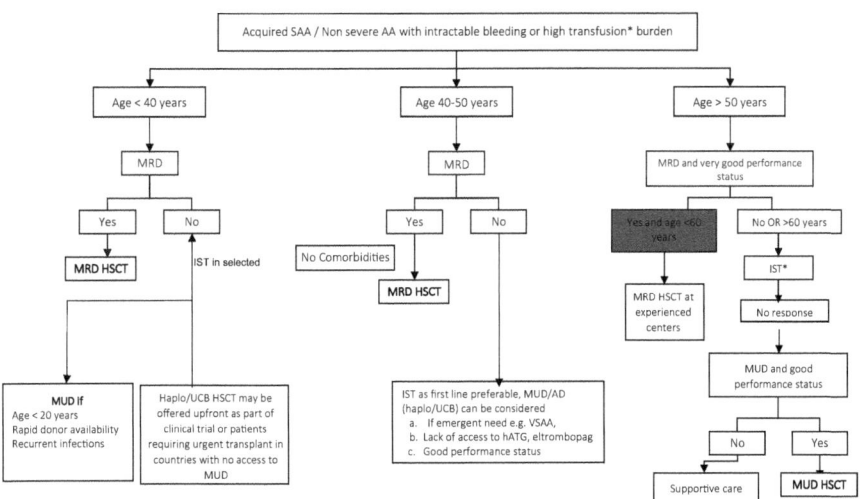

Fig. 24.2 Proposed treatment algorithm of AA management in resource-constrained countries. MRD: matched related donor, MUD: matched unrelated donor, IST: immunosuppressive therapy, haplo: haploidentical, CB: cord blood, and IST*: cyclosporine, horse antithymocyte globulin, and eltrombopag. *NSAA patients with high transfusion burden or those with intractable bleeding (young females with menorrhagia requiring repeated transfusion support) should be considered for allo-HSCT, if transplant eligible

the nonavailability of local donor registries. On the other hand, haploidentical donors are readily available, and virtually every patient has a donor, with the resultant increased interest in haploidentical transplant for patients with AA [41, 42]. Recent reports comparing haplo-HSCT with MUD transplant in children and adolescents revealed fewer differences in overall survival (OS) [43, 44]. Donor-specific antibodies may frequently be found in these heavily transfused patients, and expertise in this area is essential, as they may be associated with graft rejection [45].

Recommendations for conditioning regimens and graft-versus-host disease (GVHD) prophylaxis in resource-limited countries are summarized in Table 24.2.

Table 24.2 Considerations for managing aplastic anemia in resource-constrained countries

Donor-related:
Large family size, with a higher likelihood of finding a related sibling donor
Possibility of finding a non-sibling related donor in consanguineous pedigrees
Alternative-donor HSCT:
Related haplo-HSCT preferred
Limited number of local unrelated donor registers
Limited access to international MUD registry donors
Low likelihood of finding a match in international registries
Limited cord blood banks and limited access to international cord blood banks
Presence of donor-specific antibodies
Treatment choices:
The cost of performing related HSCT is lower in low-income countries than combined IST using hATG, CsA, and eltrombopag
Conditioning and GVHD prophylaxis:
Consider Flu/Cy conditioning where ATG is not available
Consider the use of peripheral blood as a graft source in heavily transfused patients, particularly with preexisting infections
May consider the use of CsA and MMF as GVHD prophylaxis in the presence of significant infections to avoid delay in count recovery with methotrexate administration
Viral infections:
High prevalence of CMV seropositivity in patients and donors and, hence, higher risk of CMV reactivation after HSCT: Vigilant CMV monitoring and preemptive treatment strategy are required
Higher prevalence of hepatitis B and/or hepatitis C in patients and donors: appropriate viral hepatitis treatment/prophylaxis in HSCT recipients is required in consultation with hepatology service
Non-transplant treatment:
Consider treatment with CsA alone in the absence of ATG and/or eltrombopag
Use of androgens
Use of tranexamic acid to reduce the risk or severity of mucosal bleeding episodes in patients with severe thrombocytopenia
Gynecological referral and/or hormonal therapy for menstrual bleeding in female patients
Supportive care:
Use generic azoles, antimicrobials, G-CSF, and oral chelating agents
Limiting routine platelet transfusion to a cutoff of 5×10^9/L in the absence of bleeding
Limiting routine packed red cell transfusions to a cutoff of 70 g/L

CsA cyclosporine, *MMF* mycophenolate mofetil, *ATG* antithymocyte globulin, *Flu/Cy* fludarabine and cyclophosphamide, *CMV* cytomegalovirus, *G-CSF* granulocyte colony-stimulating factor, *haplo* haploidentical, *HSCT* hematopoietic stem cell transplantation

Monitoring CsA and tacrolimus (Tac) levels is recommended, with optimal levels around 200–300 ng/mL for CsA and 10–15 ng/mL for Tac. A very slow taper of calcineurin inhibitors should be carried out, avoiding the discontinuation of calcineurin inhibitors before 9 months after HSCT, with full count recovery. This is to be followed through a very slow and extended taper, with careful follow-ups on counts at every step of dose reduction.

Comparative Outcomes of HSCT in Low- Versus High-Income Countries

Excellent outcomes have been reported following HSCT from high-income countries [46]. One of the largest single-center studies from Pakistan by Chaudhry et al. reported that 97% of patients receiving transplants had one or more high-risk features. The study included 147 high-risk patients transplanted using fludarabine-based conditioning with a reported OS of 84% [20]. George et al. reported a superior OS with a fludarabine-based regimen (82.8%) as compared to Cy200/antilymphocyte globulin (46.1%) [47]. Another study by Iftikhar et al., comparing fludarabine-based vs. conventional cyclophosphamide conditioning, documented OS (85.8% vs. 77.2%; $p = 0.15$), DFS (84.1% vs. 68.4%; $p = 0.02$), and GRFS (77.9% vs. 54.4%; $p = 0.01$) with fludarabine-based conditioning [48]. Jalılı et al. reported an OS of 82% and DFS of 75% in Iranian patients receiving MRD transplant [49]. Overall, although the reported HSCT outcomes are encouraging, they remain lower than the data reported from high-income countries. Possible explanations include the factors mentioned above.

Conclusion

The management of acquired AA remains challenging in countries with restricted resources despite recent advances worldwide. The lack of advanced healthcare facilities, essential drugs, and optimum blood component support necessitates changes in treatment protocols to improve survival outcomes. Long-term survival in the order of 70%–80% is achievable in resource-constrained countries for a disease that was historically associated with very high mortality.

References

1. Wang L, Liu H. Pathogenesis of aplastic anemia. Hematology. 2019;24(1):559–66.
2. Issaragrisil S, Kaufman DW, Anderson T, Chansung K, Leaverton PE, Shapiro S, et al. The epidemiology of aplastic anemia in Thailand. Blood. 2006;107(4):1299–307.

3. Yong AS, Goh AS, Rahman J, Menon J, Purushothaman V. Epidemiology of aplastic anemia in the state of Sabah, Malaysia. Med J Malaysia. 1998;53(1):59–62.
4. Ahamed M, Anand M, Kumar A, Siddiqui MKJ. Childhood aplastic anaemia in Lucknow, India: incidence, organochlorines in the blood and review of case reports following exposure to pesticides. Clin Biochem. 2006;39(7):762–6.
5. Ahmed P, Chaudhry QN, Satti TM, Mahmood SK, Ghafoor T, Shahbaz N, et al. Epidemiology of aplastic anemia: a study of 1324 cases. Hematology. 2020;25(1):48–54.
6. Arewa OP, Akinola NO. Survival in primary a plastic anaemia; experience with 20 cases from a tertiary hospital in Nigeria. Afr Health Sci. 2009;9(4):290.
7. Mahapatra M, Singh PK, Agarwal M, Prabhu M, Mishra P, Seth T, et al. Epidemiology, clinico-haematological profile and management of aplastic anaemia: AIIMS experience. J Assoc Physicians India. 2015;63(3 Suppl):30–5.
8. Waja M, Philip V, Lakha A, Patel M. Aplastic anaemia—a South African public sector perspective. Int J Sci Res Methodol. 2018;10(3):101–6.
9. Moore CA, Krishnan K. Aplastic anemia. In: StatPearls [Internet]. StatPearls Publishing; 2019.
10. Adil S, Kakepoto GN, Khurshid M, Burney IA. Epidemiological features of aplastic anaemia in Pakistan. J Pak Med Assoc. 2001;51:443.
11. McCahon E, Tang K, Rogers PC, McBride ML, Schultz KR. The impact of Asian descent on the incidence of acquired severe aplastic anaemia in children. Br J Haematol. 2003;121(1):170–2.
12. Chen C-H, Ferreira JC, Joshi AU, Stevens MC, Li S-J, Hsu JH-M, et al. Novel and prevalent non-East Asian ALDH2 variants; implications for global susceptibility to aldehydes' toxicity. EBioMedicine. 2020;55:102753.
13. Taj M, Shah T, Aslam SK, Zaheer S, Nawab F, Shaheen S, et al. Environmental determinants of aplastic anemia in Pakistan: a case-control study. J Public Health. 2016;24(5):453–60.
14. Marsh JCW. Aplastic anemia: what's in the environment? Blood. 2006;107(4):1250.
15. Dutta A, De R, Dolai TK, Mitra PK, Halder A. Comparative study of environmental factors and different addictions in aplastic anaemia patients in Eastern India. J Blood Disord Symptoms Treat. 2019;8:2015–8.
16. Alter BP. Inherited bone marrow failure syndromes: considerations pre- and posttransplant. Blood. 2017;130(21):2257–64.
17. Gutierrez-Rodrigues F, Munger E, Ma X, Groarke EM, Tang Y, Patel BA, et al. Differential diagnosis of bone marrow failure syndromes guided by machine learning. Blood. 2023;141(17):2100–13.
18. Han W. Health care system reforms in developing countries. J Public Health Res. 2012;1(3):199.
19. Höchsmann B, Moicean A, Risitano A, Ljungman P, Schrezenmeier H. Supportive care in severe and very severe aplastic anemia. Bone Marrow Transplant. 2013;48(2):168–73.
20. Chaudhry QUN, Iftikhar R, Satti TM, Mahmood SK, Ghafoor T, Shamshad GU, et al. Outcome of fludarabine-based conditioning in high-risk aplastic anemia patients undergoing matched related donor transplantation: a single-center study from Pakistan. Biol Blood Marrow Transplant. 2019;25(12):2375–82.
21. Jubelirer SJ. The benefit of the neutropenic diet: fact or fiction? Oncologist. 2011;16(5):704.
22. Killick SB, Bown N, Cavenagh J, Dokal I, Foukaneli T, Hill A, et al. Guidelines for the diagnosis and management of adult aplastic anaemia. Br J Haematol. 2016;172(2):187–207.
23. Quillen K, Wong E, Scheinberg P, Young NS, Walsh TJ, Wu CO, et al. Granulocyte transfusions in severe aplastic anemia: an eleven-year experience. Haematologica. 2009;94(12):1661–8.
24. Garg A, Gupta A, Mishra A, Singh M, Yadav S, Nityanand S. Role of granulocyte transfusions in combating life-threatening infections in patients with severe neutropenia: experience from a tertiary care centre in North India. PLoS One. 2018;13(12):e0209832.
25. Aljurf MD, Gluckman E, Dufour C. Congenital and acquired bone marrow failure. Elsevier; 2016.
26. Townsley DM, Scheinberg P, Winkler T, Desmond R, Dumitriu B, Rios O, et al. Eltrombopag added to standard immunosuppression for aplastic anemia. N Engl J Med. 2017;376(16):1540–50.

27. Maschan A, Bogatcheva N, Kryjanovskii O, Shneider M, Litvinov D, Mitiushkina T, et al. Results at a single centre of immunosuppression with cyclosporine A in 66 children with aplastic anaemia. Br J Haematol. 1999;106(4):967–70.
28. Mandal PK, Baul S, Dolai TK, De R, Chakrabarti P. Outcome of cyclosporine monotherapy in patients of aplastic anemia: experience of a Tertiary Care Hospital in Eastern India. Indian J Hematol Blood Transfus. 2017;33(1):144–7.
29. Khan M, Iftikhar R, Mehmood SK, Faraz T, Ghafoor T, Shahbaz N, et al. Response to immunosuppressive therapy in patients of acquired aplastic anaemia: a single center experience from a developing country. J Ayub Med Coll Abbottabad. 2022;34:S969–73.
30. Scheinberg P, Nunez O, Weinstein B, Scheinberg P, Biancotto A, Wu CO, et al. Horse versus rabbit antithymocyte globulin in acquired aplastic anemia. N Engl J Med. 2011;365(5):430–8.
31. Scheinberg P, Wu CO, Nunez O, Young NS. Predicting response to immunosuppressive therapy and survival in severe aplastic anemia. Br J Haematol. 2009;144(2):206–16.
32. Groarke EM, Patel BA, Shalhoub R, Gutierrez-Rodrigues F, Desai P, Leuva H, et al. Predictors of clonal evolution and myeloid neoplasia following immunosuppressive therapy in severe aplastic anemia. Leukemia. 2022;36(9):2328–37.
33. Champlin R, Ho W, Feig S, Winston D, Lenarsky C, Gale RJB. Do androgens enhance the response to antithymocyte globulin in patients with aplastic anemia? A prospective randomized trial. Blood. 1985;66(1):184–8.
34. Shahidi NT. Aplastic anaemia: aetiological and therapeutic dilemmas. Br J Haematol. 1979;43(2):163–5.
35. Allen DM, Fine MH, Necheles TF, Dameshek WJB. Oxymetholone therapy in aplastic anemia. Blood. 1968;32(1):83–9.
36. Najean Y, aplastic Fcgftso, Haematology raJSJo. Androgen therapy in aplastic anaemia: a comparative study of high and low-doses and of 4 different androgens. Scand J Haematol. 1986;36(4):346–52.
37. Pagliuca S, Kulasekararaj AG, Eikema D-J, Piepenbroek B, Iftikhar R, Satti TM, et al. Current use of androgens in bone marrow failure disorders: a report from the Severe Aplastic Anemia Working Party of the European Society for Blood and Marrow Transplantation. Haematologica. 2024;109(3):765.
38. Nassani M, Fakih RE, Passweg J, Cesaro S, Alzahrani H, Alahmari A, et al. The role of androgen therapy in acquired aplastic anemia and other bone marrow failure syndromes. Front Oncol. 2023;13:1135160.
39. Zhu Y, Gao Q, Hu J, Liu X, Guan D, Zhang F. Allo-HSCT compared with immunosuppressive therapy for acquired aplastic anemia: a system review and meta-analysis. BMC Immunol. 2020;21(1):10.
40. Georges GE. Consider allogeneic bone marrow transplantation for older, fitpatients with aplastic anemia. Biol Blood Marrow Transplant. 2019;25(3):e69–70.
41. Ciceri F, Lupo-Stanghellini M, Korthof E. Haploidentical transplantation in patients with acquired aplastic anemia. Bone Marrow Transplant. 2013;48(2):183–5.
42. Arcuri LJ, Nabhan SK, Cunha R, Nichele S, Ribeiro AAF, Fernandes JF, et al. Impact of CD34 cell dose and conditioning regimen on outcomes after haploidentical donor hematopoietic stem cell transplantation with post-transplantation cyclophosphamide for relapsed/refractory severe aplastic anemia. Biol Blood Marrow Transplant. 2020;26(12):2311–7.
43. Dufour C, Veys P, Carraro E, Bhatnagar N, Pillon M, Wynn R, et al. Similar outcome of upfront-unrelated and matched sibling stem cell transplantation in idiopathic paediatric aplastic anaemia. A study on behalf of the UK Paediatric BMT Working Party, Paediatric Diseases Working Party and Severe Aplastic Anaemia Working Party of EBMT. Br J Haematol. 2015;171(4):585–94.
44. Yue C, Ding Y, Gao Y, Li L, Pang Y, Liu Z, et al. Cotransplantation of haploidentical hematopoietic stem cells and allogeneic bone marrow-derived mesenchymal stromal cells as a first-line treatment in very severe aplastic anemia patients with refractory infections. Eur J Haematol. 2018;100(6):624–9.

45. Lima ACM, Bonfim C, Getz J, do Amaral GB, Petterle RR, Loth G, et al. Untreated donor-specific HLA antibodies are associated with graft failure and poor survival after haploidentical transplantation with post-transplantation cyclophosphamide in pediatric patients with nonmalignant disorders. Transplant Cell Ther. 2022;28(10):698.e1–698.e11.
46. Ruiz-Argüelles GJ, Seber A, Ruiz-Delgado GJ. Conducting hematopoietic stem cell transplantation in low and middle income countries. Hematology. 2022;27(1):809–12.
47. George B, Mathews V, Viswabandya A, Kavitha ML, Srivastava A, Chandy M. Fludarabine and cyclophosphamide based reduced intensity conditioning (RIC) regimens reduce rejection and improve outcome in Indian patients undergoing allogeneic stem cell transplantation for severe aplastic anemia. Bone Marrow Transplant. 2007;40(1):13–8.
48. Iftikhar R, Satti TM, Mahmood SK, Ghafoor T, Shamshad GU, Shahbaz N, et al. Comparison of conventional cyclophosphamide versus fludarabine-based conditioning in high-risk aplastic anemia patients undergoing matched-related donor transplantation. Clin Hematol Int. 2020;2(2):82–91.
49. Jalili M, Alimoghaddam K, Hamidieh AA, Hamdi A, Jahani M, Bahar B, et al. Hematopoietic stem cell transplantation in patients with severe acquired aplastic anemia: Iranian experience. Int J Hematol-Oncol Stem Cell Res. 2011;5(4):22–7.

Open Access This chapter is licensed under the terms of the Creative Commons Attribution 4.0 International License (http://creativecommons.org/licenses/by/4.0/), which permits use, sharing, adaptation, distribution and reproduction in any medium or format, as long as you give appropriate credit to the original author(s) and the source, provide a link to the Creative Commons license and indicate if changes were made.

The images or other third party material in this chapter are included in the chapter's Creative Commons license, unless indicated otherwise in a credit line to the material. If material is not included in the chapter's Creative Commons license and your intended use is not permitted by statutory regulation or exceeds the permitted use, you will need to obtain permission directly from the copyright holder.

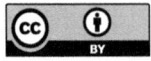

Index

A
Absolute neutrophils count (ANC), 327
Acquired aplastic anemia, 2
  age-and gender-related demographics, 9
  allogeneic bone marrow transplantation, 99
  annual incidence, 8
  and antifungal prophylaxis recommendations, 101
  associated with chemicals, 66–67
  associations with other autoimmune diseases, 14, 67
  characteristic biphasic distribution, 9
  clothing and hygienic routines, 101
  demographics, 7
  diagnosis, 8
  drug or toxin induced, 10–12
  during pregnancy, 15
  early mobilization of the patient, 101
  epidemiology, 7, 16, 21
  exposures to drugs, 11, 17
  geographical variability, 7
  hand washing and rubbing with alcohol-based disinfection solutions, 101
  hematopoietic stem cell reserve, 9
  immunosuppressive therapy, 15, 99
  incidence, 8
  low-bacterial diet, 100
  molecular pathways for therapeutic exploitation, 16
  multicenter clinical trials, 16
  neutropenic infections, 100
  optimized supportive care, 99
  passive mobilization and breathing exercises, 101
  population-based study, 16
  post-vaccination, 15–16
  prolonged period of severe neutropenia, 101
  retrospective studies, 7
  sex ratio, 9
  specific HLA genes or alleles, 13, 17
  systematic case-control studies, 15
  variability in incidence rates, 7
  viral infection, 102
Acquired bone marrow failure, 21
Acquired cytopenias, 1
Acquired neutropenia, 331
  in infancy, 332
Acute graft-versus-host disease (aGVHD), 179
Acute myeloid leukemia (AML), 22
ADA2 activity, 231
Age, per se, 139
Agranulocytosis, 80
Alemtuzumab, 93, 127
Allogeneic cell transplantation with ATG, 87
Allogeneic hematopoietic stem cell transplantation, 318
  DC, 273
  treatment algorithm for idiopathic and inherited bone marrow failure, 185
Allogeneic stem-cell transplantation (alloSCT), 37
Allosensitization, 105
AMED syndrome, 349
Amino acid leucine, 318
Androgens, 91, 258
  therapy, 258, 366
Anemia, 120
Anti-HLA antibodies, 178
Antithymoglobulin (ATG)
  allogeneic cell transplantation, 87
  potent lymphocyte-depleting agents, 92

Aplastic anemia (AA), 2, 78
  in aging, 68
  aspiration of bone marrow, 57
  autoimmune destruction of early
      hematopoietic cells, 55
  children
      diagnostic work-up, 118
      treatment algorithm, 122
  clonality and clonal evolution in, 31–33
  complete response, 69
  diagnosis, 58, 60, 61
      of exclusion, 77
      phases, 59
  differential diagnosis, 57
  geographic rate variability, 55
  and hypoplastic MDS, 64
  immune pathophysiology, 87
  with other clonal and congenital
      disorders, 82
  partial remission, 69
  pathogenic mechanisms, 57
  persistent pancytopenia, 55
  in resource-limited countries
      care considerations, 362
      clinical features, 362
      comparative outcomes, 369
      considerations, 368
      demographics, 362
      diagnostic algorithm, 364
      dysmorphic features, 363
      genetic predisposition, 363
      incidence, 362
      irradiation of blood products, 364
      specialized hematology centers and
          limited availability of genetic
          testing, 363
      supportive care, 364–365
      treatment algorithm, 367
  response criteria, 69
  severity, 69
Associated proteins, 250
Autoantibodies, 29
Autologous cellular therapy, 259
Autoregulated heme–GATA1 feedback
    loop, 293
Avatrombopag, 37, 137
Azithromycin, 8

B
Baltimore platform, 162
Benzene, 8, 10
Bleeding due to thrombocytopenia, 105

Blood cancer in SDS, 296
BMT with matched sibling donors, 33
Bone marrow aspiration and trephine
    biopsy, 60
Bone marrow biopsy, 231
Bone marrow cellularity, 117
Bone marrow examination in CAMT, 340
Bone marrow failure syndrome 3, 352
Bone marrow failure syndromes
  diagnostic and therapeutic challenges, 1
  diagnostic considerations, 2
  disease-specific discussions and treatment
      modalities, 2
  foundational concepts, 2
  research and clinical practice, 1
  supportive care and non-transplant
      treatment strategies, 2
Bone marrow, stem cell source, 148, 163

C
Camitta severity criteria, 88
Cancer predisposition with long
    telomeres, 255
Cancer risk and surveillance in DBAS, 320
CAR T-cell therapy hematotoxicity, 12
Cartilage-hair hypoplasia (CHH), 321, 322
Cell cycle study, 239
Cell metabolism and free heme overload, 293
Center for International Blood and Marrow
    Transplant Research (CIBMTR),
    161, 194
  in nonmalignant disorders, 160
Chelation therapy, 315–316
  in DBAS, 315
Children, AA
  diagnostic work-up, 118
  treatment algorithm, 122
Chimerism, 151
Chinese Epidemiologic Study Group of
    Leukemia and Aplastic Anemia
    survey, 8
Chloramphenicol, 8, 11
Chromosome Breakage Test (CBY), 239
Chronic graft-versus-host disease (cGvHD),
    34, 35, 146, 170, 175, 178, 179, 342
Chronic idiopathic neutropenia (CIN)
  clonal hematopoiesis, 333
  NGS myeloid panel, 334
  pathophysiologic mechanisms, 333
  profile of, 333
Chronic neutropenia
  classification, 329

Index 375

diagnostic algorithm according to
    International Guidelines, 328
diagnostic approach to neutropenia, 327
first-and second-line investigations, 329
Ciclosporin with eltrombopag, 95
Clonal evolution, 22, 32, 242–243
Clonal hematopoiesis, 24, 27, 77, 79, 119, 207
Clonal transformation, 37
Clonality and clonal evolution in AA, 31–33
Clozapine-induced agranulocytosis, 14
CMV-negative blood products, 107
Coats plus, 253
Complete blood count, 60
Comprehensive sequencing, 27
Conditioning and GvHD prophylaxis, 342
Congenital abnormalities, 241
Congenital amegakaryocytic
    thrombocytopenia (CAMT), 31,
    119, 193
  autosomal recessive inherited bone marrow
    failure, 337
  central nervous system (CNS)
    hemorrhages, 338
  clinical features, 338
    and amegakaryocytosis, 339
  clinical subtypes, 339
  clonal evolution, 342
  c-MPL gene, 337
  comprehensive diagnostic framework, 340
  diagnosis, 337
  fetal hemorrhage, 338
  homozygous or compound heterozygous
    c-MPL mutations, 338
  HSCT, 341
  malignant transformation, 339
  morphologic amegakaryocytosis, 339
  natural progression, 339
  structured approach to treatment and
    supportive care, 343
  TPO signaling pathway, 338
Congenital marrow failure undiagnosed, 81, 82
Congenital neutropenia (CN), 194, 329, 330
Congenital ribosomopathies, 287
Constitutional bone marrow failure
  ADA2 activity, 231
  CTLA4, 228
  DNA double-strand break repair disorders,
    228, 229
  immune dysregulation disorders, 227,
    228, 231
  STAT1, 228
  WES, 119, 228, 333
  WGS, 119, 228

Copy-number neutral loss of heterozygosity
    (CNN-LOH), 27
Cord blood transplantation (CBT), 34, 35
Corticosteroids, 89, 316
Crm1/Xpo1, 286
Cyclophosphamide (Cy), 35, 93, 161
Cyclosporin A (CSA), 342
Cyclosporine, 14
Cy-only conditioning, 152
Cytogenetic abnormalities, 61
Cytokine gene polymorphisms, 26–27
Cytomegalovirus infection, 179
Cytopenia, 108
Cytotoxic T-lymphocyte-associated Protein 4
    (CTLA4), 228

D

DADA2 mesenchymal stromal cells, 231
Danicopan, 217
Defective ubiquitylation, of RPs, 290
Deficiency of adenosine deaminase type 2
    (DADA2), 119, 231
Diamond–Blackfan anemia syndrome
    (DBAS), 193, 287, 292, 293
  associated with *GATA1* variants, 314
  clinical presentation, 311
  diagnosis, 311
  differential diagnosis, 313
  genetic counseling and family
    planning, 321
  genotype/phenotype correlations, 312
  pathophysiology, 293, 294
  red cell transfusion support, 314
  TCE pathology, 313
  transfused patient, 316
  transfusion, 314
Dichloro-diethyly-trichlorthane (DDT), 10
DKC1 mutations, 270
DNA double-strand break repair disorders,
    228, 229
DNAJC21, 352
DRB1*07 allele, 12
Drosophila neuroblasts, 289
Drug-induced AA, 66
Dual pathophysiology theory, 205–207
Dyskeratosis congenita (DC), 251–253
  abnormalities of telomere
    maintenance, 267
  androgens, 272
  clinical features, 269–270
  clinical presentation, 269
  concerns over graft failure, 274

Dyskeratosis congenita (DC) (cont.)
  conditioning regimens, 274
  crude rate of malignancy, 268
  definitive management, 277
  diagnosis, 271
  erythropoietin receptor, 272
  general rules and guidelines, 273
  identified genes, 268
  management, 271
  mechanism of action of androgens, 272
  mortality due to pulmonary
    complications, 276
  non-myeloablative conditioning
    regimen, 274
  pulmonary and hepatic toxicities, 273
  reduced-intensity conditioning (RIC)
    transplants, 273
  solid and hematological
    malignancies, 277
Dyskerin, 268
Dysplasia of erythropoiesis, 63

E
Eastern Mediterranean Blood and Marrow
  Transplantation Registry, 274
ELANE-and *HAX1*-related neutropenias, 330
Elderly, AA
  algorithm of treatment, 139
  first-line treatment, 139, 140
  HCT, 138, 139
  supportive measures, 134
  treatment decision-making
    process, 133
Eltrombopag, 21, 36–38, 90, 126, 135,
    137, 246
  monotherapy, 91
ERCC6L2-associated bone marrow failure,
    347, 348
Erythroblastopenia, 313
Erythroid differentiation, 290
Erythropoietin, 318
  resulting in pure red cell aplasia
    (PRCA), 227
ETS1 cleavage, 285
ETV6, 119
Eukaryotic ribosome, 281
  composition, 284
Eurocord and other international transplant
    consortia, 186
European Group for Blood and Marrow
    Transplantation (EBMT), 213
  retrospective analysis, 125

F
Familial AA, 31
FANCD2 test, 239
Fanconi anemia (FA), 119, 203
  carrier frequency, 238
  diagnosis, 238
  follow-up after diagnosis, 241–242
  genotype/phenotype correlation, 238
  hematological monitoring plan, 241
  HSCT, 244
  pathogenic variants, 237
  physical abnormalities, 238
  post-diagnosis hematological monitoring
    plan, 240
  testing procedures, 239
  workup for patients, 240
FARF guidelines, 239
Fever with neutropenia, 103
FLAG regimen, 243
Flow-FISH assay, 257
Flu administration, 189
Fludarabine, cyclophosphamide, and Campath
    (FCC) regimen, 162

G
GATA1 target gene expression, 293
GATA2, 119
  deficiency, 31, 229–231
  mutations, 31
  sequencing, 31
Gene editing techniques, 246
Genetic testing for telomere-related gene
    mutations, 257
Genomic instability, 22
Germline *GATA2* gene mutations, 31
GI telangiectasias, 257
Glycosyl phosphatidylinositol–anchored
    proteins (GPI–APs), 23
Gonadal function, 152
Graft engineering with selective T-cell
    depletion, 151
Graft failure, 275
Graft rejection, 33, 342
Graft-versus-host disease (GvHD), 33
  prevention, 342
  prophylaxis, 124, 151, 161, 163, 176, 178
Granulocyte-colony-stimulating factor
    (G-CSF), 121
  doses, 331
  study, 135
  therapy, 332
  to IST, 94

H

Haploidentical and cord blood HSCT, 34–35
Haploidentical donor, 177, 178
Haploidentical hematopoietic stem cell
    transplantation (haplo-HSCT),
    124–125, 244
  in SAA, 170–173
  therapeutic strategies, 179
Haploidentical stem cell transplantation,
    idiopathic AA, 178
Healthcare delivery, 364
Hematologic and immunologic anomalies, 252
Hematological outcomes in DBAS, 320
Hematologic monitoring, 258
Hematopoiesis in AA, 22
Hematopoietic cell transplantation (HCT)
  in elderly, 138, 139
  from haplo-identical donors, 276
Hematopoietic dysfunction, 254
Hematopoietic gene therapy (GT) of
    autologous hematopoietic stem
    cells, 246
Hematopoietic growth factors
  prophylaxis of infections, 103
  combination with immunosuppression, 103
Hematopoietic stem cell transplantation
    (HSCT), 2, 366, 367, 369
  allogeneic, 318
  congenital amegakaryocytic
    thrombocytopenia, 337
  decision-making process in FA, 245
  fanconi anemia, 244
  haploidentical, 124–125, 244
  from MSD, 123
  from MUD, 123–124
Hemolysis, 210
Hepatitis, 66
Hepatopulmonary syndrome, 256
High-resolution genotyping of HLA-DRB1, 14
HLA-DR2 B15 allele, 14
HLA-DRB1*08 alleles, 14
HLA-DR2 gene, 12, 27
HLA-DR typing, 67
HMGA2 overexpression, 207
Hoyeraal–Hreidarsson syndrome (HHS), 253
HSC fate-mapping analyses in mice, 22
HSC gene therapy, 231
HSP70/GATA1 complex, 293
Human leukocyte antigen (HLA), 26, 105, 121
  HLA-DR2 B15 allele, 14
  HLA-DRB1*08 alleles, 14
  HLA-DR2 gene, 12, 27
  HLA-DR typing, 67
  HLA-identical sibling donor, 33
  matching techniques, 185
  mismatched grafts, 160
  MSD for BM transplantation, 169
  system, 12–14
  typing, 62, 160
  unrelated donor and treatment
    strategies, 164
Human platelet antigens (HPA), 105
Human rRNA maturation, 286
Hypocellular leukemia, 117
Hypoplastic myelodysplastic syndrome
    (MDS), 77–79

I

Idiopathic aplastic anemia, 187
Idiopathic neutropenia (IN), 332
Idiopathic pulmonary fibrosis, 256
immune aplastic anemia, 89
Immune escape clones, 27
Immune hypothesis, 27
Immune mechanism, AA, 25
Immune-mediated attack sparing PNH
    hematopoiesis, 207
Immune-mediated BM failure mouse
    models, 29
Immune pathophysiology, 89
Immune suppressive therapy, DC, 272
Immune thrombocytopenia (ITP), 80
Immunosuppressive agents, 92
Immunosuppressive therapy (IST), 2, 10, 14,
    35–37, 102, 125–126, 134,
    169, 365–366
  efficacy, 21
  in elderly, 134–138
  immune mechanism, 21
Impaired pre-rRNA processing and ribosome
    biogenesis, 292
Inherited bone marrow failure syndromes
    (IBMFS), 2, 62–63, 117, 240, 339
  disease classification, 346
Inherited C5 polymorphism, 216
Inherited cytopenias, 1
Inherited erythroblastopenias, 313
Inherited ribosomopathies with a
    hematological phenotype, 309, 311
Innate Immunity, 28
International Agranulocytosis and Aplastic
    Anemia Study (IAAAS), 8
Invasive procedures platelet transfusions, 106
In vitro experiments, 22
Iron Chelation therapy, 107, 108
Irradiated blood products in aplastic
    anemia, 106

J
JAK1/2 inhibition with ruxolitinib, 25

L
Large granular lymphocyte (LGL) leukemia, 28, 68, 80
Large ribosomal subunit, 283
Lat-onset neutropenia (LONp), 332
Liver disease, in TBD, 255
Long-lasting neutropenias, (LLNp), 332
Long-term culture-initiating cells (LTC-ICs), 22, 26, 204
Lymphocyte count, 60
Lymphocyte-depleting agents, 93–94

M
Matched related donor stem cell transplants for bone marrow failure syndromes, 274, 275
Matched related or unrelated donors, 277
Matched sibling donor (MSD) hematopoietic stem cell transplantation
  age, 147
  history, 145
  HLA matching, 147
  immunologic reactivity, 147
  indications, 146
  optimal conditioning regimen, 161
  patient selection, 160
  pretransplant factors, 146
  severity, 147
  survival rates, 152
Matched unrelated donor (MUD), 33
Matched-related UCBT for BMF, 194
Mathé and Schwarzenberg, immunosuppression with ATG, 89
MECOM gene (MDS1 and EVI1 complex locus), 348
Methotrexate, 342
Methylprednisolone, 89
Metoclopramide, 318
MicroRNA (miRNA), 28
Molecular analysis, 61
Monosomy 7 and/or complex karyotype, 32
Mouse models of chemical and drug hematopoietic toxicity, 29, 30
Multi-lineage differentiation, 231
Mycophenolate mofetil, 92
Myelodysplastic syndrome (MDS), 22
Myeloid PNH, 209
MYSM1 deficiency, 346

N
Neonatal alloimmune amegakaryocytosis, 340
Neutropenic AA anemia, 102
Neutropenic fever, 103, 104
Neutropenic subjects, 331
Next generation sequencing (NGS) panels, 119, 228
Next-generation sequencing (NGS), 61
Next-generation sequencing (NGS) technology, 345
NFKB1 haploinsufficiencies, 228
Non transplant therapy, 245, 246
Non-cirrhotic liver disease, 255
Nonhomologous end Joining (NHEJ) mechanisms, 228
Nonmyeloablative (NMA) conditioning, 175
Non-severe forms (NSAA), 121
Noonan syndrome, 340
NOP10, 268
Nucleophosmin (NPM1), 290

O
Oligoclonal skewing of the T-cell repertoire, 25
Oncostatin M-related BMF syndrome, 354
Oral iron chelators, 37
Oral leukoplakia and excessive ocular tearing, 251

P
p53 tumor suppressor protein, 292
Pancytopenia, 60
Pancytopenia with persistent and unexplained reduced marrow hematopoietic cellularity, 203
PAPD5 inhibitor, 259
Paroxysmal nocturnal hemoglobinuria (PNH), 21–23, 27, 65, 81
  allogeneic hematopoietic stem cell transplantation, 212–214
  cells, 79, 81
  chronic hemolysis, 210
  clinical and biological follow-up, 211
  clone analysis, 119
  clone, hemolysis, 214–216
  complement inhibitors, 211
  diagnosis, 209
  disease subcategories, 208–209
  "escape" theory, 206
  glycosylphosphatidylinositol, 205
  hematopoiesis, 206

homologous TCR-beta sequences, 205
immune-mediated pathophysiology of bone marrow failure, 204
immunosuppressive therapy, 211–212
intravascular hemolysis, 211
management of marrow failure, 211
manifestations, 204
oligoclonality of T cell pool, 205
persistent and unexplained reduced marrow hematopoietic cellularity, 209
proximal complement inhibitors, 216, 217
relative advantage, 206
risk of thrombosis, 210
tests, 65
Pathophysiological p53-dependent anemia, 292
Patient care and surveillance, 322–323
PCRA, 80
Pegcetacoplan, 216
PIGA mutant cells, 24
PIGA mutations and HLA loss, 32
Platelet transfusions, 105
Pneumocystis pneumonia prophylaxis, 121
Post-hepatitis AA, 9, 10
Post transplant cyclophosphamide (PTCy), 170–175, 178
Post-transplant immunosuppression, 151
Pre-HSCT blood product transfusion, 148
Pre-HSCT infection, 148
Pre-40S particles, 285
Primary anti-mold prophylaxis, 90
Primary autoimmune neutropenias (pAIN), 332
Primary immunodeficiencies (PIDs), 227
Primary immunoregulatory disorders (PIRDs), 227
Prolonged neutropenia, 100
Psychological support, 108
Pulmonary disease, 256
Pulmonary fibrosis, 256
and shortened telomeres, 256
Pure red cell aplasia (PRCA), 80, 227

R
Rabbit ATG (r.ATG, Thymoglobuline®, Sanofi), 93
Radioulnar synostosis with amegakaryocytic thrombocytopenia type 2, 348
Randomized RACE study, 136
Rapamycin, 92

Rapid telomere loss, 32
Recombinant hematopoietic growth factors, DC, 272
Recurrent somatic mutations, 78
Red blood cell (RBC), 60
transfusions, 105
Reduced-Intensity Conditioning (RIC) regimen, 322
Regulatory T cells (Treg), 25
Restrictive transfusion policy, 105
Retinal telangiectasias, 257
Revesz syndrome, 253
Ribosomal dysfunctions, 287
Ribosomal proteins, 290
nomenclature, 282–284
Ribosomal RNAs, 291
Ribosome biogenesis, 289
and translation, 289
Ribosome heterogeneity, 289
Ribosome-associated protein (RAP), 290
Ribosomes, protein synthesis, 282
Ribosomopathy, 309
cancer, risk and associated mutations, 288
clinical characteristics, 288
diminished quantity or quality of ribosomes, 289
IBMFSs, 287
pathophysiological mechanisms, 291
ribosome assembly machinery, 287
ribosome dysfunction and bone marrow failure, 287
structural variations of the ribosome, 290
tissue specificity and proclivity, 289
Ribosomopathy-associated bone marrow failure, 352
RNA polymerase I (RNA Pol I), 284
RNA polymerase II (RNA Pol II), 285
Romiplostim, 36, 37, 94, 127
RP gene mutations, 293
18S rRNA, 285
rRNA modifications, 289

S
SAMD9-related disorder, 350–352
SAMD9/SAMD9L, 119
Secondary malignancies following AA transplant, 152
Secondary neutropenias, 331
Seronegative hepatitis, 117
Serum thrombopoietin (TPO) levels in CAMT, 340

Severe aplastic anemia (SAA), 90
  without an HLA-matched related donor, 187
Severe combined deficiency phenotype, 322
Severe congenital neutropenia (SCN), 119
Severe hepatic disease, 255
Severe (SAA) or very severe aplastic anemia (VSAA), 117
Shelterin, 249
Short telomeres, 22, 268
Shwachman–Diamond syndrome (SDS), 30, 192, 287, 295
Signal transducer and activator of transcription 1 (STAT1) genes, 228
Single-cell studies, 23
Single lineage cytopenias, 80
Sirolimus, 92
Small ribosomal subunit, 282
Solid organ transplantation, TBD, 259
Solid tumors, 243–244, 255
Somatic genetic rescue (SGR), 295
Somatic reversion, 257
Splice site mutations in the *GATA1* gene impair production, 293
STAT3 clones, 28
Stem cell choice, 176
Stem cell source, 150
  and dose, 342
  in haploidentical transplants in SAA, 176, 177
Stem-cell stimulation, 36, 37
Steroids, 126
Steroid therapy, 316
Subclinical PNH, 209
Supportive care, 163
Syngeneic HSCT, 150
Syngeneic transplantation, 140
Synthetic androgens, 245

T

TBI-sparing regimen, 175
T-cell attack on BM, 26
T cell co-stimulation blockade with abatacept, 175
T-cell depleted and T-cell replete haploidentical strategies, 176
T cell depletion (TCD), 244
T-cell large granular lymphocytes, 80–81
T cells, 25

TCR-αβ-depletion, 244
Telomerase, 250
  clinical ramifications, 250
  pathogenic variants, 250
  repair mechanism, 249
Telomere, 30, 250
  attrition, 62
  biology, 249, 250
  biology and ribosomopathies in hematologic dysfunction and malignancy, 2
  community, 260
  diseases, 191
  dynamics, 32
  dysfunction, 250
  length, 271
Telomere biology disorder (TBD), 32, 251
  clinical manifestations, 252
  HSCT, 259
  inheritance, 251
Telomere length (TL) measurement, 257
Telomere shortening, 250, 254, 255
Telomeropathy, 270, 276
Telomeropathy/ribosomopathy
  X-linked Dyskeratosis congenita, 296–297
TERC oligoadenylation and increased TERC, 259
Th1 and Th17 cells, 26
Th-17 polarized CD4+ CAMK4+ T cells, 23
Thionamide-induced AA, 14
Third immunosuppressive agent, 92
Thrombocytopenia, 121
  in CAMT, 340
Thrombocytopenia with Absent Radii (TAR) Syndrome, 339
TINF2 affecting shelterin, 268
T-LGL, 81
Toll-like receptor 8 (TLR8), 228
TP53 activation syndrome, 353, 354
TP53 IBFMS due to germline gain-of-function TP53 mutations, 353
TP53-mutated cancer evolution, 295
TPO mimetics, 36
Tranexamic acid, 341
Transcriptional analysis of T cells, 28
Transfusion management, 341
Transfusion therapy, 105
Transplant-related mortality, 342
Treacher Collins syndrome (TCS), 297, 298, 314

U

Umbilical cord blood transplantation (UCBT), 187, 188
   historical indication, 186
   unrelated in
      FA, 190
      SAA, 188–189
      telomere disorders, 191–192
Unrelated donor transplants, 159

V

Vaccination strategies for aplastic anemia, 104
Vascular anomalies, 256–257
Viruses, 65

W

Watch and wait, 88

WHO provisional entities of idiopathic cytopenias of undetermined significance, 78
Whole exome sequencing (WES), 119, 228, 333
   in AA, 21
Whole genome sequencing (WGS), 119, 228
Wiskott–Aldrich syndrome, 339

X

X-linked phosphatidylinositol glycan class A gene (*PIGA*), 23

Z

Zinsser–Cole–Engman syndrome, 267

GPSR Compliance

The European Union's (EU) General Product Safety Regulation (GPSR) is a set of rules that requires consumer products to be safe and our obligations to ensure this.

If you have any concerns about our products, you can contact us on ProductSafety@springernature.com

In case Publisher is established outside the EU, the EU authorized representative is:

Springer Nature Customer Service Center GmbH
Europaplatz 3
69115 Heidelberg, Germany

Batch number: 09768224

Printed by Printforce, the Netherlands